The SOCIAL and STRUCTURAL DETERMINANTS of HEALTH

The SOCIAL and STRUCTURAL DETERMINANTS of HEALTH

Educating Nurses to Advance Health Equity

Teri A. Murray, PhD, PHNA-BC, RN, ANEF, FAAN
Professor, Dean Emerita, Chief Diversity and Inclusion Officer
Trudy Busch Valentine School of Nursing, Saint Louis University
St. Louis, Missouri

ELSEVIER

Elsevier
3251 Riverport Lane
St. Louis, Missouri 63043

THE SOCIAL AND STRUCTURAL DETERMINANTS OF HEALTH: ISBN: 978-0-443-12681-9
EDUCATING NURSES TO ADVANCE HEALTH EQUITY

Executive Content Strategist: Lee Henderson
Director, Content Development: Ellen Wurm-Cutter
Content Development Specialist: Dominque McPherson
Publishing Services Manager: Deepthi Unni
Senior Project Manager: Manchu Mohan
Design Direction: Margaret Reid

Printed in India.

Last digit is the print number: 9   8   7   6   5   4   3   2   1

Working together to grow libraries in developing countries

www.elsevier.com • www.bookaid.org

The editor wishes to dedicate this book to her loving family for their unwavering commitment and support, and to her friends, colleagues, and all those who wish to advance health equity.

CONTRIBUTORS

Lisa Anderson-Shaw, DrPH, MA, MSN, HEC-C
Assistant Professor
Niehoff School of Nursing and Neiswanger Institute
for Bioethics
Loyola University Chicago;
Assistant Professor
University of Illinois College of Medicine at Chicago
Chicago, Illinois

Lena Hatchett, PhD
Associate Professor
Director, Community and University Partnerships
Neiswanger Institute for Bioethics
Loyola University Chicago Stritch School of Medicine
Chicago, Illinois

Mary Ann Lavin, ScD, RN, ANP-BC (retired), FNI, FAAN
Professor Emerita
Trudy Buch Valentine School of Nursing
Saint Louis University
St. Louis, Missouri

Priscilla Limbo Sagar, EdD, RN, ACNS-BC, CTN-A, FTNSS, FAAN
Professor Emerita
Mount Saint Mary College;
Fellow
Transcultural Nursing Society Scholars
Newburgh, New York

Vanessa Loyd, DNP, PhD, RN
Dean's Fellow for Diversity, Equity, & Inclusion
Teaching Professor
College of Nursing
University of Missouri–St. Louis
St. Louis, Missouri

Teri A. Murray, PhD, PHNA-BC, RN, ANEF, FAAN
Professor
Dean Emerita
Chief Diversity and Inclusion Officer
Trudy Busch Valentine School of Nursing
Saint Louis University
St. Louis, Missouri

Deena A. Nardi, PhD, PMHCNS-BC, FAAN
Psychotherapist
Cathedral Counseling Center
Chicago, Illinois

Sabita Persaud, PhD, RN, APHN-BC
Associate Professor
School of Nursing
Notre Dame of Maryland University
Baltimore, Maryland

Diana Ruiz, DNP, RN, CNE, PHNA-BC, CCTM, CWOCN, NE-BC
Medical Surgical Division Manager
Midland Memorial Hospital
Midland, Texas

Vetta L. Sanders Thompson, PhD
E. Desmond Lee Professor of Racial and Ethnic Studies
Brown School at Washington University
St. Louis, Missouri

Pamela Talley, MSN, APRN-BC
Director of Clinic and Outreach Services
CHIPS Health and Wellness Center
St. Louis, Missouri

Roberta Waite, EdD, PMHCNS, ANEF, FAAN
Dean
School of Nursing
Georgetown University
Washington, DC

Carolyn Hart, PhD, RN, CNE
Dean, College of Health Professions and Associate
    Professor of Nursing
Coker University
Hartsville, South Carolina

Jill Peltzer, PhD, APRN-CNS
Associate Professor, Tenured
University of Kansas School of Nursing
Kansas City, Kansas

Ruth Elizabeth Politi, PhD, MSN, RN, CNE
Senior Contributing Faculty
College of Nursing
Walden University
Minneapolis, Minnesota

As a board-certified public health nurse, I often reflect on the early days of public health nursing when public health nurse pioneers such as Lilian Wald and Mary Brewster embraced social reform by seeing the connections between the social environment and health. Wald and Brewster advocated for policies that reflected social justice and promoted health. Today, the clinical education of nurses leans toward individualized care in the acute or primary care setting, despite mounting evidence that the social environment is more responsible for health than the provision of clinical services. It is critical that students understand the relationship between the social environment and health.

Few nursing education programs integrate the social determinants of health (SDOH) into the curriculum in progressive and pervasive ways. Given the lack of intentionality, leading professional organizations have issued calls to do so. In 2019, the National League for Nursing (NLN) released the national report, *Vision for Integration of the Social Determinants of Health into Nursing Education Curricula,* which called for nursing education to integrate the SDOH. The NLN recognized that multiple social and environmental factors have a lifelong impact on health and contribute to health inequities and subsequent health disparities among various population groups. Thus, the NLN admonished nurse educators to ensure students have a deep understanding of the health threats posed by the SDOH. In 2020, the US Department of Health and Human Services, National Advisory Council on Nurse Education and Practice (NACNEP) released its report, *Integration of the Social Determinants of Health in Nursing Education, Practice, and Research.* Recognizing the critical need for the nursing profession to address the SDOH, the NACNEP recommended that the US Secretary of Health and Human Services and US Congress provide funding support for educational and research initiatives that addressed the SDOH to advance health equity. In 2021, two major reports were released. First, the American Association of Colleges of Nursing's document, *The Essentials: Core Competencies for Professional Nursing Education,* identified the SDOH as a concept essential to nursing practice. This concept was recognized as central to the extent that it should be integrated throughout curricula at undergraduate and graduate levels of nursing education. Second, the landmark report, *The Future of Nursing 2020-2030: Charting a Path to Achieve Health Equity,* made eight recommendations to help the nursing profession realize a culture of health for all. Seven of the eight recommendations focused on SDOH and health equity. Additionally, the *Future of Nursing Report* highlighted the need to integrate the SDOH and health equity into nursing education. The desire to write this book originated before these recent reports, although the reports substantiated the need for a book of this nature.

This book provides context for the health disparities seen at the population level, both in terms of structural and social determinants. It describes how the disparities seen in marginalized and minoritized populations can be attributed to structural determinants such as the distribution of wealth, power, social and cultural norms, and economic and political factors. It further describes the SDOH, the environmental conditions where people are born, live, learn, work, play, worship, and age, and how these conditions lead to systemic disadvantage in health and all aspects of life.

Unit I of the book is titled *Understanding the Social and Structural Determinants of Health* and comprises six chapters. The initial five chapters are patterned after the framework used by Healthy People 2030, *Social Determinants of Health.* Healthy People 2030 identifies five specific domains of the SDOH: Healthcare access and quality; economic stability; education; educational access and quality; physical, natural, and built environments; and social and community environments. Chapter 6 looks at the impact of the historical context of race and racism on health and how it is an underlying factor for the inequities that lead to health disparities. Unit 2, *Strategies to Address Health Equity,* details strategies that would help to achieve health equity and contains four chapters. The final four chapters address the political environment; social justice and health equity; culture, cultural competemility, and health equity; and action-oriented models of community research and partnerships, which are strategies and approaches nurses could employ to advance health equity.

Chapter 1 presents an overview of the SDOH, recognizing that broader social and structural contexts impact individual and population health far more than the provision of clinical services. Frameworks are introduced that provide a conceptual understanding of the SDOH. The levels of interventions nurses can use to address the health of populations to advance health equity are described. Lastly, this chapter discusses becoming structurally aware and the development of structural competence.

Chapter 2 presents an overview of the interconnectedness among income, the SDOH, and health. It points out the social gradient between income and health relative to socioeconomic status. The chapter presents information on the relationship between income and housing, food, access to healthcare, and a host of other health-promoting resources. The levels of interventions nurses can use to address the health of populations to advance health equity related to income and income inequality are described. It further explains the nurse's role as a social justice advocate in pursuing health equity.

Chapter 3 focuses on the dynamic and complex relationship between education, educational access and quality, and health at individual and population levels. Information is presented on this relationship. The chapter concludes by addressing upstream, midstream, and downstream interventions that could promote educational equity, recognizing that multisector engagement and collaboration are needed.

Chapter 4 presents the impacts the physical, natural, and built environments have on health, quality of life, and well-being. Key components of the physical, natural, and built environment are discussed, including health-promoting goods, housing limitations, infrastructure, environmental justice, climate change, and access to broadband internet service. It concludes by identifying the role nurses can play in promoting health-enhancing environments.

Chapter 5 addresses the influence of the social environment on health, including the physical environment. Specific features of the social environment are presented, including how social networks, capital, and cohesion within communities can build resilience to achieve health-promoting outcomes. The chapter concludes with an example of how nurses can implement downstream, midstream, and upstream interventions in social and community contexts.

Chapter 6 focuses on understanding the origins of race and racism and their intersection with health, along with the associated direct and indirect influences racism has on the physical and mental well-being of individuals and populations. The *groundwater approach* is applied to understand the need for individual and population-level (upstream) interventions to create sustainable change toward health equity. Finally, antiracism efforts are shared to advance healthcare practice and improvements toward racial and health justice.

Chapter 7 presents information on the relationship between policy and health. It points out how the political determinants of health are the drivers of the SDOH, and how these processes create inequities in health, leading to health disparities. As the largest group of health professionals, and deemed the most trusted and ethical, nurses must use their individual and collective voices to advocate for health policies that promote the health and well-being of the population to achieve health, particularly for the most marginalized people. The chapter concludes by discussing upstream strategies to improve the population's health.

Chapter 8 examines the social and structural determinants of health from a social justice perspective. First, the history of social justice in the United States is explored, including the principles and practices of social justice, structural competence, social inclusion and exclusions, health activism, advocacy, and the politics of society and social justice. The chapter concludes with examples of how nurses can implement downstream, midstream, and upstream interventions related to social justice.

Chapter 9 addresses the concept of culture and its relationship to health. The chapter presents a discussion of culture through the lens of social identities and intersectionality. It describes how an intersectional lens allows nurses to analyze how individuals can have multiple social identities that impact inequities and disparities. The chapter looks at cultural frameworks and the synergistic relationship between cultural humility and cultural competence—competemility—as a framework for strategies to provide culturally responsive care to individuals, families, organizations, and communities to achieve health equity. The chapter concludes with upstream measures that could be implemented to advance health equity.

Chapter 10 provides a brief history of community-engaged research. It describes the frameworks that inform community-engaged research and the categories on the community engagement continuum. It further describes the implementation of community-engaged research strategies. Special attention is given to community-based participatory research and its key concepts and principles. The chapter ends with a discussion of strategies to develop sustainable community partnerships.

This book offers a holistic framework of the structural and social processes influencing health. It is intended to help students understand that multisector engagement outside the traditional healthcare arena is critical to remedying the root causes of ill health in marginalized populations. Some concepts are interwoven into several chapters and are presented within the context of the specific chapter. The book promotes the notion that health disparities seen in marginalized populations are connected to the allocation of resources and that differences in health are unjust and preventable. Lastly, the book discusses how the health status of marginalized populations extends beyond their personal healthcare choices and is rooted in the processes and policies promulgated by society.

Teri A. Murray
St. Louis, Missouri

ANCILLARIES

For the Instructor
The Evolve site offers answer guidelines for in-text case studies and reflection questions, PowerPoints with case studies and questions for each chapter, and access to the image collection for further review.

ACKNOWLEDGMENTS

I am grateful to my family, friends, and colleagues who supported me through the long and arduous process of writing this book. Their encouragement and belief in me sustained me and fueled my determination to see this project through to completion, despite the many hurdles along the way. I appreciate the knowledge brokers and leaders in public health, population health, and health equity. Their insights, wisdom, and expertise taught me much. Their commitment to justice in health was the inspiration for writing this book. I will forever be indebted to the chapter contributors, whose expertise prevailed in each of their chapters. I offer my heartfelt thanks to the contributors for enriching this book and persevering throughout the process. I appreciate the reviewers' thoughtful feedback and suggestions, which further refined and strengthened the book. Finally, I am thankful for Elsevier and the editorial team, whose expertise and support were indispensable in bringing this book to fruition. This book is a testament to our collective commitment to advancing health equity. To all who have contributed to this endeavor, thank you.

CONTENTS

Understanding the Social and Structural Determinants of Health

Health, Health Status, and the Social Determinants of Health

Teri A. Murray

By any measure, the United States has a level of health inequity rarely seen among developed nations. The roots of this inequity are deep and complex, and are a function of differences in income, education, race and segregation, and place.
—*José Escarce, MD, PhD*

CHAPTER OUTLINE

LEARNING OBJECTIVES

1. Analyze the relationships among health, health status, and the determinants of health.
2. Distinguish nuances among the terms health inequities, health disparities, and health equity.
3. Contrast US healthcare expenditures with the healthcare expenditures and outcomes in other countries.
4. Describe conceptual models and frameworks that advance understanding of the social and structural determinants of health.
5. Explain the relationships among social, structural, and political determinants of health in advancing health equity.

INTRODUCTION

The United States differs significantly from other industrialized countries when it comes to healthcare. It has been simultaneously praised and criticized. The United States is highly acclaimed for its well-trained healthcare workforce, expansive range of healthcare specialists, subspecialties, world-class healthcare institutions, and cutting-edge research, yet disparaged for its sizeable uninsured population, healthcare expenditure levels that far exceed those of other countries, poor measures of performance on critical health outcomes, and inequitable distribution of resources and health outcomes among specific populations (Rice et al., 2020). It also has the dubious distinction of paying more for healthcare and having far worse results than other high-income countries in the Organization for Economic Cooperation and Development (OECD), an international organization representing 37 countries (Tikkanen & Fields, 2021). The United States spent more on healthcare than 10 high-income countries in the OECD, Switzerland, Germany, France, Sweden, Canada, Norway, the Netherlands, the United Kingdom, Australia, and New Zealand.

The spending trends in any given country can be determined by what percentage of the economy is dedicated to health. Health spending is calculated as a percentage of the gross domestic product (GDP) or per capita. The GDP is the total monetary or market value of all the finished goods and services produced in the country. Health expenditure per capita is the measure of the final consumption of health goods and services. It is the amount a country spends on health goods and services from public and private funding sources, including public health, prevention programs, and such programs' administration (OECD, 2020). Both the GDP and the total health expenditures per capita are measured annually. Each varies in response to changes in demographic, social, and economic factors such as the total spending in the economy.

In 1970, the United States spent 6.9% of GDP on health, which correlated to $1848 per resident. This 6.9% is in contrast to 2019, where the United States spent 17.7% of GDP on health or $11,852 per resident (OECD, 2020; Tikkanen & Abrahms, 2020 (Fig. 1.1). When adjusted for different purchasing power within countries, this amount was higher than the other countries in the OECD by a considerable margin (OECD, 2020). Between 2008 and 2019, the US GDP for

healthcare spending rose from 8% to nearly 18%, while the average for the 37 countries in the OECD was 9% (Martin et al., 2021; Schneider et al., 2017; Tikkanen & Abrahms, 2020). The United States spent twice as much as the average country in the OECD (Tikkanen & Abrahms, 2020). Switzerland was the second-highest spender in the OECD, and it spent an average of $7300 per resident. However, considering all 37 OECD member countries, the average spent per resident was $3994 (OECD, 2020). Given the current economic and demographic trends, it is anticipated that national health expenditures will represent nearly 20% of US GDP in 2027 (Sisko et al., 2019).

There is no doubt that the cost of US healthcare is high and has steadily increased over the decades. The growth in US spending is primarily due to the greater use of advanced medical technologies, better healthcare coverage, higher utilization of healthcare services, rising prices of healthcare services, and an aging population (Tikkanen & Abrams, 2020). Despite the higher levels of health spending, the United States ranked lower than its high-income peers on the most common measures of population health.

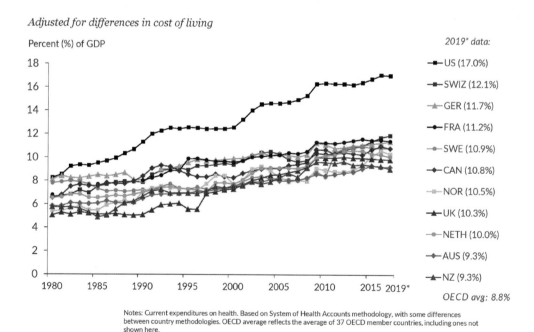

Fig. 1.1 Healthcare spending as a percent of gross domestic product 1980–2019. (From: Roosa Tikkanen and Katharine Fields, *Multinational Comparisons of Health Systems Data, 2020* (Commonwealth Fund, Feb. 2021).)

MEASURES OF HEALTH

Population health is a term that has evolved over the years. Initially defined by Kindig and Stoddart (2003) as "the field of study that examines the health outcomes of a group of individuals, including the distribution of such outcomes within the group" (p. 380). Understood within this definition is that the field of study includes studying not only the health outcomes and patterns of health determinants but also the policies and interventions that link the outcomes to the determinants (Kindig & Stoddart, 2003). Population health attends to the system of influences that interact to create differences in health outcomes for various groups (Silberberg et al., 2019). The systems of influence can be social, environmental, economic, or healthcare system–related factors. These and other factors influence a person's health and create differences in health status and health outcomes (Silberberg et al., 2019). The novel coronavirus disease 2019 (COVID-19) is an example of how systems of influence create health disparities. Racialized populations, those from racial and ethnic minority groups, were affected by higher rates of infection, sickness, disease, and death than the dominant white, non-Hispanic population (CDC, 2020a). This difference in risk and exposure to COVID-19 could be due to household composition (overcrowding), social and economic inequities, increased numbers of frontline workers versus the ability to work from home (public-facing factors), food insecurity, and limited access to healthcare. Experts agree that social and structural conditions shape a population's health to a greater extent than biological factors or the services provided by clinicians (Silberberg et al., 2019). Thus population health as a framework is used to conceptualize why some populations are healthier and have different outcomes than other populations.

A population can be defined in a variety of ways. The population can be defined as a geographic area such as a community, state, region, or country, or some shared identity, such as race or ethnicity. A population can also refer to groups or subgroups, such as incarcerated individuals, veterans, level of ability, socioeconomic status, or those with specific health conditions. Population health focuses on the lived experiences of individuals within particular groups, their patterns of health, health outcomes, and the determinants that influence those outcomes. To effectively assess the health of a population, traditional metrics or measures are used

for comparison (Table 1.1). The traditional measures of population health include life expectancy at birth, maternal mortality, infant mortality, suicide, functional limitations, chronic disease burden, and obesity.

Life expectancy at birth measures how long a newborn is expected to live considering age-specific death rates. In 2018, life expectancy at birth in the United States was 78.7 years (National Center for Health Statistics [NCHS], 2021). The 78.7 years is 2.0 years less than the OECD average life expectancy of 80.7 years and the lowest life expectancy out of the 10 high-income countries in the OECD (Tikkanen & Abrahms, 2020) (Fig. 1.2).

This considerably lower life expectancy in the United States has been attributed to the rise in unintentional injuries, Alzheimer disease, and suicide in recent years. COVID-19 rapidly became the number-one cause of death in the United States in 2020, averaging more than 3000 people per day (CDC, 2021a). This number of deaths per day far exceeded the mortality rate for heart disease, which causes approximately 2000 deaths per day, while cancer claims approximately 1600 lives per day (CDC, 2021a). The other leading causes of death in the United States are heart disease, cancer, accidents (unintentional injuries), chronic respiratory diseases, cerebrovascular diseases, Alzheimer disease, diabetes, kidney disease, influenza and pneumonia, and suicide (CDC, 2021a).

Years of potential life lost (YPLL) is another measure of mortality that estimates the average time a person would have lived had the person not died prematurely (CDC, 2021a; OECD, 2020). In 2014, the United States ranked seventh highest in potential years of life lost and, of those countries that ranked higher, each had a lower average per capita income than the United States (Rice et al., 2020). Methods to calculate YPLL vary, but YPLL is counted as the number of years of life lost due to death before the age of 70, although some references indicate before 75 (CDC, 2020b; Rice et al., 2020). YPLL is used to document the different causes of premature death in a given population and compare early mortality rates within and between populations. The relevance of this measure is mainly to draw comparisons in life expectancy between groups within population subsets, often as it relates to race and ethnicity.

The infant mortality rate (IMR), defined as the death of an infant before the first birthday, is measured as the number of deaths per 1000 live births. This rate is a standard public health measure that reflects the health of an entire population, including living conditions, morbidity rates, access to healthcare, and maternal health

TABLE 1.1 Measures of Health

Core Measures of Health	Definition
Life expectancy	Typically, this is calculated as the life expectancy at birth, although it may be calculated as the remaining life expectancy for any given age. Life expectancy at birth is one of the most frequently used health status indicators.
Healthy life expectancy	The expected number of remaining years of life spent in good health from a particular age, typically birth or age 65, assuming current rates of mortality and morbidity.
Mortality rate	The number of deaths that occur in a population during a period (usually 1 year) divided by the size of the population is the population's crude mortality; the measure of the frequency of occurrence of death in a defined population during a specified interval.
Infant mortality rate	The infant mortality rate is the number of infant deaths for every 1000 live births. In addition to giving us key information about maternal and infant health, the infant mortality rate is an important marker of the overall health of a society.
Chronic disease burden	Burden of disease is a concept that describes death and loss of health due to diseases, injuries, and risk factors for specific regions or countries.
Health functional status	Methods to assess and classify the health, function, and disability of members of a population, for example, the International Classification of Functioning, Disability, and Health, and methods to estimate the overall health of populations.
Morbidity	An illness, disease, or condition. Incidence and prevalence rates are terms commonly associated with morbidity. *Prevalence* is the proportion of a population that has a health condition at a point in time or allows us to determine a person's likelihood of having a disease. *Incidence* conveys the sense of speed with which a condition occurs in a population and allows us to determine the probability of being diagnosed with a specific disease during a specific time.
Health-related quality of life	Indices used to quantify health and analyze cost-effectiveness. These indices are based on interviewer- or self-administered questionnaires that address various health dimensions or domains, such as mobility, ability to perform certain activities, emotional state, sensory function, cognition, social function, and freedom from pain.
Years of potential life lost	Years of potential life lost is a summary measure of premature mortality (early death). It represents the total number of years not lived by people who die before reaching a given age.

From: https://www.healthypeople.gov/2020/about/foundation-health-measures/General-Health-Status; Cdc.gov; who.it.

(NCHS, 2021). In 2018, the IMR for the United States was slightly under 6% but still much higher than the comparable OECD country average of 3.4–3.5%. The United States had a higher infant mortality rate than Canada, France, the United Kingdom, Belgium, the Netherlands, Switzerland, Australia, Germany, Austria, Sweden, or Japan (Kamal et al., 2019; Rice et al., 2020). In addition, notable differences exist in the IMRs among the subpopulations within the United States. For example, the IMRs for Whites, Hispanics/Latinos, and Asian/Pacific Islanders are significantly lower than for Blacks/African Americans by almost twice as much (NCHS, 2021). The US states with the highest populations of African Americans have higher IMRs and have 3- to 4-year differences in life expectancy for adults (Rice et al., 2020).

The United States has higher rates of obesity, chronic disease burden, and suicide than Switzerland, Germany, France, Sweden, Canada, Norway, the Netherlands, the United Kingdom, Australia, or New Zealand (Tikkanen & Abrahms, 2020). Of these 10 OECD countries, the United States has the highest obesity rate, 40%. This 40% obesity rate is twice as high as the OECD average of 21% (Rice et al., 2020; Tikkanen & Abrahms, 2020). Overweight and obesity are determined by a higher weight than what is considered a healthy weight for the person's height and are calculated using the body mass index (BMI) (CDC, 2021b). The BMI is calculated as a person's weight in kilograms divided by the square of height in meters (CDC, 2021b). For example, if a person is 5 feet, 9 inches and weighs 170 pounds, the BMI is 25.1, slightly

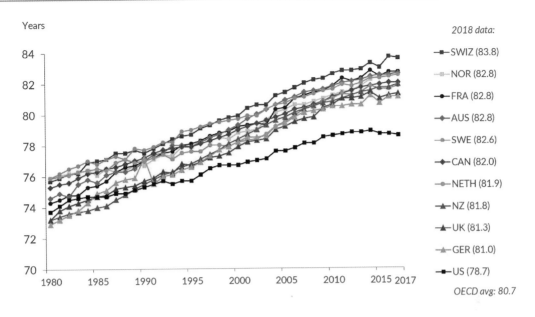

Years

2018 data:
- SWIZ (83.8)
- NOR (82.8)
- FRA (82.8)
- AUS (82.8)
- SWE (82.6)
- CAN (82.0)
- NETH (81.9)
- NZ (81.8)
- UK (81.3)
- GER (81.0)
- US (78.7)

OECD avg: 80.7

OECD average reflects the average of 37 OECD member countries, including ones not shown here.

Source: OECD Health Data 2020.

Fig. 1.2 Life expectancy at birth. (From: Roosa Tikkanen and Katharine Fields, *Multinational Comparisons of Health Systems Data, 2020* (Commonwealth Fund, Feb. 2021).)

overweight. If a person's BMI is between 18.5 and 25, the weight is within the normal range. If the BMI is in the 25 to 30 range, the person is considered overweight. If the BMI is 30 or higher, the person is obese (CDC, 2021b). Obesity contributes to the burden of chronic disease. In the United States, chronic diseases are both prevalent and costly. Nearly 60% of all adults in the United States suffer from at least one chronic disease, and 40% suffer from two or more chronic conditions (CDC, 2021a) (Fig. 1.3).

Chronic conditions cause more than 66% of deaths in the United States, which occurs despite the vast amount of money spent on healthcare. Most of the major chronic diseases in the United States, such as heart disease, cancer, chronic lung disease, stroke, Alzheimer disease, diabetes, and chronic kidney disease, could be prevented with modifications to lifestyle and health-related behaviors. Suicide, death by self-injury with the intent to die, is the 10th leading cause of overall death in the United States (CDC, 2021a). Over the last 20 years, the suicide rate has increased from 10.5% to 14.2% (CDC, 2021a).

Another measure of health often used is self-rated health. Self-rated health is an individual's assessment of their physiological and psychological status. Eighty-eight percent of the US population describe their self-rated health as good or better. This rating is higher than other countries in the OECD, although Canada and New Zealand residents ranked near the US rate (Rice et al., 2020). Self-rated health ratings vary by subpopulation and socioeconomic status. This variation is consistent with many conditions and measures of health in the United States.

The poor performance of the United States on standard measures of health is in stark contrast to its high spending on healthcare. Considering the international comparison against the 10 high-income countries in the OECD, the United States ranked last in access, equity, and healthcare outcomes, and next to last in administrative efficiency (Schneider et al., 2021). In this context, access and equity measures refer to affordability, access to care, timeliness of care, the financial burden or barrier in receiving care, and the ability of healthcare providers to render patient-centered care (Schneider et al., 2021). Healthcare outcomes include the standard measures of health (Schneider et al., 2021). The US measures are alarming with the realization that the United States has the highest per capita health expenditures of any country and spends a more significant percentage of its GDP on healthcare than any other

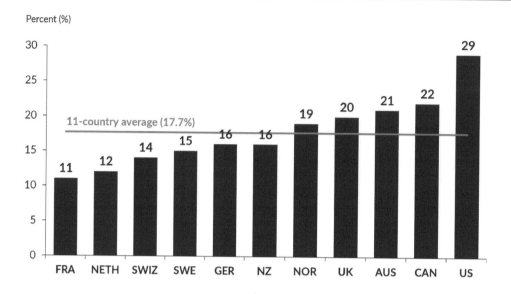

Percent (%)

Fig. 1.3 Adults with multiple chronic conditions, 2020.

Definition: Adults age 18 years or older who have ever been told by a doctor that they have two or more of the following chronic conditions: joint pain or arthritis; asthma or chronic lung disease; diabetes; heart disease, including heart attack; or hypertension/high blood pressure. Average reflects that of the 11 countries shown on the slide that take part in the Commonwealth Fund's International Health Policy Survey, all of which are shown here.
Source: 2020 Commonwealth Fund International Health Policy Survey.

country (Schneider et al., 2021). Given the comparison of the United States with other countries in the OECD on standard health measures and based on the healthcare dollars spent, there is little doubt that efficiencies could be achieved by providing a comparable level of service at lower cost.

HEALTHCARE FINANCING

National health expenditures are based on the types of goods or services delivered and the source of funding for those services. Typical health care spending is spread across services such as hospital care, provider/physician services, clinical services, prescription drugs, nursing care facilities, home care, personal health-related costs, governmental administrative costs, the net costs of health insurance, public health initiatives, and investment spending, but the bulk of expenditures is for the care provided by hospitals and physicians (American Medical Association, 2019). Healthcare insurance covers these expenditures with substantial variations in coverage across the different categories of care. The major sources of funding for healthcare are from private health insurance or federal and state taxpayer-funded

programs such as Medicare, Medicaid, the Children's Health Insurance Program (CHIP), the military, or other health coverage programs.

Health Insurance Programs

Private health insurance is coverage offered by a private company instead of through the state or federal government. Most Americans are enrolled in private healthcare insurance through an employer-based benefits plan, most often financed through employee- and employer-based contributions. Employer-based insurance plans may be through contracts with Blue Cross and Blue Shield, United Health Care, or health maintenance organizations (HMOs). Considerable variations exist in private health insurance plans as related to costs and coverage. There are two major types of private health insurance: preferred provider organizations (PPOs) and HMOs. The major differences between the two types are cost and network coverage. A network is a group of providers who have agreed to provide healthcare services to members of a specified insurance plan. The services provided can be categorized as in-network or out-of-network. The PPO is a more flexible health plan that costs less if your providers are in-network but covers the cost of services for out-of-network care at a higher price. The HMO offers coverage for in-network care at reduced costs and does not provide coverage for healthcare services that occur out-of-network.

Medicare is a federal health insurance program that pays for healthcare services for individuals 65 and older and individuals with specific disabling conditions. There are four major parts to Medicare: A, B, C, and D. Medicare Part A pays for hospitalization; Part B pays for physician services; Part C includes payment for hospital and physician services with the option for pre-scription drugs, vision, hearing, and dental coverage; and Part D pays for outpatient medications. Medicaid is a combined federal and state insurance program that finances the delivery of healthcare services and sup-port to low-income individuals, including children, pregnant women, adults, individuals with disabilities, and individuals over the age of 65, although the eligi-bility varies by state (Congressional Research Service, 2021; Rice et al., 2020). CHIP provides insurance cov-erage for low-income children and pregnant women who have an annual income above the Medicaid eli-gibility levels but do not have health insurance cov-erage through other healthcare plans (Congressional Research Service, 2021). Military health care programs are for military service members and veterans through the Department of Veteran Affairs (VA) and their dependent families (TRICARE). Other health insur-ance programs can be any combination of private or public plans. Despite these health insurance programs, many American citizens, 30 million or nearly 10%, remain uninsured (Congressional Research Service, 2021). Uninsured individuals often go without medi-cal care or visit hospital emergency departments when ill because they have no access to primary healthcare services.

The Patient Protection and Affordable Care Act of 2010 (ACA), the most groundbreaking compre-hensive piece of legislation passed to date, brought health insurance coverage to millions of Americans. The ACA legislation was intended to expand access to insurance coverage, increase consumer health insur-ance protections, promote prevention and wellness, improve health quality and healthcare system per-formance, decrease rising healthcare costs, and pro-vide states the opportunity to expand their Medicaid program.

Before the ACA, Medicaid eligibility was limited to specific low-income groups, such as the elderly, people with disabilities, children, pregnant women, and some parents. A provision in the ACA allowed for the expan-sion of Medicaid; the expansion would increase eligi-bility to cover more low-income people, that is, adults who earned up to 138% of the federal poverty level. With this expansion, the federal government would be responsible for the bulk of the cost for the newly cov-ered individuals, 90%, while the individual states would be responsible for the remaining 10% (Price & Eibner, 2013). This program, known as the Medicaid Expansion or the Exchange program, would allow states to partic-ipate voluntarily. Unfortunately, the states that did not participate or expand their coverage left many of their citizens unable to afford health insurance (Kaiser Family Foundation, 2021).

Conversely, the states that expanded Medicaid through the Medicaid Expansion program enabled many uninsured poor and near-poor individuals to receive health insurance coverage (Rice et al., 2020). The Medic-aid Expansion program allowed individuals and families whose incomes were too high to meet Medicaid eligibil-ity requirements to receive subsidies to purchase private health insurance on what is known as a health insurance marketplace. With the advent of the ACA, significant gains in healthcare coverage were realized by racial and ethnic minorities primarily due to the implementation of the Medicaid Expansion and health insurance market-places (Guth et al., 2020). The ACA improved access to coverage and services for many individuals.

The ACA also made provisions for funding com-munity health centers. The funding of such centers would improve access to healthcare for many under-served racial and ethnic minorities. Disparities stem from limited access, differential treatment, and clini-cian biases in the provision of services (Boyd et al., 2020). Evidence demonstrates that diverse providers are more likely to serve diverse people and advocate for their needs. Patients who see providers who look like them are more likely to have increased provider trust and improved communication with the provider due to language concordance (LeVeist & Pierre, 2014; Neff et al., 2020). In the ACA, there was support for having a diverse and culturally competent workforce that could positively impact the health of minority populations. Cultural and linguistic competency was an added provision in the ACA to help with cultural and linguistic differences, improve cultural competence, and strengthen data collection and research efforts (Guth et al., 2020). The relationship between culture and health equity is presented in more detail in Chapter 9 (Section: Understanding Culture and Why it Matters in Achieving Health Equity).

Despite the provisions initially included in the ACA that afforded insurance to many uninsured Americans, the federal policy priorities under the Trump administration led to substantial rollbacks of the provisions, causing the rates of uninsured Americans to soar from 10% to 15.5% (Congressional Research Service, 2021). This climb occurred when Congress removed the individual mandate for insurance coverage. The restrictive policies on immigration under the Trump administration made immigrants fearful of seeking healthcare through Medicaid and CHIP for fear of deportation, which led to many uninsured in the immigrant population. The effect of the Trump rollbacks increased the number of uninsured individuals and perpetuated health disparities (Guth et al., 2020).

However, the federal government made health equity a priority under the Biden administration. In 2021, President Biden issued executive orders to advance health equity. First, Biden issued an executive order on *Advancing Racial Equity and Support for Underserved Communities*. Second, the National Institutes of Health launched the UNITE initiative to address structural racism and racial inequities in biomedical research. Third, the CDC declared racism a serious threat to the public's health (CDC, 2021c). Lastly, the Office of Minority Health launched initiatives designed to (1) sustain health equity–promoting policies, programs, and practices; (2) provide community health workers to address the health and social needs of communities of color; and (3) strengthen cultural competencies among healthcare workers (Ndugga & Artiga, 2021).

Payment Models

The primary healthcare payment models are fee-for-service and value-based care. The fee-for-service model was the dominant payment model through the early 1990s. This model paid healthcare providers for the services rendered; the more services provided, the more the provider would be paid. These models would pay providers for the number of services, every test, procedure, or service rendered each time the patient visits the healthcare provider. There was no regard for the quality of the service or the outcomes of care. The fee-for-service model has been criticized because many believed it served the self-interests of providers, offered no incentive to decrease healthcare costs, and contributed to unnecessary services. Not only did this reimbursement model disregard the cost of services; it also created a strong incentive to increase the healthcare services rendered to individuals. In addition, the fee-for-service model could lead to the duplication and fragmentation of provider and diagnostic services. As a result, the fee-for-service model significantly contributed to the overprovision of services, inefficiency, and uncontrollable healthcare expenditures (Ikegami, 2015). These concerns, coupled with rising healthcare costs and worries about quality of care, were the impetus to consider alternative payment models that could reduce costs, improve the patient experience, and improve healthcare outcomes.

Value-based care encompasses a reimbursement model that focuses on the outcomes of the healthcare services provided instead of the fee-for-service model that renders payment regardless of care outcomes. Value-based models advance the quadruple aim of healthcare by improving healthcare services, implementing population health management, lowering healthcare costs, and increasing healthcare worker satisfaction (Bodenheimer & Sinky, 2014). Value-based care is based on the quality rather than the quantity of services (Revcycle Intelligence, 2023). The intent is to ensure that healthcare organizations perform at the highest level, although there is little agreement on how that highest performance is measured (Revcycle Intelligence, 2023). Aside from the lack of a clear definition of high performance, perspectives vary in terms of whether quality, cost, outcomes, or access measure the value.

Moreover, where the responsibility and accountability for ensuring value lie is unclear. These different views on the "value in healthcare" perpetuate the current healthcare model and impede the adoption of models of care where value is based on outcomes rather than output (Pendleton, 2018). Despite these discrepant views, most stakeholders would agree that the current model and costs of healthcare are unsustainable.

The pay-for-performance (P4P) model is intended to improve the quality of services rendered to individuals. This model attaches a financial incentive to provider performance. P4P measures provider performance against a set of predetermined quality and efficiency measures used to gauge the provider's performance. In a P4P model, the healthcare provider would receive a financial incentive if the provider met a range of objectives, including delivery efficiencies, submission of data and measures to payers, and improved quality and safety of patient care (Rice et al., 2020). For example, if a certain percentage of the provider's patients had cholesterol levels within the standard limit, the P4P would financially reward the provider for attaining high performance on the cholesterol measure compared to the prior year (Rand Corporation, n.d.). The positive aspects are that the P4P model stresses quality over quantity of care and allows payors to redirect funds to encourage best practices that promote positive health outcomes. The criticisms associated with P4P are the harm these models could cause for low-income populations. Since health and wealth follow a social gradient, it is plausible that providers who serve low-income people would be at a financial disadvantage. Thus the physician could elect not to serve low-income populations. In addition, patients of lower socioeconomic statuses tend to be challenged by various circumstances that can influence their health outcomes. For example, the patient may not have the money for prescriptions or may lack transportation for needed follow-up care, affecting health status and care outcomes. Because of these challenges, risk adjustments and modifications were made allowable to P4P plans to avoid the disadvantage to providers for providing services to patients at the lower rungs of the socioeconomic ladder. Despite the modification, providers who treat low-income patients may still not perform well and ultimately decide not to treat low-income patients despite adjustments. Critics of the P4P model believe this model reduces provider job satisfaction due to the costly administrative systems required to gather the data for the necessary metrics and submission requirements (NEJM Catalyst, 2018).

Bundled payment models cover multiple healthcare services previously paid for separately. A healthcare bundle approximates the total cost of services a patient would receive during one episode of care over a specific time for one event. For example, a bundled payment model would calculate the price based on all the anticipated services needed within a 30-day time period for a cardiac bypass. If that cost is estimated to be $97,000 and the providers reduce the price by 5%, the provider receives the difference. On the other hand, if the costs exceed the allotted amount, the provider is responsible for the overage. This payment method encourages the team to coordinate care to avoid potential complications such as rehospitalization or other costly services. Thus this model would result in better patient care management.

Accountable care organizations (ACOs) are healthcare providers across different settings that improve an individual's health while reducing costs. This model rewards providers for cost reductions because they recognize that poorly coordinated care and uncoordinated transitions in care lead to increased costs. ACOs are designed to integrate the various care components, such as primary care, specialists, hospitals, home care, and so on, to ensure that all parts of the system work together collaboratively (Rand Corporation, n.d.; Rice et al., 2020). As a result, care is coordinated across a range of healthcare services. By having the providers work collaboratively, the care is better coordinated and focuses on prevention, which prevents the patient from having costly procedures due to unanticipated complications. In addition, the participating providers and organizations are financially rewarded with the savings that accrue through improved coordination and quality of care (Rice et al., 2020). ACOs are growing in numbers, increasing across the nation with public and private health insurers. Healthcare systems that have moved toward value-based care models are making significant investments in addressing the health-related social needs of the population while tracking the health outcomes, cost, patient experiences, and numbers of social services utilized by the people.

HEALTH AND THE SOCIAL DETERMINANTS

The US healthcare system has historically emphasized clinical intervention over interventions aimed at the broader circumstances in life that influence health. This continued emphasis on clinical interventions occurs despite the understanding that clinical care only accounts for 20% of a person's health outcomes, especially compared to the social and economic factors that account for 40–50% of health outcomes (National Academies of Sciences, Engineering, and Medicine [NASEM], 2019). Other factors shape health far more than clinical interventions, although the healthcare system is not structured to respond to the nonclinical matters that influence health. If the goal is to improve health for Americans at lower costs, then waiting for people to get sick and treating them is not the most appropriate approach. Health is more closely tied to physical and socioeconomic environments than to the clinical services rendered for healthcare.

Factors such as income and wealth, education, employment and occupation, family and social support, the built environment, the food environment, community safety and culture, media and information, and environmental pollution significantly influence health. It is now known that a person's zip code or place of residence is more strongly associated with life expectancy than their genetic code. The fact that the zip code impacts health more than the genetic code highlights the limited role the provision of healthcare services has in overall health (Daniel et al., 2018; NASEM, 2019). Why does zip code matter? Residential segregation is a form of structural racism in the housing market. Structural racism is a system in which public policies, institutional practices, cultural representations, and other norms work in various, often reinforcing ways to perpetuate racial group inequity (The Aspen Institute, 2016; Murray & Loyd, 2020). The place of residence is associated with the social and economic resources of an individual and the entire community. One's residence is a significant variable that accounts for differences in health status across populations. Neighborhoods are often divided by race, ethnicity, and socioeconomic status (a combination of income, education level, and occupation), all of which significantly impact health. Racism has a significant impact on health. The CDC declared racism a serious threat to the public's health (CDC, 2021c). Experiences of interpersonal racism and other acts of oppression can lead to poor health outcomes. The chronic stress of being treated differently and unfairly (racism) compared to others and having inequitable access to resources causes biological aging (Gee et al., 2019). Frequent activation of the stress response can happen when individuals and communities are confronted with repeated inequities and discrimination, resulting in chronic cortisol elevations, also known as allostatic load. Allostatic load is the biological wearing or the "wear and tear" on the body that occurs over time as individuals are exposed to repeated episodes of racism at the interpersonal, systemic, or structural levels. When allostatic load occurs,

the body's cardiovascular, metabolic, nervous, and immune systems lose their ability to adapt and function normally (California Health in All Policies Task Force, 2018; Gee et al., 2019; Williams & Mohammed, 2013).

A person's health is influenced by various individual factors such as age, sex, race, genetic makeup, and health-related behaviors such as smoking, physical activity, alcohol use, and diet. Health is also influenced by social, economic, and cultural environments, level of education, financial status, and social and community contexts. The conditions in the physical environment that impact health include air and water quality, housing conditions, and transportation systems. The location of the healthcare system within the environment determines the type of healthcare services available and the quality of those services. These environmental factors lie outside the provision of clinical services yet shape health. Approximately 50% of health and health outcomes are related to the community context in which the person lives and thrives (Fig. 1.4).

For this reason, the Centers for Medicare and Medicaid Services (CMS) launched its Accountable Health Communities Model (CMS, 2020). This innovative model allowed dozens of healthcare system providers to act as conduits between clinical and community services. The hope is these CMS innovative project demonstrations will determine the promising practices needed for healthcare systems to expand beyond clinical care provision and address health more broadly and holistically.

The WHO has defined health as a state of "complete physical, mental, and social wellbeing" (WHO, 2021). The WHO affirms health as a fundamental right that should be afforded to individuals regardless of race, religion, partisan politics, or socioeconomic status (WHO, 2021). For years, the responsibility for health was placed solely on the individual. Much of healthcare in the United States focused on attending to the conditions and behaviors of the individual. This approach emphasized individual responsibility for health. Within the last two decades, there has been the growing realization that an individual's health results from a combination of experiences and circumstances that unfold over time within distinct political, social, environmental, and physical contexts (Short & Mollborn, 2015). This newer perspective suggests that conditions for health extend beyond

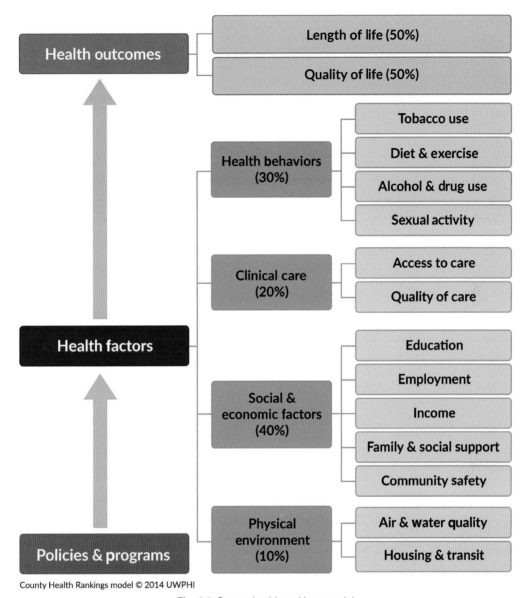

Fig. 1.4 County health rankings model.

the individual and are influenced by multiple factors and at various levels (personal [biological, behavioral, physiological, spiritual, and resiliency], organizational [healthcare system, healthcare quality, and healthcare access], environmental [housing, air quality, transportation, and employment] and policy) (US Department of Health and Human Services [USDHHS], n.d.). Ndduga & Artiga (2021) detail the complex and interrelated set of individual, provider, health system, societal and environmental factors that contribute to differences in health outcomes (Fig. 1.5).

HEALTH DISPARITIES

Considering the many factors that influence health, it is now known that certain factors create differences in the health and health outcomes of groups. The differences, known as health disparities, are the differences in health

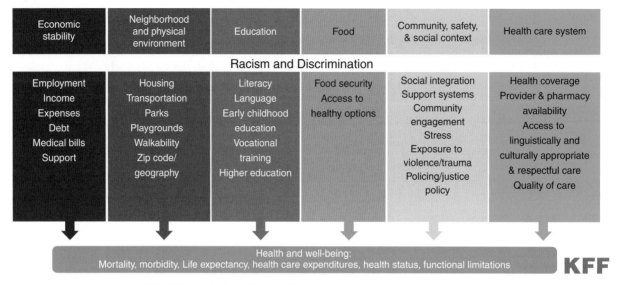

Economic stability	Neighborhood and physical environment	Education	Food	Community, safety, & social context	Health care system
		Racism and Discrimination			
Employment Income Expenses Debt Medical bills Support	Housing Transportation Parks Playgrounds Walkability Zip code/ geography	Literacy Language Early childhood education Vocational training Higher education	Food security Access to healthy options	Social integration Support systems Community engagement Stress Exposure to violence/trauma Policing/justice policy	Health coverage Provider & pharmacy availability Access to linguistically and culturally appropriate & respectful care Quality of care

Health and well-being:
Mortality, morbidity, Life expectancy, health care expenditures, health status, functional limitations

KFF

Fig. 1.5 Health disparities are driven by social and economic inequities.

status associated with social, economic, and environmental disadvantage, including characteristics linked to historical patterns of discrimination and exclusion (Braveman, 2014; Braveman & Gottlieb, 2014; Institute of Medicine, 2003; Ndugga & Artiga, 2021). Health disparity refers to the higher burden of illness, injury, disability, or mortality across groups or when comparing one group to another (Braveman, 2022; Ndugga & Artiga, 2021). Disparities are the disproportionate differences manifested in groups of people who have systematically experienced more significant obstacles to health based on racial or ethnic group, religion, socioeconomic status, sex, age, mental health, ability, sexual orientation or gender identification, geographic location, or other characteristics historically linked to discrimination or exclusion (Artiga, 2020; Braveman, 2022; Ndugga & Artiga, 2021). Health disparities are seen in the morbidity and mortality rates between groups. Disparities are also noted in the ability to access healthcare; these differences can be traced to specific populations when aggregated by factors such as socioeconomic status, sex, residence, and race and ethnicity (Braveman, 2014; Braveman & Gottlieb, 2014; Institute of Medicine, 2003). These differences in health, or disparities, persist and pose a significant economic burden to the affected individuals and all Americans. Disparities are rooted in the environmental contexts and conditions in which people live, most often shaped by structural realities such as the distribution of wealth and

power, social mores and cultural norms, and economic and political forces (WHO Commission on the Social Determinants of Health [CSDH], 2010; Artiga & Hinton, 2018). Unfortunately, until recently, little attention has been given to understanding the myriad of factors, systems, and structures that create and perpetuate differences in health. Many of the circumstances that make the differences are unjust and preventable (Braveman, 2022).

Marginalized Populations
Health in the United States has two vastly different realities when comparing specific populations. The burden of illness, premature death, and disability disproportionately affects marginalized populations (Zuckerman et al., 2016). Marginalized populations have often suffered discrimination, exclusion, or disregard by society and from the health-promoting resources it has to offer. These populations have been pushed to society's margins, with inadequate access to opportunities for better health. They are economically and socially disadvantaged. Historically excluded and marginalized or disadvantaged groups include people racialized as Black or Brown; people living in poverty, particularly those who have experienced intergenerational poverty; religious minorities; people with physical or mental disabilities; those with variations in sexual orientation and gender identification (lesbian, gay, bisexual, transexual, queer, questioning, intersexual, asexual [LGBTQ+]), and women. It is important to note that

these identities do not exist in isolation. Identity is complex and best explained through the concept of intersectionality. Intersectionality holds that a person can occupy more than one marginalized identity, such as a bisexual African American male. Whenever a person belongs to two or more marginalized identities, the concept of *intersectionality* provides a view of the person's lived experience in totality. Intersectionality is a theoretical framework that explains experiences of privilege and oppression at the individual level. The theory describes the intersectionality of multiple and complex aspects of a person's social identity. These interlocking forms of oppressed identities interrelate, making the two forms of oppression greater than the sum of each form, creating a multiplier effect. Another way to comprehend intersectionality is to view it as layered forms of bias held against a person because of multiple aspects of their identity.

HEALTH INEQUITIES AND HEALTH EQUITY

Health inequities are the systemic differences in a population's health status that are patterned, unfair, unjust, and actionable instead of random or caused by those who become ill (Michigan Department of Health and Human Services, 2019; WHO, n.d.). In other words, inequity is produced by social norms, policies, and practices that tolerate or promote the unfair distribution of and access to power, wealth, and other social resources. It is these inequities that lead to disparities in health. Health equity is achieved when everyone has a fair and just opportunity to be as healthy as possible (Braveman, 2022). No one is disadvantaged based on a socially defined identity or circumstance. A focus on health equity calls for a focus on the root causes of health disparities that expands beyond healthcare.

Obstacles (poverty, discrimination, and their consequences, including powerlessness and lack of access to jobs with fair pay and livable wages, quality education and housing, safe environments, and inaccessible healthcare) must be removed to achieve health equity. Health equity means reducing and ultimately eliminating disparities in health and the determinants that adversely affect excluded or marginalized populations. Health equity is the ethical and human rights principle that motivates us to eliminate health disparities (Braveman, 2014; Braveman & Gottlieb, 2014; USD H HS, Office of Minority Health, 2019). Health equity involves social justice. Social justice, like action, is a form of justice that consists of analysis, critique, and change in the social structures,

policies, laws, customs, power, and privileges that disadvantage or harm marginalized, excluded, exploited, and voiceless populations (Fawcett, 2019). Nurses have a long history of social justice. The commitment to social justice and health equity is rooted in nursing practice's ethical foundations and advocacy for vulnerable and marginalized populations.

Social justice is embedded in the code of ethics for nurses. According to Buettner and Lobo (2011), attributes of social justice include the following:

- Elements of fairness
- Equity in the distribution of resources
- Just institutions, systems, structures, policies, and processes
- Equity
- Sufficiency of well-being

There is a difference between equality and equity. Equality provides the same resources and opportunities for everyone without considering their specific needs, even when everyone is not situated the same in life (Michigan Department of Health and Human Services, 2019). Equity consists of fair and just treatment. Equity involves access to resources and opportunities for all people while building better outcomes for historically and currently disadvantaged populations. Equity requires targeted strategies. Equity recognizes that marginalized groups may need more resources, not equal resources, to account for the toll that has been taken by being a member of a historically excluded group.

THE SOCIAL DETERMINANTS OF HEALTH

Although there is no single definition of the social determinants of health (SDOH), the widely accepted definition is the conditions in which people are born, live, learn, work, play, worship, and age coupled with the broader set of forces and systems that shape the conditions of daily life that affect health and well-being (USDHHS, n.d.; WHO, 2010). These nonmedical conditions greatly influence health and contribute to the differences or disparities in health and health outcomes for particular groups (NASEM, 2019). The resources needed for health extend beyond access to medical care but include health-promoting physical and social conditions in homes, neighborhoods, and workplaces (Braveman, 2014; Braveman, 2022). The acknowledgment that the social and structural determinants of health are the root causes of disparities in health among marginalized populations is the initial step in a trajectory toward social justice (Fawcett, 2019).

UPSTREAM, MIDSTREAM, AND DOWNSTREAM

It is essential to note the distinction between two separate but related concepts, the nonmedical, health-related social needs of an individual and the SDOH. The terms upstream, midstream, and downstream are used to draw distinctions between the two concepts (Fig. 1.6) (upstream and downstream concepts). Upstream actions aim to reduce inequity by looking at the system issues that created the inequities resulting in health disparities. Midstream actions address the nonmedical social needs of an individual. Downstream actions provide the individual clinical care needed to treat a person once problems arise or a health condition occurs.

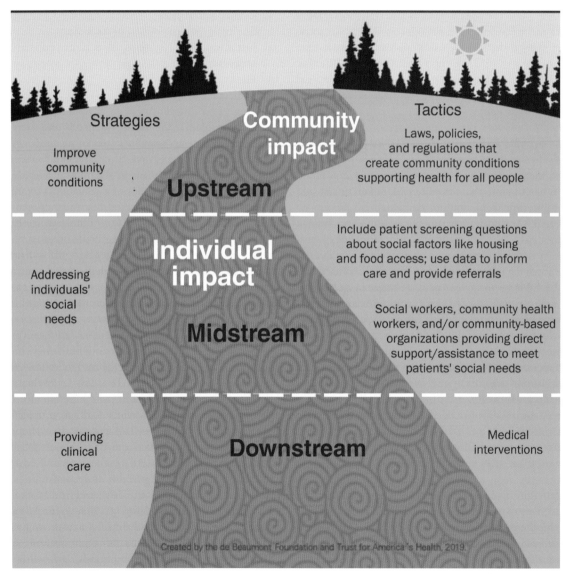

Fig. 1.6 Social determinants and social needs: Moving beyond midstream. (From: Castrucci, B. C., & Auerbach, J. (2019). Meeting individual social needs falls short of addressing social determinants of health. *Health Affairs Blog/Health Affairs.* 10.1377/hblog20190115.234942.)

Nonmedical health-related needs have also been referred to as health-related social needs. These health-related social needs are addressed at the individual level. However, the SDOH should be addressed at the population level since policy is involved because the conditions being addressed impact populations or entire communities (Castrucci & Auerbach, 2019). An example of a health-related social need is when an individual lacks food and needs assistance to purchase food. In this case, the nurse would refer the individual to social services to be connected to the Supplemental Nutrition Assistance Program (SNAP) for assistance. Another example might be a person who needs protection from an abusive partner. The nurse would get social services involved and refer that person to a shelter for abused partners. Lastly, the nurse learns that a person has had many missed appointments due to unaffordable or unreliable transportation to get to clinic appointments. In this case, the nurse would refer the person to a social service agency to connect to a transportation service. Other examples of meeting individual health-related social needs include getting social service assistance for housing insecurity, utility needs, food insecurity, education, or financial aid. These are examples of the nonmedical health-related social needs of individuals that impact the individual's health. Addressing a person's social needs has historically not been part of medical and healthcare practices, but an increasing amount of evidence supports that addressing social needs can produce improved health outcomes. For this reason, many healthcare providers have now incorporated screening for health-related social needs as a routine part of their practice (Castrucci & Auerbach, 2019). Screening for social needs enables the nurse to address the individual-level needs through referrals to social service and community organizations. The Structural Vulnerability Assessment Tool (Fig. 1.7) is a tool used to guide the clinician in learning more about the nonmedical social needs of individuals. Additionally, the movement toward value-based care has incentivized healthcare providers to address needs that traditionally fell outside of the realm of provider-based healthcare services. These types of nonmedical, health-related social needs are midstream interventions.

Solutions that address the SDOH are systemic, upstream, and impact the broader community or population. The new *Future of Nursing 2020–2030: Charting a Path to Health Equity Report* (2021) concluded,

"students should have learning opportunities to gain experience with interprofessional collaboration and multisector partnerships to enable them to address social needs comprehensively and drive structural improvements" (Agency for Healthcare Research and Quality [AHRQ], 2019 p. 9; NASEM, 2019). Upstream interventions tend to be policy oriented and often involve advocacy, engagement with community partners, and involvement with policymakers. To adequately address the SDOH, changes in laws, policies, or practices are required, and those changes affect entire communities or populations. One example of nurses engaged in upstream interventions is when a public health nurse works with municipal officials to advocate for laws and codes that make housing more affordable for an entire community. For example, US Representative Cori Bush notified a nurse constituent that President Biden signed the American Rescue Plan into law. The law ensured safe housing throughout the COVID-19 pandemic. The nurse constituent shared the information regarding the American Rescue Plan with the local Black Nurses Association to spread the word to nurses caring for patients who might need those services. The American Rescue Plan, an upstream intervention, provided emergency rental assistance to help millions of families keep up the rent on their homes and remain housed. It also called for a moratorium on evictions. Implementing the new law provided those who feared becoming house insecure with details on how to stay housed. Furthermore, it offered those unhoused the needed information to secure noncongregate shelter space.

There are several ways in which nurses and students can engage in upstream interventions. Advocacy is one way for nurses to become involved. Engaging in upstream interventions can occur at the individual level or through professional networks and organizations such as the state nurses associations, student nurses associations, and specialty nursing organizations with a health policy focus or governmental affairs arm. Health policy committees are aimed at social change and address community-level concerns. Laws directed at raising minimum wages to a livable wage and requiring health insurance benefits are examples of upstream interventions. Nurses, as advocates for the socioeconomically disadvantaged, can work through their professional nursing organizations and networks as advocates to advance policies aimed at social justice.

Assessment domain	Sample questions
Financial security	1. Do you have enough money to meet your daily living expenses? 2. Do you run out of money before your next pay day? 3. Do you receive income from other sources? 4. Are you dependent on others to meet your needs of daily living?
Housing	1. Do you have a stable place to live? 2. Do you ask to sleep over at your friends or family's home because you have nowhere to sleep?
Risk environment	1. Do you consider your environment safe? 2. Do you have adequate green space and walk paths for exercise? 3. Are you exposed to violence in your home or neighborhood environments? 4. Is your environment free of toxins or pollutants?
Food security	1. Do you eat healthy foods daily? 2. Can you describe your normal daily/weekly intake? 3. Are there adequate places to purchase healthy nutritious foods in your neighborhood?
Social cohesion and networks	1. Do you have friends or family members that you can count out should you need assistance? 2. Do you feel supported by friends and family? 3. Is there someone you can talk to when needed?
Legal status	1. Do you have or fear you may have legal problems? 2. Are you concerned about your legal status?
Literacy	1. What is your highest level of education? 2. Can you read, write, and comprehend most of what you read? 3. Is English your primary language?
Discrimination and bias	1. Do you feel you have been treated differently based on some aspect of your identity?

Fig. 1.7 Structural Vulnerability Assessment Tool.

Similarly, upstream interventions occur when the nurse is working with city officials or through the local school board to help levy a property tax increase for revenue for the local school district to improve educational services and opportunities for students in an underserved district. The nurse recognizes the relationship between education and health. These poorly funded schools place poor communities at a disadvantage in terms of educational attainment. Additionally, nurses can discuss zoning laws with elected and municipal officials through neighborhood associations, pointing out the negative impact

of predatory lending agencies such as payday loans and check-cashing companies on a community. These stores, often concentrated in underresourced communities, establish significantly higher fees and interest rates than traditional banks or credit unions, taking advantage of underserved and marginalized communities and their financial vulnerability. Consider the law that requires an individual to reveal their criminal background on an employment application. The law limits gainful employment for those incarcerated or convicted of a felony. Through various organizations and networks, nurses could advocate for changing laws of this nature to allow gainful employment for those who have paid their debt to society by serving time in a penal system.

Upstream interventions are viewed as outside the realm of traditional nursing practice. Economic power, politics, policy, and societal values influence structural factors, such as affordable housing, livable wages, commercial lending agencies, and employment requirements. These factors affect health and must be addressed if we are ever to minimize the disparities seen in disadvantaged populations (Braveman, 2022; Braveman & Dominguez, 2021; Murray, 2018). A narrow focus on the SDOH without a focus on the structural factors (policies and politics) would perpetuate inequities since these issues are tied to laws or policies that could be addressed through legal remedies (Dawes, 2020). Unless the structural problems are addressed, the risk of perpetuating a cycle of inequity and disparity will remain for generations to come (NASEM, 2019). To effectively address the upstream health measures, there must be an understanding of the role structural factors play in individual and population health. In addition, there must be advocacy for public policies that reach the disadvantaged and marginalized while targeting individuals' day-to-day needs.

CONCEPTUAL MODELS AND FRAMEWORKS

Conceptual models or frameworks detail the connection between and among concepts or constructs to explain a given phenomenon. There are several models or frames that can be used to advance the understanding of the social and structural determinants of health. These models provide a visual representation of concepts or constructs and their relationship to the determinants of health. They provide a conceptual view of the interrelated concepts used to explain health's social and structural determinants. The concepts are assembled by their relevance to the common theme and, when brought together in a rational or explanatory way, illuminate the relationships among the concepts to the overall phenomenon. The models provide perspective on the interrelatedness of the concepts to advance an understanding of the structural and SDOH. The concepts are represented through symbols, boxes, and diagrams that integrate the concepts into a whole.

Four conceptual models were selected to advance understanding of the social and structural determinants of health. Each model highlights the critical concepts that make up the social and structural determinants of health, although there is considerable variation among the models. The models illustrate how the various components of the social or structural environments (where people are born, live, learn, work, play, and age) have direct, indirect, and interactive effects on health. Within each model, consideration should be given to how the various concepts influence individual, family, and community levels of health and the progressive permanence of these factors throughout the life course. The models explain how the different determinants affect and interact with each other to impact health and well-being. The four models described in this section are the Healthy People 2030 Social Determinant of Health Framework, the National Institute of Minority Health and Health Disparities Research Framework, the WHO Commission on Social Determinants of Health Conceptual Framework, and the Future of Nursing 2020–2030, Nurse's Role in Addressing Health and Health Care Equity Conceptual Model. Each of these models describes the various concepts connected to health determinants. Two models, the National Institute of Minority Health and Health Disparities Research Framework and the WHO Commission on Social Determinants of Health Conceptual Framework, specifically highlight the complex, interrelated social, political, and economic structures that shape and influence the determinants.

Healthy People 2030 Social Determinant of Health Framework

Healthy People is a national effort aimed at improving the health and well-being of the American people. The Healthy People vision is for "a society in which all people can achieve their full potential for health and wellbeing across the lifespan" and the mission is "to promote, strengthen, and evaluate the Nation's efforts to improve the health and well-being of all people (USDHHS, Office of Disease Prevention and Health Promotion [ODPHP], paragraph 5, n.d.)." To accomplish this mission and vision, Healthy People 2030 identified five overarching goals:

1. Attain healthy, thriving lives and well-being, free of preventable disease, disability, injury, and premature death.
2. Eliminate health disparities, achieve health equity, and attain health literacy to improve the health and well-being of all.

3. Create social, physical, and economic environments that promote attaining full potential for health and well-being for all.
4. Promote healthy development, health behaviors, and well-being across all life stages.
5. Engage leadership, key constituents, and the public across multiple sectors to take action and design policies that improve the health and well-being of all.

The Framework by Healthy People 2030 has health equity and well-being at its center and highlights how social, economic, and environmental conditions produce health inequities that lead to health disparities. Healthy People 2030 provides a simple framework that categorizes the SDOH into five distinct domains: economic stability (employment, poverty, housing instability, and food insecurity), education access and quality (early childhood education and development, high school graduation, enrollment in higher education, and language and literacy), healthcare access and quality (access to health care, access to primary care, and health literacy), neighborhood and built environment (access to foods that support healthy eating patterns, crime and violence, environmental conditions, and quality of housing), and social and community context (civic participation, discrimination, incarceration, and social cohesion) (USDHHS, ODPHP, n.d.) (Fig. 1.8).

The five domains of Healthy People 2030 illustrate how health is determined by access to social and economic opportunities; the resources and supports available in our homes, neighborhoods, and communities; the quality of our schooling; the safety of our workplaces; the quality and cleanliness of our water, food, and air; and the nature of social interactions and relationships (USDHHS, ODPHP, n.d.). Examples from each of the five domains follow to illuminate the relationship of that domain to health. The examples are not an exhaustive list but rather an introduction to each of the five components introduced in the Health People 2030 Framework and the impact those factors have on health.

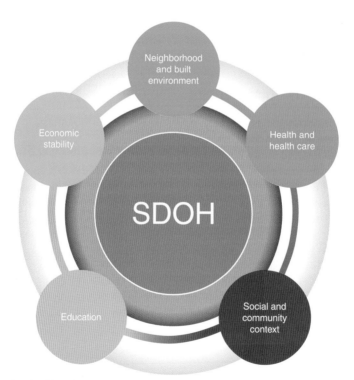

Fig. 1.8 Healthy People 2030 Framework for the Social Determinants of Health. (From: US Department of Health and Human Services, Office of Disease Prevention and Health Promotion. (n.d.). *Healthy People 2030: Social determinants of health.* Retrieved from https://health.gov/healthypeople/objectives-and-data/social-determinants-health.)

Economic Stability

Unemployment contributes to the inability to purchase food. Food insecurity is a critical issue in the economic stability domain. Healthy People 2030 defines food insecurity as a disruption in food intake or eating patterns due to the lack of money or resources (USDHHS, ODPHP, n.d.). There are two levels of food insecurity: low food security and very low food security. Low food security is when the individual has a reduction in the quality, variety, and desirability of the diet. Low food security is not necessarily associated with a decrease in food consumption. Very low food security is when the individual has disrupted eating patterns and a reduced amount of food consumed. Food insecurity can be short or long term, depending on the circumstances that led to the insecure state. The ability to purchase food is influenced by income and employment. Additionally, factors such as the availability of food resources such as grocery stores and fresh food markets and transportation also play a significant role in accessing food sources. Many neighborhoods, specifically in rural and urban areas, have limited places to buy food. These neighborhoods are known as food deserts. Food deserts are defined as communities that lack affordable and nutritious food and have an overabundance of convenience stores with higher food prices, lower-quality foods, less variety, and lacking fresh vegetables and fruits. Transportation is also a factor for food-insecure individuals because the closest full-service supermarket or grocery store may not be within walking distance. Transportation infrastructure is lacking in rural and urban communities, thus further limiting access to grocery stores. Reduced frequency, quality, variety, and quantity of health-producing foods will negatively affect health.

Education Access and Quality

High school graduation is a crucial issue in the education access and quality domain. A high school diploma is an essential requirement for most jobs, and most employers seek individuals with a college education. Individuals lacking a high school diploma are set up for a sequence of life circumstances that impact health, such as limited employment opportunities, lower wages than those who completed high school, and a higher incidence of poverty. Disparities in high school graduation rates exist between Whites and racialized and ethnically minoritized individuals. These disparities

are due to factors associated with the educational experience (teacher quality, educational resources in the school district, student behaviors, violence or bullying in the school setting, discipline in the school system, parental involvement, and parental participation in the educational process). Programs that encourage students to complete high school have been found helpful in improving the graduation rates of high-risk students. Evidence has shown that a student's lifetime wealth increases with each consecutive year of high school completion. Advances in educational attainment provide individuals with improved living conditions, better jobs with benefits, and subsequent access to healthcare services.

Social and Community Context

Discrimination is a vital issue in the social and community context domain. Discrimination is an action that results in the unfair and unjustified treatment of individuals or groups (USDHHS, ODPHP, n.d.). Discrimination comes into play when the power and privileges of one group are exercised over another group that has been deemed subservient based on some aspect of their identity (race, gender, sexual orientation, etc.). Discrimination can occur at the interpersonal level (between two individuals) or at the societal level, which is considered systemic or structural. At times, the words "systemic" and "structural" are both used to describe discrimination at the societal level. Discrimination at the individual level refers to the negative and differential treatment of an individual.

In contrast, structural discrimination refers to the societal-level conditions that limit the opportunities, resources, and overall well-being of the less privileged group. Both types of discrimination are harmful and can be intentional or unintentional. Both types of discriminatory acts create stress and take a toll on the physiological and psychological health of the person or group on the receiving end. Structural discrimination can be observed in residential segregation, disparities in access to quality education, criminalization of racial minorities, and healthcare. Residential segregation is a major cause of differences in health status between minoritized individuals and White people. Confinement to specific neighborhoods limits where a parent can send their child to school and perpetuates the cycle of exclusion from opportunities for upward mobility that have enabled many poor Whites to receive a better education. Residential segregation determines the social and economic resources of a community and the type and quality of education received in the community. For example, most school districts generate their income from local personal property taxes, so residential segregation and the valuation of homes translate into quite different possibilities for funding across school districts. Evidence supports that children who enroll in low-quality schools with limited health resources, increased safety concerns, and low teacher support are more likely to have poorer physical and mental health (Braveman & Dominguez, 2021). Structural discrimination is manifested in the variations in incarceration rates between Whites and minoritized groups. Disparities in incarceration rates are seen with the different sentencing levels between crack cocaine, which was primarily used by low-income racial minorities, and powdered cocaine, often branded as the drug of choice for high-income professionals. This differential sentencing has led to much higher arrests, convictions, and incarceration rates among minority populations than the White population (Braveman & Dominguez, 2021). Routine discrimination can be a chronic stressor that leads to increased vulnerability and generalized "wear and tear" on the body (Braveman & Dominguez, 2021; Gee et al., 2019).

Neighborhood and Built Environment

Environmental conditions are key issues in the neighborhood and built environment domain. Air, water, and heat are three environmental conditions that can have a significant impact on health. Poor water quality places the public's health at risk, as seen with the Flint, Michigan water crises. Flint is a predominantly African American city, and 41% of residents live below the federal poverty level. The state of Michigan authorized switching the source of tap water for the approximately 99,000 residents of Flint from the Detroit Water and Sewerage Department to the Flint River. The Flint Water Treatment Plant did not use corrosion control, resulting in increased lead contamination in the water supply. After several parents and community healthcare workers heard about elevated levels of lead and noticed health problems affecting citizens after the switch, testing was done and revealed that blood lead levels had increased among children in the city. Lead ingestion is serious, and the effects are sometimes irreversible. As with water, outdoor and indoor air quality influences

health. Chronic exposure to air pollutants increases the risk of cardiovascular and respiratory disease. Air temperature also influences health, as seen with sickness and deaths related to extreme heat or cold temperatures. The distribution of biohazards, toxic waste sites, sewage treatment plants, and other environmental toxins, pollutants, and dangers has been disproportionately located in or near low-income and minority communities. Environmental components such as proximity to hazardous waste sites, exposures to air and water pollution, high levels of ambient noise, residential crowding, quality of the housing stock, quality of the neighborhood schools, and the local employment opportunities lead to situations where communities of color and impoverished people bear a disproportionate burden of exposure to suboptimal and unhealthy environment conditions (Brulle & Pellow, 2006).

Health Care Access and Quality

Healthcare access is one of the key issues in the Health Care Access and Quality domain. Access to health care is defined as the timely use of health services to achieve the best health outcome. However, many people experience significant barriers to healthcare. The lack of health insurance or inadequate health insurance coverage poses a substantial barrier to healthcare access. Many individuals will forgo needed care because they lack health insurance or cannot afford the copayments required to have health insurance. Uninsured individuals are less likely to receive preventive care or screening for early detection of specific conditions.

Transportation is a barrier to health care access. The lack of transportation can lead to missed appointments, skipped appointments, the inability to get prescriptions for needed medications, or the postponement of care. Many neighborhoods located in low-income areas have limited healthcare facilities available. The lack of neighborhood healthcare services exacerbates issues with the lack of transportation.

Other factors that affect access to healthcare include a shortage of healthcare providers. Rural and urban areas typically have what is known as health professions shortage areas (HPSAs), and the residents live in what are known as medically underserved areas (MUAs). The lack of providers in certain regions further limits access to healthcare and often results in prolonged waiting to see the provider or even to obtain an appointment, which ultimately impacts health.

National Institute on Minority Health and Health Disparities Framework

The National Institute on Minority Health and Health Disparities Framework conceptualizes the factors relevant to understanding minority health and reducing disparities (National Institute of Minority Health and Health Disparities [NIMHD], 2017). The framework identifies specific domains and levels of influence. The domains of influence are biological, behavioral, physical/built environment, sociocultural, and the healthcare system. The levels of influence extend from the micro level to the macro level and include individual, interpersonal, community, and societal. Health outcomes can be at the individual, family/organizational health, community health, or population health levels (Fig. 1.9).

Alvidrez and colleagues (2019) illustrate how the racial/ethnic disparities in lung cancer result from a combination of the concepts in the NIMHD Framework. Lung cancer mortality may be driven by genetic risk (individual-biological), smoking behavior (individual-behavioral), exposure to secondhand smoke in the

home (physical and built environment–interpersonal), neighborhood-level exposure due to environmental toxins (physical and built environment–community), engagement in early screening (healthcare system–individual), access to high-quality cancer treatment (healthcare system–community), state policies related to Medicaid health insurance coverage (healthcare system–societal), and state laws regarding cigarette taxes and smoking bans (behavioral-societal). The NIMHD framework illustrates the complex and multifaceted nature by which factors across different spheres and levels can influence health and health disparities.

WHO Commission on Social Determinants of Health Conceptual Framework

The WHO conceptual model identifies two broad determinants that impact health and lead to health disparities (Fig. 1.10). The two categories of determinants are (1) the Structural Determinants, Social Determinants of Health Inequities and (2) the Intermediary Determinants of Health, Social Determinants

		Levels of influence*			
		Individual	**Interpersonal**	**Community**	**Societal**
Domains of influence (Over the life course)	**Biological**	Biological vulnerability and mechanisms	Caregiver–child interaction family microbiome	Community illness exposure Herd immunity	Sanitation immunization Pathogen exposure
	Behavioral	Health behaviors Coping strategies	Family functioning School/work functioning	Community functioning	Policies and laws
	Physical/built environment	Personal environment	Household environment School/work environment	Community environment Community resources	Societal structure
	Sociocultural environment	Sociodemographics Limited English Cultural identity Response to discrimination	Social networks Family/peer norms Interpersonal discrimination	Community norms Local structural discrimination	Social norms Societal structural discrimination
	Healthcare system	Insurance coverage Health literacy Treatment preferences	Patient–clinician relationship Medical decision-making	Availability of services Safety net services	Quality of care Healthcare policies
Health outcomes		Individual health	Family/ organizational health	Community health	Population health

National Institute on Minority Health and Health Disparities, 2018
*Health disparity populations: Race/ethnicity, Low SES, rural, sexual and gender minority
Other fundamental characteristics: Sex and gender, disability, geographic region

Fig. 1.9 National Institute on Minority Health and Health Disparities Framework.

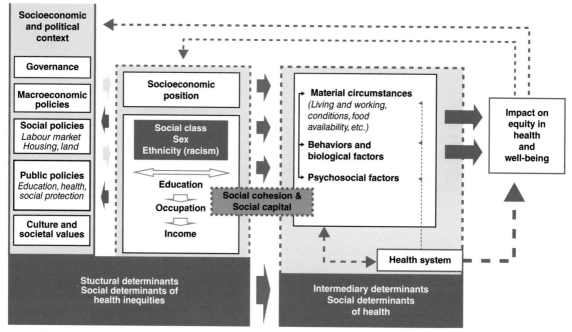

Fig. 1.10 WHO International Commission on the Social Determinants of Health Framework. (From: Solar, O., & Irwin, A. (2010). A conceptual framework for action on the social determinants of health. Social determinants of health discussion. Paper 2 (Policy and Practice), WHO.)

of Health. The Structural Determinants, Social Determinants of Health Inequities category contains the socioeconomic and political contexts, the structures that maintain and reinforce the social hierarchies such as the social, economic, and political contexts in which a person lives that include governance, how the society organizes itself, economic and social and public policies, and social and cultural values of the community (WHO, 2010). Socioeconomic and political contexts can lead to inequities in health based on the distribution of resources. These resources, in turn, shape the socioeconomic position, which determines the person's status in society. Socioeconomic position is influenced by ethnicity and race (due to racism), education, occupation, and income. These factors influence the intermediary determinants of health. The intermediary determinants of health are the material circumstances (housing and living conditions, working conditions, food availability, etc.). Living and working conditions reflect social position and are based on social class; a person can be exposed to health-enhancing or health-inhibiting behaviors. Behavioral, biological, and psychosocial factors are intermediary determinants that influence health, as are access to healthcare

and the types of services provided through the health system. Social cohesion and social capital are crosscutting concepts between structural and intermediary determinants. The linkages between concepts are complex, bidirectional, and illustrate the cyclical nature of a given social position and its impact on health. Structural determinants work together with intermediary determinants (material, behavioral, and biological factors, and psychosocial factors) to influence health outcomes. For example, income and education can impact health. Still, poor health can affect the ability to work or get an education, and the political contexts, including macroeconomic policies such as sick pay or unemployment, impact health. The model is complex and dynamic but a valuable framework to understand health's structural and social contexts.

Nurses' Role in Addressing Health and Health Equity Care Model

The *Future of Nursing Report 2020–2030* identified a conceptual model that illustrates nursing's role in addressing health at both the social and structural levels (NASEM, 2021) (Fig. 1.11). The model depicts five key areas to strengthen nursing as a profession: workforce,

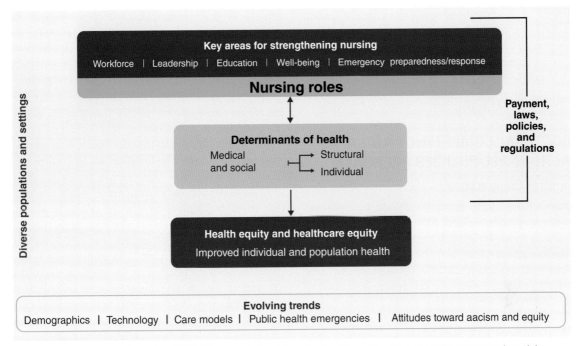

Fig. 1.11 Future of Nursing 2030: Nurses role in addressing health and healthcare equity conceptual model. (From: National Academies of Sciences, Engineering, and Medicine, 2021. The Future of Nursing 2020–2030: Charting a Path to Achieve Health Equity. https://doi.org/10.17226/25982. Reproduced with permission from the National Academy of Sciences, Courtesy of the National Academies Press, Washington, D.C.)

leadership, education, well-being, and emergency preparedness and response (NASEM, 2021, p. 5). Nurses are expected to function in various roles to impact the health needs of individuals and populations to advance health equity. The profession must develop a much more robust and diverse workforce; leadership capacity at all levels; relevant programs for entry; advanced, scientific, and continuing education; workforce resilience; and the ability to respond to disasters. These opportunities, like levers, can enhance the nursing profession's ability to address the SDOH and advance health equity along with focused attention on demographic trends, technological advances, innovative care models, public health emergency preparedness, and the ubiquitous nature of attitudes toward racism that is at the heart of the inequities and results in health disparities. Both the opportunities and trends depicted in this model will impact the nurse's role in promoting health equity.

The Life Course Perspective

While not a model, the life course perspective explains how a person's health status is shaped by physical, environmental, and psychosocial factors and how these factors affect health throughout the lifetime (Jones

et al., 2019). The perspective recognizes the importance of the causal links between exposures and outcomes within a person's life course, across generations, and in populations. It looks at life experience for patterns of health and disease with the recognition that current health and past health are shaped by social, economic, and cultural contexts (WHO, 2000). The life course view connects how the SDOH influences every level of individual development, immediately and later in life (WHO, 2010).

There are two ways of looking at the life course perspective through critical periods or the accumulation of risk. Critical periods, known as biological programming, are when exposure occurs during a specific period and has lifelong lasting effects on the bodily structures and functions of organs, tissues, and body systems that are not moderated by later life experiences (Ben-Shlomo & Kuh, 2002). The accumulation of risk view suggests that factors that promote or impede disease risk accumulate over the life course. This accumulation of risks adds to the notion that as the intensity, number, and duration of exposures increase, there will be a corresponding increase in the cumulative damage to the biological system (WHO, 2010). The life course perspective purports that biological and social risks are not limited to individuals within a single generation but extend across generations. This is commonly seen with adverse childhood experiences (ACEs). Nurius and colleagues (2019) conclude that reducing early ACEs will benefit early health but is also essential in preventing health disorders over the life course.

STRUCTURAL COMPETENCY AND A HEALTH-IN-ALL-POLICIES APPROACH

Structural Competence

Nurses and healthcare providers should be equipped with the knowledge, skills, and abilities to envision how the broader structural contexts are responsible for the conditions seen in patients and populations (Woolsey & Narruhn, 2018). Understanding how broader structural issues impact health is critical to advancing health equity. To have this understanding, the nurse must recognize that disparity is due to the allocation of resources, that differences in health outcomes are unjust and preventable, and not make the assumption that marginalized populations have made bad choices or poor lifestyle decisions (Murray 2021; WHO, 2019). The term *structural violence* addresses how political structures and social hierarchies lead to unnecessary suffering in marginalized populations. For example, structural violence occurs when social structures perpetuate inequity, causing preventable suffering, but yet is naturalized (Rylko-Bauer & Farmer, 2017). Naturalizing inequality refers to ways in which health disparities are often attributed to the behaviors or innate characteristics of individuals or groups of people most affected by the disparities. Naturalization causes the social and political origins of the disparities to be overlooked (Neff et al., 2020). Nurses must be aware that many of the health-related factors previously attributed to culture or ethnicity represent the downstream consequences of many upstream decisions made within larger structural contexts about matters related to healthcare access, food sources, residential living, zoning, and urban and rural infrastructures (Braveman, 2022; Metzl & Roberts, 2014; Murray 2021; Ndugga & Artiga, 2021; Neff et al., 2020). Nurses must become structurally competent to advance health equity.

Structural competency is the capacity for health professionals to recognize and respond to health and illness as the downstream effects of broad social, political, and economic upstream decisions about matters related to food delivery systems, zoning laws, urban and rural infrastructures, and even the very definition of health and illness (Metzl & Hansen, 2014; Neff et al., 2020). This competency enables the nurse to examine the SDOH frameworks and shift their attention to the forces that influence health at levels above individual interactions and contextualize disparities within the broader, social, political, and economic structures that impact health (Neff et al., 2020). A structurally competent approach enables the nurse to think more clearly, critically, and practically about how social structures create illness and disparities in health (Bourgois et al., 2017; Neff et al., 2020). Equally important is to understand how racism has been embedded in the institutions and laws of society and how racism influences health at all levels: interpersonal, systemic, and structural (Braveman & Dominguez, 2021). Nurses should frequently engage in self-reflection, collaboration, and advocacy to address the complexities of the inequities that produce disparities and adverse health outcomes.

Structural awareness and competence can provide nurses with an understanding of the interconnectedness between the individual clinical level and the sociopolitical structures that impact health. One way to understand this complexity is to understand that all policies impact people's health, yet nurses may not always consider the impact before the laws are enacted. Health in All Policies (HiAP) is an approach that integrates health considerations into the policymaking process to improve the health of individuals, communities, and populations (CDC, 2016). This approach recognizes that many factors beyond the scopes of traditional medical or public health services are needed to advance health equity. The HiAP approach calls for a multisectoral approach where policymakers are informed of the relationship between policies developed outside of the healthcare arena, such as housing, education, food security, transportation, and how those policies impact health. To achieve health equity and mitigate the disparities seen in marginalized populations, nurses must develop the structural awareness to work across sectors for policies that promote health. This frame of reference will encourage nurses to engage in social, political and policymaking processes that affect individual and population health and to advocate for policy transformation (Orr & Unger, 2020).

CONCLUSION

This chapter presents an overview of the SDOH, recognizing that broader social and structural contexts impact individual and population health more than the provision of clinical services. It points out how specific determinants are responsible for the disparities often seen in marginalized populations, and that the conditions for health extend beyond an individual. The connection is made that health disparities represent the downstream consequences of the many upstream decisions made in society. The frameworks introduced can provide a conceptual understanding of the totality of the conditions that impact health and how those conditions are embedded within policies and practices in society. Examining the social and structural determinants of health from a structural framework allows nurses to recognize the complexities associated with the myriad factors that contribute to disparities in the distribution of illness, the biases that undergird attributions about health and disease in marginalized groups, and that these disparities are unjust, avoidable, and preventable. This chapter also distinguishes between the levels of interventions—downstream, midstream, and upstream—that can be used to address the health of populations.

▌ CASE STUDY

J.X., a 19-year-old woman, has had several miscarriages. She gave birth to an infant 9 weeks early, weighing less than 3 pounds, but J.X. almost died during the delivery. As a premature infant, the baby was taken to the neonatal intensive care unit because she was severely underdeveloped. Diagnostic tests revealed several contaminants and toxins in the baby's system.

J.X. left her parents' home due to her father's substance use disorder. Ten years before that, her dad could access the health services and treatment he needed to maintain sobriety. Still, healthcare policies were changed, resulting in the closure of the neighborhood mental health and substance use centers. As a result, the dad was unable to access healthcare services, and he ended up in an altercation at work, badly beating a coworker, resulting in his termination and arrest.

Her mother could not secure a job with livable wages because she lacked skills and became depressed. She, like her husband, could not access mental health services because the community mental health centers had been closed.

J.X. moved into an apartment in a low-income neighborhood. The neighborhood had convenience stores and fast-food restaurants on every corner. Sidewalks were scarce. City buses did not run through the community. Schools were failing, and healthcare providers refused to operate in the community due to poor reimbursement rates from Medicaid.

1. What social determinants are at play in this situation?
2. What are the political implications that impacted J.X.'s and her baby's health in this situation?
3. Were the neighborhood conditions politically determined? If so, how?
4. To what extent does this situation show the compounding effect of the political determinants of health over personal responsibility?
5. What could you as the nurse do as upstream, midstream, and downstream measures to impact J.X.'s health?

Adapted from: Dawes, D. (2020). *The political determinants of health*. John Hopkins University Press.

▌ STUDENT REFLECTION QUESTIONS

1. Why is it necessary to screen patients for the SDOH?
2. What are some of the inequities embedded in societal structures that lead to poor health for marginalized populations?
3. You have encountered a patient in a community health clinic that communicates he is hungry and does not regularly eat because he has little resources to purchase food. You are aware that having access to nutritious and healthy food is essential for health. What are examples of downstream-, midstream-, and upstream-level interventions you can do as a nurse?
4. Does the information in this chapter cause you to think differently about the health problems of certain populations and the needed solutions to address them? Please explain.
5. Go to the Healthy People 2030 website, Social Determinants of Health Workgroup webpage, https://health.gov/healthypeople/about/workgroups/social-determinants-health-workgroup (ODPHP, n.d. b). Review the seven SDOH workgroup objectives. For example, six of the seven objectives aim to reduce parental incarceration and people living in

poverty, increase employment in working-age people and the proportion of children with at least one parent working full-time, reduce the proportion of families that spend 30% of income on housing, and increase the proportion of high school graduates in college the October after graduation. Reflect on the relationship that these objectives have to health. What role do you think nurses could have in reducing health disparities related to these objectives? How can that role be enacted in your nursing practice?

KEY POINTS OF REFLECTION

1. The unmet social needs of hospitalized patients and persons living in the community have a significant impact on health. Screening provides the nurse with an awareness of the person's living situation. Screening enables nurses to identify individuals or families who have unmet social needs, such as being food or housing insecure. Screening allows the nurse to know if the patient may have transportation challenges that would prohibit them from getting to their medical appointments.

2. The conditions in which people live can produce health inequities, such as housing, food, and the quality of their neighborhoods (physical environments). Concentrated poverty can create unhealthy living conditions. The tax base associated with school districts is maldistributed. School funding is dependent upon the property taxes of a community. This puts school districts in impoverished communities at a disadvantage. These schools would have fewer resources than higher-resourced communities. Education is closely linked to health.

3. Downstream: Provide health education to teach the person how to improve dietary behavior, including the selection of food. Provide counseling regarding daily nutrition guidance. Midstream: Make appropriate social service referrals to organizations such as Meals on Wheels, Women's, Infants, and Children's (WIC) Supplemental Food Program, and SNAP. Upstream: Address policy issues with legislators and town councilpersons, such as supplemental income, the establishment of local food banks, and the need to lower income thresholds to qualify for food assistance programs.

4. Think about structural competence, structural violence, and a health in all policies approach.

5. Reflect on the various roles nurses could play in meeting these objectives.

REFERENCES

Agency for Healthcare Research and Quality. (2019). *2018 National healthcare quality and disparities report*. Retrieved from https://www.ahrq.gov/research/findings/nhqrdr/nhqdr18/index.html.

Alvidrez, J. A., Castille, D., Laude-Sharp, M., Rosario, A., & Tabor, D. (2019). The National Institute on Minority Health disparities research framework. *American Journal of Public Health, S1*(109), S16–S20.

American Medical Association. (2019). *Trends in healthcare spending*. Retrieved from https://www.ama-assn.org/about/research/trends-health-care-spending.

Artiga, S. (2020). *Health disparities are a symptom of broader social and economic inequities*. Retrieved from https://www.kff.org/policy-watch/health-disparities-symptom-broader-social-economic-inequities/.

Artiga, S., & Hinton, E. (2018). *Beyond health care: The role of social determinants in promoting health and health equity*. KFF Henry J Kaiser Family Foundation. Retrieved from https://www.kff.org/disparities-policy/issue-brief/beyond-health-care-the-role-of-social-determinants-in-promoting-health-and-health-equity/.

Ben-Shlomo, Y., & Kuh, D. (2002). A life course approach to chronic disease epidemiology: Conceptual models, empirical challenges and interdisciplinary perspectives. *International Journal of Epidemiology, 31*(2), 285–293. https://doi.org/10.1093/ije/31.2.285.

Bodenheimer, T., & Sinsky, C. (2014). From triple to quadruple aim: Care of the patient requires care of the provider. *Annals of Family Medicine, 12*(6), 573–576. doi:10.1370/afm.1713.

Bourgois, P., Holmes, S. M., Sue, K., & Quesada, J. (2017). Structural vulnerability: Operationalizing the concept to address health disparities in clinical care. *Academic Medicine, 92*(3), 299–307. https://doi.org/10.1097/ACM.0000000000001294.

Boyd, R. W., Lindo, E. G., Weeks, L. D., & McLemore, M. R. (2020). On racism: A new standard for publishing on racial health inequities. *Health Affairs, Health Affairs Blog*. doi:10.1377/hblog20200630.939347.

Braveman, P. (2014). What are health disparities and health equity? We need to be clear. *Public Health Reports, 129*(Suppl. 2), 5–8. https://doi.org/10.1177/00333549141291S203.

Braveman, P. (2022). Defining health equity. *Journal of the National Medical Association, 114*(6), 593–600. https://doi.org/10.1016/j.jnma.2022.08.004.

Braveman, P., & Gottlieb, L. (2014). The social determinants of health: It's time to consider the causes of the causes. *Public Health Reports, 129*(Suppl. 2), 19–31. https://doi.org/10.1177/00333549141291S206.

Braveman, P., & Parker Dominguez, T. (2021). Abandon "race." Focus on racism. *Frontiers in Public Health, 9*, 689462. https://doi.org/10.3389/fpubh.2021.689462.

Brulle, R. J., & Pellow, D. N. (2006). Environmental justice: Human health and environmental inequalities. *Annual Review of Public Health, 27*, 103–124. https://doi.org/10.1146/annurev.publhealth.27.021405.102124.

Buettner, K., & Lobo, M. L. (2011). Social justice: A concept analysis. *Journal of Advanced Nursing, 68*(4), 948–958.

California Health in All Policies Task Force. (2018). *HiAP equity in government practices.*

Castrucci, B. C., & Auerbach, J. (2019). *Meeting individual social needs falls short of addressing social determinants of health.* doi:10.1377/hblog20190115.234942. Health Affairs Blog/Health Affairs.

CDC. (2016). *Health in All Policies.* Retrieved from https://www.cdc.gov/policy/hiap/index.html.

CDC. (2020a). *Coronavirus disease 2019: Health equity considerations & racial & ethnic minority groups.* Retrieved from https://www.cdc.gov/coronavirus/2019-ncov/community/health-equity/race-ethnicity.html.

CDC. (2020b). *WISQARS tutorials: Years of potential life lost.* Retrieved from https://www.cdc.gov/injury/wisqars/fatal_help/ypll.html.

CDC. (2021a). *National Center for Chronic Disease Prevention and Health Promotion: About chronic diseases.* Retrieved from https://www.cdc.gov/chronicdisease/about/index.htm.

CDC. (2021b). *Overweight & obesity.* Retrieved from https://www.cdc.gov/obesity/adult/defining.html.

CDC. (2021c). *Racism and health: Racism is a serious threat to the public's health.* Retrieved from https://www.cdc.gov/minorityhealth/racism-disparities/index.html.

Centers for Medicare & Medicaid Services. (2020). *National health expenditures 2019 highlights.* Retrieved from https://www.cms.gov/files/document/highlights.pdf.

Congressional Research Service. (2021). *US health care coverage and spending.* Retrieved from https://crsreports.congress.gov.

Daniel, H., Bornstein, S. S., Kane, G. C. & Health and Public Policy Committee of the American College of Physicians. (2018). Addressing social determinants to improve patient care and promote health equity: An American College of Physicians position paper. *Annals of Internal Medicine, 168*(8), 577–578. https://doi.org/10.7326/M17-2441.

Dawes, D. (2020). *The political determinants of health.* John Hopkins University Press.

Fawcett, J. (2019). Thoughts about social justice. *Nursing Science Quarterly, 32*(3), 250–255. https://doi.org/10.1177/0894318419845385.

Gee, G. C., Hing, A., Mohammed, S., Tabor, D. C., & Williams, D. R. (2019). Racism and the life course: Taking time seriously. *American Journal of Public Health, 109*(S1), S43–S47. https://doi.org/10.2105/AJPH.2018.304766.

Guth, M., Artiga, S., & Pham, O. (2020). *Effects of the ACA Medicaid expansion on racial disparities in health and health care.* Retrieved from .org/report-section/effects-of-the-aca-medicaid-expansion-on-racial-disparities-in-health-and-health-care-issue-brief/.

Ikegami, N. (2015) Fee-for-service payment—An evil practice that must be stamped out? *International Journal of Health Policy and Management, 4*(2), 57–59. https://doi.org/10.15171/ijhpm.2015.26.

Institute of Medicine. (2003). *Unequal treatment: Confronting racial and ethnic disparities in health care.* Retrieved from http://www.nap.edu/openbook.php?record_id=10260&page=R1.

Jones, N. L., Gilman, S. E., Cheng, T. L., Drury, S. S., Hill, C. V., & Geronimus, A. T. (2019). Life course approaches to the causes of health disparities. *American Journal of Public Health, 109*(S1), S48–S55. https://doi.org/10.2105/AJPH.2018.304738.

Kaiser Family Foundation. (2021). Who could get covered under Medicaid expansion? State fact sheets. Retrieved from https://www.kff.org/medicaid/fact-sheet/uninsured-adults-in-states-that-did-not-expand-who-would-become-eligible-for-medicaid-under-expansion/.

Kamal, R., Hudman, J., & McDermott, D. (2019). *What do we know about infant mortality in the US and comparable countries?* Retrieved from https://www.healthsystemtracker.org/chart-collection/infant-mortality-u-s-compare-countries/#item-start.

Kindig, D., & Stoddart, G. (2003). What is population health? *American Journal of Public Health, 93*(3), 380–383. https://doi.org/10.2105/ajph.93.3.380.

LeVeist, T. A., & Pierre, G. (2014). Integrating the 3Ds—Social determinants, health disparities, and health-care workforce diversity. Nursing in 3D: Workforce diversity, health disparities, and social determinants of health. *Public Health Reports, 129*(Suppl. 2), 45–50.

Martin, A. B., Hartman, M., Lassman, D., Catlin, A. & The National Health Expenditure Accounts Team. (2021). National health care spending in 2019: Steady growth for the fourth consecutive year. *Health Affairs, 40*(1), 14–24.

Metzl, J. M., & Hansen, H. (2014). Structural competency: Theorizing a new medical engagement with stigma and inequality. *Social Science & Medicine (1982), 103*, 126–133. https://doi-org.ezp.slu.edu/10.1016/j.socscimed.2013.06.032.

Metzl, J. M., & Roberts, D. E. (2014). Structural competency meets structural racism: Race, politics, and the structure of medical knowledge. *The Virtual Mentor, 16*(9), 674–690. https://doi-org.ezp.slu.edu/10.1001/virtualmentor.2014.16.09.spec1-1409.

Michigan Department of Health & Human Services. (2019). *Health inequities.* Retrieved from https://www.michigan.gov/mdhhs/0,5885,7-339-71550_2955_2985_79566—,00.html.

Murray, T. A. (2018). Overview and summary: Addressing social determinants of health: Progress and opportunities. *The Online Journal of Issues in Nursing, 23*(3). http://doi.org/10.3912/OJIN.Vol23No03MANOS.

Murray, T. A. (2021). Teaching the social and structural determinants of health: Considerations for faculty. *Journal of Nursing Education, 60*(2), 63–64.

Murray, T. A., & Loyd, V. (2020). Dismantling structural racism in academic nursing. *Journal of Nursing Education, 59*(11), 603–604.

National Academies of Sciences, Engineering, and Medicine. (2019). *Investing in interventions that address non-medical, health-related social needs: Proceedings of a workshop,* Washington DC: The National Academies Press. http://doi.org/10.17226/25544.

National Academies of Sciences, Engineering, and Medicine. (2021). *The future of nursing 20202030: Charting a path to achieve health equity.* The National Academies Press. https://doi.org/10.17226/XXXXX.

National Center for Health Statistics. (2021). *Health, United States, 2019.*

National Institute of Minority Health and Health Disparities. (2017). *NIMHD Minority Health and Health Disparities Research Framework.* Retrieved from https://www.nimhd.nih.gov/about/overview/research-framework/.

Ndugga, N., & Artiga, S. (2021). *Disparities in health and health care: 5 key questions and answers.* Retrieved from https://www.kff.org/racial-equity-and-health-policy/issue-brief/disparities-in-health-and-health-care-5-key-question-and-answers/.

Neff, J., Holmes, S. M., Knight, K. R., Strong, S., Thompson-Lastad, A., McGuinness, C., Duncan, L., Saxena, N., Harvey, M. J., Langford, A., Carey-Simms, K. L., Minahan, S. N., Satterwhite, S., Ruppel, C., Lee, S., Walkover, L., De Avila, J., Lewis, B., Matthews, J., & Nelson, N. (2020). Structural competency: Curriculum for medical students, residents, and interprofessional teams on the structural factors that produce health disparities. *MedEdPORTAL: The Journal of Teaching and Learning Resources, 16,* 10888. https://doi.org/10.15766/mep_2374-8265.10888.

NEJM Catalyst. (2018). What is lean healthcare? Retrieved from https://catalyst.nejm.org/topic/catalyst-article-type/brief-article.

Nurius, P. S., Fleming, C. M., & Brindle, E. (2019). Life course pathways from adverse childhood experiences to adult physical health: A structural equation model. *Journal of Aging and Health, 31*(2), 211–230. https://doi.oreg/10.1177/0898264317726448.

Organization for Economic Co-operation and Development. (2020). *Health at a glance 2019: OECD indicators.* Paris: OECD Publishing. Retrieved from https://doi.org/10.1787/4dd50c09-en.

Orr, Z., & Unger, S. (2020). The TOLERance model for promoting structural competency in nursing. *Journal of Nursing Education, 59*(8), 425–432. https://doi.org/10.3928/01484834-20200723-02.

Pendleton, R. C. (2018). We won't get value-based health care until we agree on what "value" means. *Harvard Business Review, 2,* 2–5.

Price, C. C., & Eibner, C. (2013). For states that opt out of Medicaid expansion: 3.6 million fewer insured and $8.4 billion less in federal payments. *Health Affairs, 32*(6), 1030–1036.

Rand Corporation. (n.d.). *Paying for care: In depth.* Retrieved from https://www.rand.org/health-care/key-topics/paying-for-care/in-depth.html.

RevCycle Intelligence. (2023). *What is value-based care, what it means for providers.* Retrieved from https://revcycleintelligence.com/features/what-is-value-based-care-what-it-means-for-providers.

Rice, T., Rosenau, P., Unruh, L. Y., & Barnes, A. J. (2020). United States: Health system review. *Health Systems in Transition, 22*(4), 1–441.

Rylko-Bauer, B., & Farmer, P. (2017). Structural violence, poverty, and social suffering. *The Oxford Handbook of the Social Science of Poverty.* Oxford University Press. doi:10.1093/oxfordhb/9780199914050.013.4.

Schneider, E. C., Sarnak, O., Squires, D., Shah, A., & Doty, M. M. (2017). *Mirror, mirror 2017: International comparison reflects flaws and opportunities for better US health care.* The Commonwealth Fund.

Schneider, E. C., Shah, A., Doty, M. M., Tikkanen, R., Fields, K., & Williams, R. D., II. (2021). *Mirror, mirror 2021–Reflecting poorly: Health care access in the US compared to other high-income countries.* The Commonwealth Fund.

Short, S. E., & Mollborn, S. (2015). Social determinants and health behaviors: Conceptual frames and empirical advances. *Current Opinion in Psychology, 5,* 78–84. https://doi.org/10.1016/j.copsyc.2015.05.002.

Silberberg, M., Martinez-Bianchi, V., & Lyn, M. J. (2019). What is population health? *Primary Care, 46*(4), 475–484. https://doi.org/10.1016/j.pop.2019.07.001.

Sisko, A. M., Keehan, S. P., Poisal, J. A., Cuckler, G. A., Smith, S. D., Madison, A. J., Rennie, K. E., & Hardesty, J. C. (2019). National health expenditure projections, 2018–27: Economic and demographic trends drive spending and enrollment growth. *Health Affairs (Project Hope), 38*(3), 491–501. https://doi.org/10.1377/hlthaff.2018.05499.

The Aspen Institute. (2016). *Racial equity: 11 terms you should know to better understand structural racism.* https://www.aspeninstitute.org/blog-posts/structural-racism-definition/.

Tikkanen, R., & Abrams, M. K. (2020). *US health care from a global perspective, 2019: Higher spending, worse outcomes.* The Commonwealth Fund.

Tikkanen, R., & Fields, K. (2021). *Multinational comparisons of health systems data, 2020.* The Commonwealth Fund. https://doi.org/10.26099/tc4h-db02.

US Department of Health and Human Services, Office of Disease Prevention and Health Promotion. (n.d.). *Healthy People 2030 Framework.* Retrieved from https://health.gov/healthypeople/about/healthy-people-2030-framework.

US Department of Health and Human Services, Office of Disease Prevention and Health Promotion. (n.d.a). *Healthy People 2030: Social determinants of health.* Retrieved from https://health.gov/healthypeople/objectives-and-data/social-determinants-health.

US Department of Health and Human Services, Office of Disease Prevention and Health Promotion. (n.d.b). *Social determinants of health workgroup.* Retrieved from https://health.gov/healthypeople/about/workgroups/social-determinants-health-workgroup.

US Department of Health and Human Services, Office of Minority Health (OMH). (2019). *Think cultural health.* Retrieved from https://thinkculturalhealth.hhs.gov/education/behavioral-health.

Williams, D. R., & Mohammed, S. A. (2013). Racism and health I: Pathways and scientific evidence. *American Behaviorist Scientist, 57*(8), 1152–1173.

WHO. (n.d.) *Health inequities and their causes.* Retrieved from https://www.who.int/news-room/facts-in-pictures/detail/health-inequities-and-their-causes.

WHO. (2000). *A life course approach to health.* Retrieved from https://www.who.int/ageing/publications/lifecourse/alc_lifecourse_training_en.pdf.

WHO. (2010). *Commission on Social Determinants of Health: A conceptual framework for action on the social determinants of health.*

WHO. (2019). *Social determinants of health.* Retrieved from https://www.who.int/social_determinants/en/.

WHO. (2021). *WHO remains firmly committed to the principles set out in the preamble to the constitution.* https://www.who.int/about/who-we-are/constitution#:~:text=Health%20is%20a%20state%20of,absence%20of%20disease%20or%20infirmity.&text=The%20achievement%20of%20any%20State,is%20of%20value%20to%20all.

Woolsey, C., & Narruhn, R. A. (2018). A pedagogy of social justice for resilient/vulnerable populations: Structural competency and bio-power. *Public Health Nursing (Boston, Mass.), 35*(6), 587–597. https://doi.org/10.1111/phn.12545.

Zuckerman, D., Duncan, V., & Parker, K. (2016). Building a culture of health equity at the federal level. *NAM Perspectives.* Discussion Paper, National Academy of Medicine. https://doi.org/10.31478/201603a.

Income, Income Inequality, Poverty, and Health

Teri A. Murray

> *Overcoming poverty is not a gesture of charity. It is an act of justice.*
> —*Nelson Mandela*

CHAPTER OUTLINE

LEARNING OBJECTIVES

1. Describe the social gradient between health and income.
2. Explore the relationships between poverty, environmental resources, and health.
3. Examine the impact of low SES on health.
4. Analyze the structural factors that produce poverty leading to food and housing insecurity, low educational attainment, and poor health.

INTRODUCTION

The SDOH, the conditions in which people are born, grow, live, work, and age, include factors such as SES, education, occupation, and social environment and networks (US Department of Health and Human Services [USDHHS], n.d.). These conditions of daily life are significantly affected by the socioeconomic position one occupies in society and have a collective impact on the health of individuals over the life course. The SDOH have the capacity to augment or reduce the requisite resources to promote health, including the availability of food, housing, economic and social relationships, transportation, employment, criminal justice, education,

and healthcare (Beech et al., 2021). The SDOH determine the length and quality of life. Inequities that result from the maldistribution of resources result in unjust and avoidable differences in health outcomes. Poverty, income inequality, housing insecurity, and food insecurity pose grave health risks and significantly impact health and health outcomes. Many illnesses and diseases have complex origins but are often deeply rooted in social and economic inequities.

Income and wealth are entwined and part of a complex web of social conditions that impact health (The Urban Institute and Center on Society and Health, 2015). A sufficient income allows one to purchase the resources necessary to maintain a healthy lifestyle.

Higher-level incomes are associated with having better nutritional intake, better living conditions, increased access to healthcare, better quality of healthcare services, and higher educational attainment, including knowledge of health-enhancing and health-promoting behaviors. A higher income allows people to reside in neighborhoods with less crime, fewer fast-food restaurants and liquor stores, and more green spaces and recreational parks. Wealthier neighborhoods have less air pollution and fewer environmental toxins and other respiratory hazards often seen in poor communities.

Lower-income Americans face significant barriers when accessing healthcare and are less likely to have health insurance, receive new drugs and technologies, and have access to primary and specialty healthcare services (Khullar & Chokshi, 2018). Healthcare services can be unaffordable for those below certain income levels. Lower-income individuals are more likely to be employed by companies without employer-sponsored health insurance programs. This lack of employer-sponsored health insurance makes it more challenging to seek healthcare because of the lack of resources necessary to pay for provider fees, prescriptions, or even transportation to receive care. Inadequate health insurance coverage is the major barrier to healthcare access; this insufficient coverage leads to healthcare disparities (Yearby et al., 2022).

THE SOCIAL GRADIENT IN HEALTH

The *social gradient in health* refers to the phenomenon whereby individuals who are financially disadvantaged in income and socioeconomic position have worse health than those who have higher incomes and are better off financially. Individuals who are better off financially have better health and health outcomes than their poorer counterparts. A classic example is the Whitehall study of British civil servants (Marmot et al., 1991). The study revealed an inverse association between social class and health and mortality. Males in the lower levels with low-status employment positions were more likely to die prematurely than those in higher-status employment positions. Glymour and colleagues (2014) found that even when comparing societies across periods of time and where the leading causes of death varied, the socioeconomic pattern of mortality was consistent; the poor will not live as long as those who are more economically advantaged.

Socioeconomically disadvantaged populations bear a disproportionate burden of chronic diseases and are least likely to receive care leading to optimal health outcomes (Beech et al., 2021). Higher disease rates among low-income Americans have also been associated with higher incidences of behavioral risk factors, such as smoking, high consumption of alcoholic beverages, drug use, overeating, and sedentariness. Social factors and health behaviors contribute to the growing number of noncommunicable diseases, such as obesity, diabetes, hypertension, and behavioral health problems, seen in low-income individuals (Beech et al., 2021). Better health for higher-income individuals can be attributed to factors such as exercising, wholesome eating habits, better stress management, and healthy relationships (Wang & Geng, 2019). The higher the income, the lower the risks of chronic sickness, disease, and death. The evidence is clear: those with lower incomes have higher incidences of morbidity and mortality (Krisberg, 2016). Even incremental increases in income correspond to improved health. Individuals at the bottom of the economic ladder have worse health than individuals in the middle, and individuals in the middle experience worse health than individuals at the top. This difference in health based on economic position is known as the social gradient in health and validates that income is a driving force behind health inequities.

INCOME INEQUALITY

Income inequality is the measure used to highlight disparities in income distribution between individuals, groups, populations, social classes, or countries (Howard & Carter, n. d., Organization for Economic Co-operation and Development [OECD], 2021) (Fig. 2.1). Income inequality describes how income is concentrated among the wealthiest few rather than equally shared by all individuals. The social gradient, the relationship between income and health, is connected stepwise at every level of the economic ladder (The Urban Institute and Center on Society and Health, 2015). Middle-class Americans are healthier than those living in or near poverty but less healthy than upper-class Americans. Even wealthy Americans are less healthy than Americans who are more affluent than them. Income and wealth are linked to the differences in health outcomes for the various populations and life expectancy across the income distribution. Chetty and colleagues (2016b) found the

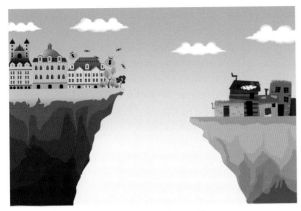

Fig. 2.1 Income inequality.

difference in life expectancy between the wealthiest 1% and poorest 1% in the United States was 14.6 years for males and 10.1 years for females. Income inequality in the United States has increased dramatically over the last 5 decades causing widening gaps in health and longevity between rich and poor Americans (Bor et al., 2017). The United States has the most significant income-based health disparities globally and these disparities seem to grow over time (Khullar & Chokshi, 2018).

WEALTH AND THE INTERGENERATIONAL TRANSFER OF WEALTH

There is a clear distinction between income and wealth. Income refers to the sum of wages, salaries, and other earnings in a given period, whereas wealth encompasses the total value of assets after subtracting debts (Box 2.1). Wealth is more comprehensive than income but is also more challenging to measure. For example, two households can earn the same income, but the one with fewer expenses will have more wealth. Wealth affords personal choice and provides stability in most aspects of life. Wealth cushions individuals from the throes of shock when dealing with unexpected emergencies, such as unanticipated medical expenses, involvement in the criminal justice system, or unexpected unemployment (South et al., 2022). Having wealth can also buffer the effects of having insufficient resources and the associated stressors.

A startling contrast exists between the net worth of Blacks and Whites in the United States. The net worth of a typical White family is nearly 10 times greater than that of a Black family, at $171,000 for Whites compared with $17,150 for Blacks (The Brookings Institute, 2020).

BOX 2.1   Income Revenue Streams

Earnings
Unemployment compensation
Worker's compensation
Social security
Supplemental security income
Public assistance
Veteran's payments
Survivor benefits
Disability benefits
Pension or retirement income
Interest
Dividends
Rents, royalties, and estates and trusts
Educational assistance
Alimony
Child support
Financial assistance from outside the household
Other income

From: US Census Bureau. (2021). Income and poverty in the United States 2019. https://www.census.gov/library/publications/2020/demo/p60-270.html.

On average, White families have eight times the wealth of Black families and five times that of Hispanic families (Board of Governors of the Federal Reserve System, 2020). The median family wealth is $188,200, $24,100, and $36,100 for Whites, Blacks, and Hispanics, respectively (Board of Governors of the Federal Reserve System, 2020). Many factors contribute to an individual's or family's wealth accumulation, such as intergenerational wealth transfers, homeownership opportunities, employer-based tax-sheltered savings plans, and other investment decisions (Board of Governors of the Federal Reserve System, 2020).

Gaps in the wealth between these groups reflect the accumulated inequities, discriminatory practices, and imbalances in power and privilege that date back to the nation's origin (The Brookings Institute, 2020). These policies began with the enslavement of Blacks through the Jim Crow Era and remain part of institutional structures to this day. These policies, known as *structural racism*, operate within work settings, academic institutions, housing markets, lending practices, criminal justice systems, and healthcare arenas. For example, discriminatory housing policies excluded Blacks from homeownership. Residential areas with high concentrations of Blacks were redlined. Historically, redlining was the practice where banks and other investors drew a red line on a map around areas with high concentrations of Blacks, low-income individuals, and other minorities. The red line signified not to invest in those areas, with no loans, insurance, and so on. This action effectively devalued the property in those neighborhoods. This devaluing of Black and poor communities, coupled with residential segregation, formed the platform for broad social disinvestment, especially in neighborhood infrastructure (e.g., green space, housing stock, and roads), services (e.g., transportation, schools, and sanitation), and employment (Bailey et al., 2021). These practices offer an explanatory view of why Blacks are overrepresented among the poor and low-wage earners compared with Whites. The Black-White wealth gap has been undergirded by policies that favored Whites over Blacks. Racial segregation is usually accompanied by concentrated socioeconomic disadvantages and limited upward mobility, such as worse employment and school options (Braveman et al., 2022).

Discriminatory policies such as redlining and racial segregation led to the differences in the homeownership rates between Blacks and Whites today. These policies, discrimination, and racial segregation impacted homeownership and account for a significant portion of the racial wealth gap. The historical practice of discrimination matters because it influences monetary inheritances. Wealth is passed down from generation to generation. The disparities in wealth between Blacks and Whites, in part, result from inheritances through housing. Housing is a significant component of wealth and is the major source of wealth accumulation and transfer in the United States. A typical White family's home value is $230,000 compared with $150,000 and $200,000 for Blacks and Hispanics, respectively (Board of Governors of the Federal Reserve System, 2020). Wealth begets wealth. The inheritance of wealth allows for the intergenerational accumulation of wealth in families. Wealth provides the resources to pay for children's college education, buy a house, start a business, or relocate for upwardly mobile professional opportunities. For example, families can support the next generation by providing a down payment for housing or investing in the children's education by paying for college or private school attendance before college. Wealth or the lack of wealth crosses generations. The current wealth gap reflects a legacy of unequal treatment in housing, education, and labor markets (Board of Governors of the Federal Reserve System, 2020). Participation in employer-sponsored retirement accounts and pension plans is an additional way to build and maintain wealth through retirement. Whites are more likely to have pension accounts than Blacks or Hispanics. These retirement accounts can be transferred from generation to generation through inheritance.

Whites have much larger professional and social networks. These networks, also known as social capital, enable individuals and families to function more effectively. For example, the professional network allows individuals to readily seek out colleagues for career advice and opportunities for themselves and their children. Wealthier families typically see education as a necessary tradition for making and maintaining connections with colleagues who may be influential in paving the way for future opportunities. Social capital is an intangible asset obtained through relational ties. Thus individuals within professional and social networks serve as conduits for information, resources, ideas, and expertise to advance careers. Intellectual capital is also created in professional networks through exchanging knowledge within groups. The many types of assets accumulated within families can be passed on to children in various ways. This financial, social, and intellectual capital transfer places future generations in a better position to have better educational, economic, professional, and social opportunities.

SOCIOECONOMIC STATUS

SES is typically characterized by three dimensions: education, employment, and money. The lower the occupational status, the worse the health outcomes. The lower the individual's educational attainment, the worse the health outcomes. The more resourced individuals are in terms of money, power, prestige, privilege, and knowledge, the more likely they will use these resources to promote and enhance their health. The relationship between SES and health is complex. Whether SES is measured by education, income, occupation, racial or ethnic background, or geographic location, low SES is associated with adverse health outcomes, shorter life expectancy, poor mental health, increased morbidity, risky health behaviors, and higher mortality; this was well established during the recent coronavirus disease 2019 (COVID-19) pandemic (Donahoe & McGuire, 2020).

There is a strong correlation between income and behavioral and environmental risk factors. Low-income Americans are more likely to smoke, be overweight or obese, use substances, and have low physical activity levels, all of which are influenced by the residential environment. Despite higher levels of environmental stress, lower SES individuals are less likely to receive medication to deal with environmental stressors (Khullar & Chokshi, 2018). These environmental stressors, even at low levels, can harm health. Chronic stressors, such as insufficient funds for daily needs, precipitate a hormonal stress response. The frequent activation of the stress response, which happens when individuals are confronted with daily stressors and inequities repeatedly and in multiple aspects of their lives, can result in a chronic elevation of stress hormones, referred to as allostatic load. Allostatic load is the general wear and tear on the body over time as individuals are exposed to repeated chronic stress. When allostatic load occurs, the body's cardiovascular, metabolic, nervous, and immune systems lose their ability to adapt and function normally. Mounting evidence links chronic stressors to changes in the DNA mechanisms that create higher hormone (cortisol and adrenaline) levels, increasing the risk for chronic disease throughout life (Commonwealth of Australia, 2012). Wealth shields against the weathering effects of the chronic stress associated with insufficient income.

Neighborhoods with less green space and fewer parks and sidewalks are less conducive to walking, exercising, or engaging in physical fitness activity, which could help reduce stress. Neighborhood conditions influence the health of individuals through the quality of local services and businesses, socialization and social networks, crime and violence, physical environment, and proximity to services (Table 2.1). The ample availability of predatory lending services disproportionately impacts low-income

TABLE 2.1 Income, Environment, and Health

Income-Based Neighborhood Characteristic	Health Impact
Food supply	Lower-resourced neighborhoods have limited access to sources of nutritious food, such as grocers that sell fresh produce and other healthy food options. Lower-resourced neighborhoods tend to have an oversupply of convenience and fast-food stores and a shortage of restaurants that offer healthy food options. For this reason, they are said to be food deserts.
Built environment	Lower-resourced neighborhoods have limited green space, therefore walking or bike paths are often nonexistent. The lack of green and open spaces discourages exercise and other health-promoting activities. Neighborhoods are often near busy highways with vehicle emissions, have factories with pollutants, and are on bus routes with high vehicle emissions, creating respiratory and environmental pollutants.
Marketing predators	Lower-resourced neighborhoods, specifically in minoritized communities, are often targets of advertising for tobacco products, fast-food chains, liquor stores, and predatory lending agencies.
Public transportation	Lower-resourced neighborhoods often have inadequate public transportation infrastructures making it difficult for residents to find employment outside the community, adequate daycare services, supermarkets, or access to healthcare services.
School systems	Lower-resourced neighborhoods have a lower tax base; thus schools lack the resources often provided by higher-resourced schools, which means fewer enrichment opportunities for those children attending school.
Employment opportunities	Because there are fewer businesses located in less-resourced communities, residents have fewer choices for employment opportunities unless they have adequate personal transportation.
Neighborhood disrepair or decay	Lower-resourced neighborhoods tend to be isolated due to practices such as redlining. Public policies coupled with the lack of revenue growth opportunities have led to disinvestment in these neighborhoods, creating more despair, persistent segregation, fewer economic opportunities, and increased crime.

Adapted from: The Urban Institute & Center on Society and Health (2015).

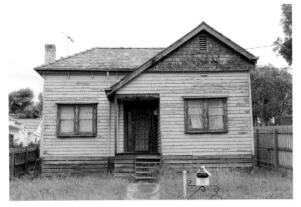

Fig. 2.2 Low resource community-dwelling. (iStock.com/ Slovegrove.)

communities, adding to the difficulty of accumulating wealth, since these lenders typically charge exorbitant fees and interest (Braveman et al., 2022). The dependence on personal property taxes to finance public schools usually leaves schools in low-resourced communities underfunded (Fig. 2.2). Underfunded schools expose students to substandard education. Additionally, low-resourced communities, particularly those of color, experience damaging effects of environmental injustice such as hazardous waste and other environmental toxins (Braveman et al., 2022). SES and neighborhood are intertwined, since the local economies determine access to jobs, commerce, schools, and other resources that enable families to enjoy economic success and place-based amenities that contribute to health (The Urban Institute and Center on Society and Health, 2015).

EMPLOYMENT AND HEALTH

Employment is inextricably linked to health; income and employment impact life expectancy, quality of life, healthcare costs, and healthcare outcomes. Being gainfully employed provides the income, benefits, and stability necessary for good health. A well-paying job brings the luxuries of living in better neighborhoods with better school districts, grocers, and other amenities like playgrounds and parks that lead to good health. Good jobs tend to provide employer-sponsored health insurance. Job-related benefits such as health insurance, paid sick leave, and parental leave influence the health of individuals and families.

Most working adults have health insurance through an employer-sponsored health insurance program. Health insurance provides access to affordable healthcare and protects individuals from unexpected healthcare costs. Paid leaves allow individuals and family members to seek healthcare when needed without the added burden of lost wages. Parental leaves are associated with positive health outcomes for babies and parents, although these leaves are not as widely available in the United States as in other wealthy nations. The United States is the only prosperous nation that does not have a national policy for paid parental leave (Burtle & Bezruchka, 2016).

In employer-sponsored health insurance programs, the employer purchases health insurance for the individual and family, if applicable, and the employer and employee jointly finance the insurance program's costs. Health insurance programs provide the insurance coverage necessary so the individual or family can maintain health, allowing the program participants to seek healthcare services as needed. Workers who have lost their jobs can continue employer-sponsored insurance through the Consolidated Omnibus Budget Reconciliation Act, but this is very expensive and only available to workers who can afford to pay for it.

Factors that impact employment include educational status, sex, and race. The educational background, level of education, and amount of specialized training or expertise required all influence salary, opportunities for advancement, and job security. Males are more likely to be employed, have higher-status positions, and have more labor-intensive jobs than females. White people are more likely to work in higher-income positions, such as managerial positions, than African Americans, who are more likely to work in service-sector areas holding blue-collar jobs. African Americans are more likely to be unemployed than Whites. African Americans who completed high school were 72% more likely to be voluntarily unemployed than White people with the same educational background (USDHHS, n.d.). The connection between unemployment and poor health is clear. Laid-off workers are more likely to have poor health, stress-related conditions such as heart disease and strokes, and greater depression and feelings of sadness than employed workers (Robert Wood Johnson Foundation [RWJF], 2013).

COVID-19 and Employment

The COVID-19 pandemic and the resultant economic crisis increased the number of unemployed individuals

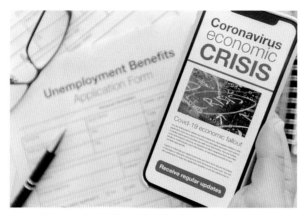

Fig. 2.3 Covid-19 and the rise in unemployment.

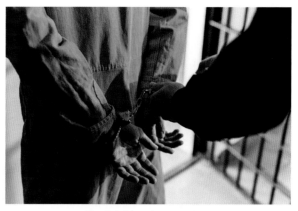

Fig. 2.4 Mass incarceration.

by more than 14 million between February and May 2020, raising the unemployment rate from 3.8% to 13.0% (Kochhar, 2020) (Fig. 2.3). As of August 2021 the civilian labor force participation rate was 61.7%. The total unemployment rate was 8.4%, rates greatly influenced by the COVID-19 pandemic, as can be seen, compared with the pre-COVID-19 rates of 62.8% and 3.8%, respectively (US Department of Labor, Bureau of Labor Statistics; 2019, 2021).

During the COVID-19 pandemic, lower-income individuals had higher rates of infection and mortality, higher rates of unemployment, less access to healthcare, and a greater risk of eviction than those in higher-income groups (Benfer et al., 2020). Emerging data suggest that socioeconomic factors such as poverty were significant predictors of infection and death rates during the COVID-19 pandemic (Benfer et al., 2020). The lower the SES, the greater the chance of suffering from chronic diseases, heart and lung ailments, and diabetes, which all increase the mortality risk of COVID-19 (Benfer et al., 2020). When the United States shut down to curb the spread of the pandemic, as the unemployment rate increased, so did the poverty rate, resulting in many families being unable to meet their basic needs, thus widening health disparities. The Families First Coronavirus Response Act provided flexibility for state unemployment insurance agencies and funding for those agencies to respond to the COVID-19 pandemic by providing unemployment insurance for workers impacted, including paid sick leave, or expanded family and medical leave for conditions related to COVID-19. In addition, the Coronavirus Aid, Relief, and Economic Security (CARES) Act enabled unemployed individuals

impacted by the pandemic to receive expanded unemployment insurance benefits, including workers who would not ordinarily receive them.

Mass Incarceration and Employment

The United States has the highest incarceration rate in the world. Mass incarceration is a threat to wealth building and employment. Those behind bars in this country are mainly among the poorest members of society. Many people are incarcerated because they lack the funds to afford bail or cannot pay the court-imposed fees, fines, and restitution that are often mandatory, regardless of their economic status (Fig. 2.4).

Members of racial and ethnic minority groups represent 42% of the population nationally but make up more than 60% of the incarcerated population (The Sentencing Project, 2020). Black Americans are most affected, representing at least one-third of the prison and jail populations. This mass incarceration of Black Americans is attributed to the overpolicing of communities of color, harsher sentencing laws such as the three-strikes provision that mandated life sentences for offenders convicted of a violent crime after two or more prior convictions, and mandatory sentencing. Additionally, the "war on drugs" resulted in harsher sentencing with mandatory minimum sentences (The Sentencing Project, 2020).

Incarceration has lifelong effects on individuals after they are released. Once released, previously incarcerated people are more likely to be unemployed or face substantial barriers to employment. Many standard employment applications have a set of common questions. For example, one question on the employment application asks, "Have you ever been convicted of a crime?" For those who check "yes," employers often use the response to weed out applicants with criminal records, thus preventing the newly released inmate from being gainfully employed. The stigma or the knowledge by prospective employers that a person has been incarcerated restricts economic opportunities for them and their families throughout life (Braveman et al., 2022). Some states have enacted what are known as "ban-the-box" laws, which help previously incarcerated individuals get jobs by encouraging employers to evaluate the applicant's skills and qualifications before denying employment. Some employers review the application and consider the circumstances of the crime, the time since the crime, and what activities the jobseeker has engaged in since their release to determine employability.

Minimum Wages, Livable Wages, and Health

The livable wage is the income necessary to provide a decent standard of living and ensure that full-time workers earn enough to live above the federal poverty level. The minimum wage is mandated by law to keep employees out of poverty. It is considered the wage necessary to meet the employee's basic needs, such as housing, food, healthcare, and other essentials. The terms *livable* and *minimum* wages are sometimes interchanged, since the original intent of the minimum wage was to provide a livable wage. Minimum wages vary by state. Lawmakers consider the overall economy, the needs of businesses, and the needs of employees when setting the dollar value for the minimum wage. Factors considered when making minimum wage adjustments include whether the increased pay results in reduced employee hours or worker displacement. The relationship between health and minimum wage increases is unclear but, in general, increased earnings have been associated with better health outcomes (Buszkiewicz et al., 2021).

Universal Basic Income

One of the 2020 US presidential election candidates, Andrew Yang, advocated for a universal basic income (UBI). A UBI guarantees everyone a basic income regardless of their status. It is a regular monetary allotment for all citizens. UBI, unlike other welfare programs, is the unconditional transfer of funds to an individual. It is a periodic cash payment unconditionally delivered to all persons without a means test or work requirement (Howard, 2023).

In contrast, other federal welfare programs are tied to work, such as the Social Security program or programs based on your willingness to work. Opponents of UBI believe the unconditional receipt of income should be tied to workforce participation, like the earned income credit on income taxes; otherwise, it creates a disincentive to work. To get the earned income tax credit, you must participate in the labor market. Most government-assisted programs require workforce participation, such as the Supplemental Nutrition Assistance Program or Temporary Assistance for Needy Families.

UBI, in its purest form, is unconditional, not based on marital status or employment. Unlike the safety net welfare programs designed to help during financial distress, UBI is meant to provide basic income before the person gets into a dire situation. It provides a solid foundation for individuals rather than a safety net to catch them when they hit rock bottom. It is considered an antipoverty measure, especially for economically vulnerable people. It ensures a minimum standard of income for everyone. However, the concept of UBI is highly controversial. Some politicians view it as an unnecessary program that would be expensive to administer. There are concerns about how a plan of this nature would be financed. Advocates believe UBI would have helped the millions of individuals who lost their jobs because of the pandemic and would help those who become displaced because of technological advances. Although UBI does not help with income equality, it can be an antipoverty measure. Another criticism of UBI is that not every individual should receive UBI, specifically individuals gainfully employed. The ultimate answers to these concerns depend on how the UBI is financed and who becomes the beneficiaries.

POVERTY

Poverty is a major determinant of health and is defined as insufficient resources to meet the needs of daily living. The United States sets poverty guidelines based on the dollar value of income and family size and composition. According to the 2022 Federal poverty level an income of $12,880 or less for an individual or $26,500 or less for a family of four constitutes poverty (Healthcare.gov, n.d.). The poverty rates vary when aggregated by population, demonstrating considerable variation by race and ethnicity (Tables 2.2 & 2.3).

SES can also define poverty, although SES is often determined by income, educational level, and occupation. Despite differences in the definitions of SES and poverty, there is a general acknowledgment of the relationship

TABLE 2.2 Poverty Rate by Population Group	
Population Group	**Poverty Rate**
Males	10.6%
Females	12.9%
Married couples	4.7%
Single-parent families with no wife present	12.7%
Single-parent families with no husband present	24.9%
People living with disability	25.7%
Children living in poverty	16.2%
Older adults living in poverty	9.7%–14.1%

Adapted from: Poverty USA (2021).

TABLE 2.3 Poverty Rates by Ethnicity and Race	
Racial/Ethnic Group	**Poverty Rate**
Native American	25.4%
African American/Black	20.8%
Hispanic	17.6%
White	10.1%
Asian	10.1%

Adapted from: Poverty USA (2021).

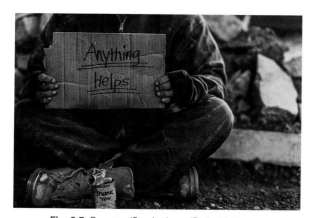

Fig. 2.5 Poverty. (Stock photo ID: 859898068.)

between SES and health. Poverty and low-income status are associated with adverse health outcomes, including shorter life expectancy, increased infant mortality rates, and increased morbidity (American Academy of Family Physicians, 2021). Although poverty is often described in terms of income level, one's quality of life should be considered. Living in poverty usually means a life of struggle and deprivation (Fig. 2.5). Poverty affects health by limiting one's ability to afford adequate, wholesome, nutritious foods, shelter or safe housing, safe neighborhoods, and other elements contributing to health-enhancing behaviors and outcomes. Approximately 10.5% of individuals, or 34 million people living in the United States, live in poverty and cannot buy the necessities for health (US Census Bureau, 2021). As such, poverty in the United States is a significant public health issue.

Legacies of racism, segregation, and systematic economic disenfranchisement have led to intergenerational and multigenerational poverty in families of color, further limiting their economic mobility and opportunity (Cheng et al., 2016). Females have higher poverty rates than males. Blacks and Hispanics tended to be overrepresented in poverty rates compared with their Non-Hispanic White counterparts. Married couples fare much better than singles and better than families. Poverty rates also vary geographically, with higher concentrations in southern states, specifically Mississippi and Louisiana. US poverty rates are higher in rural versus urban areas, at 15.4% compared with 11.9% (US Department of Agriculture [USDA], 2020).

EMERGENCY SAVINGS

Savings and checking accounts are helpful in emergencies. The typical White family has more savings and checking accounts than Black or Hispanic families and more money saved in both accounts. An emergency savings plan can be the difference between housing and food security and insecurity. During the COVID-19 pandemic, when there was unprecedented and unanticipated job loss, many people did not have an emergency savings plan. Without the CARES Act, many families would have become impoverished and home and food insecure.

Children Living in Poverty

Children living in poverty are more likely to become lower-SES adults who accumulate less wealth to pass on to their children, thus creating an intergenerational cycle of poverty. Intergenerational poverty is the relentless cycle of passing down poverty from one generation to the next. In addition, children living in poverty often lack access to quality education. Without an education, children are not prepared for higher-income positions, thus creating a cycle of intergenerational poverty.

Moreover, children growing up in poverty face additional burdens that children from higher-income families do not encounter. Impoverished children are likelier to experience multiple family transitions, move frequently, and change schools. Research shows that children who grew up in poverty experience a greater incidence of acute and chronic psychological stressors, family conflict, child abuse, single-parent families, and violence (Price et al., 2018). The stress associated with social and economic deprivation when growing up can have lasting effects, making it more difficult for children in low-income households to escape poverty (Wagmiller & Adelman, 2009). Adverse childhood experiences (ACEs) are traumatic events or experiences that occur in childhood, such as violence, abuse, neglect, substance use in the home, incarcerated parents, and other events that are linked to trauma (Centers for Disease Control and Prevention [CDC], 2021). ACEs are linked to chronic health problems in later life, mental illness, and substance use disorders in adulthood (CDC, 2021). In addition, ACEs negatively impact educational attainment, job opportunities, and earning potential (CDC, 2021).

The effects of poverty on families include the immediate physical effects of deprivation, such as inadequate housing; lack of food, clothing, and other needed resources; and chronic stress. As mentioned earlier in this chapter, exposure to chronic stress increases the allostatic load. Allostatic load leads to health disparities, including morbidity and decreased mortality, over the life course. Additionally, communities experiencing high levels of poverty have more neighborhood disorder and experience higher incidences of crime, violence, and other environmental stressors (Chetty et al., 2016a; Price et al., 2018).

HOUSING SECURITY AND HOMELESSNESS

Despite the United States being one of the wealthiest countries, it has a large homeless population (Fig. 2.6). Homelessness is structural despite the frequent focus on homelessness as a failure of the individual. Structural causes of homelessness include the inability to afford existing housing stock, gentrification, unemployment, and poverty (Chattoo et al., 2021). Access to safe and decent housing is tied to one's economic status in the United States and thus poverty prevents access to housing. Many homeless people suffer from various problems simply because they have nowhere to live. Households are considered housing insecure if more than 30% of the income is spent on housing. Housing insecurity can lead to homelessness.

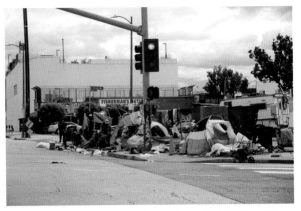

Fig. 2.6 Homelessness. (Stock photo ID: 1218467987.)

Homelessness

As of January 2020 the United States had more than 500,000 people experiencing homelessness on any given night, with 65% staying in shelters for the homeless while 35% are in unsheltered locations such as encampments (Chattoo et al., 2021). Most were individuals, but nearly one-third of the homeless were families with children. The US Department of Housing and Urban Development (HUD) defines homelessness as:

1. An individual or family who lacks a fixed, regular, and adequate nighttime residence, such as those living in emergency shelters, transitional housing, or places not meant for habitation, or
2. An individual or family who will imminently lose their primary nighttime residence within 14 days, provided that no subsequent housing has been identified and the individual/family lacks support networks or resources to obtain housing, or
3. Unaccompanied youth under 25 years of age, or families with children and youth who qualify under other Federal statutes, such as the Runaway and Homeless Youth Act, have not had a lease or ownership interest in a housing unit in the last 60 days or more, have had two or more moves in the previous 60 days, and who are likely to continue to be unstably housed because of disability or multiple barriers to employment, or
4. An individual or family fleeing or attempting to flee domestic violence, has no other residence, and lacks the resources or support networks to obtain other permanent housing (Substance Abuse and Mental Health Services Administration [SAMSA], Soar Works, n.d., paras 2–5).

A person is at risk of homelessness if the individual's or family's annual income is below 30% of the median family income for the geographic area; the person or family does not have sufficient resources or support networks immediately available to prevent them from moving into an emergency shelter or a place not designated for human habitation, and the person or family exhibits one or more risk factors of homelessness, including recent housing instability or exiting a publicly funded institution or system of care such as foster care or a mental health facility (SAMSA, Soar Works, n.d.).

The Social Security Administration's (SSA) definition of homelessness tends to be more literal than HUD's and is what most people commonly refer to as homelessness. According to SSA, a person is said to be homeless if they sleep in doorways, overnight shelters, parks, bus stations, or other public places not designated for sleep or the person does not have permanent living arrangements and stays with a succession of friends or relatives just to have a place to sleep at night (SAMSA, Soar Works, n.d.).

Homelessness is a complex issue that involves a myriad of factors such as SES, housing costs, and the degree of external and social support. According to "Healthy People 2030" (U.S. Department of Health and Human Services [USDHHS], Office of Disease Prevention and Health Promotion [ODPHP], 2021), housing instability is a primary component in the economic stability domain of the SDOH. Unfortunately, there is no standard definition for housing instability. Housing instability could include individuals who have difficulty paying rent or a mortgage, frequently move, live with others in overcrowded conditions, or spend the bulk of their income on housing with little left for other daily living expenses.

Eviction

Eviction is the forcible removal of a tenant from a property. Without a safety net, evictions lead to the need to double up at another's residence, couch surf, stay in a shelter, or be transient or homeless (Fig. 2.7). The impact of eviction on health cannot be understated. The mere threat of eviction increases stress levels, anxiety, and depression (Benfer et al., 2020). In addition, individuals who have been evicted experience increased emergency room usage, sexually transmitted infections, mental health hospitalizations, suicide, violence, and other poor health outcomes (Benfer et al., 2020). During the COVID- 19 pandemic, many families struggled to pay rent due to job loss, resulting in a heightened risk of eviction. Thus during the pandemic the federal administration called for a moratorium on eviction to prevent

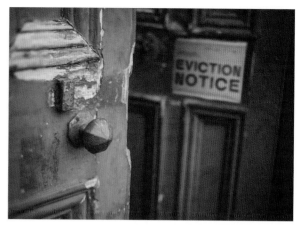

Fig. 2.7 Eviction notice. (Stock photo ID: 1032261264.)

residential crowding, a potential outcome of eviction, which could also have increased the spread of COVID-19.

Gentrification

Gentrification (social, cultural, and economic transformation) revitalizes urban neighborhoods for economic growth and is a major cause of housing insecurity and homelessness. Gentrification transforms impoverished neighborhoods with historical disinvestment into an areas of urban renaissance (Rosell, 2019). The gentrification process involves three components: (1) displacement of the current lower-income residents from a neighborhood or community; (2) renovation, transformation, and revitalization of the neighborhood; and (3) the influx of higher-income individuals shifting the balance of the socioeconomic and social statuses within the community resulting in increased property values. Gentrification causes an excessive rise in housing costs that usually attracts high-income, college-educated White persons. Gentrification further oppresses minoritized and marginalized groups, forcing many to become housing insecure. Gentrification harms those at the lower rungs of the socioeconomic ladder. The outcome of gentrification is a lack of affordable housing, extensive displacement of marginalized groups, and higher eviction rates (Rosell, 2019).

Renters and Affordable Housing

Rental costs have continued to escalate over recent decades. Combined with income insufficiency, the lack of affordable housing is a leading cause of homelessness. For 25% of renters, housing and utility costs comprise more than half the family income, up 26% since the

Great Recession in 2007 (Chattoo et al., 2021). More than 20 million families struggle to pay rent.

Income inequality, rising housing costs, and the lack of affordable housing have placed a significant burden on low-income workers in the United States. The United States has a reported shortage of nearly 7 million affordable homes for low-income renters. According to the National Low Income Housing Coalition (NLIHC), low-income renters lack affordable housing in every state, including the District of Columbia (2021). A full-time minimum wage job does not guarantee everyone can afford a place to live; there is nowhere in America where an individual who earns the minimum wage can rent a two-bedroom apartment without paying more than 30% of their income (NLIHC, 2021). In addition, unaffordable or overly expensive housing costs reduce the available money to meet other responsibilities and needs, such as healthcare. Increased housing costs create an imbalance in financial obligations, causing individuals to make difficult food, transportation, and health choices. Affordable housing near metropolitan transportation areas can help low-income individuals save money on housing costs, have transportation to better jobs, and boost the local economy because individuals will have more discretionary spending money.

The COVID-19 pandemic exacerbated the lack of affordable housing for many individuals and families. Lower-income workers were more likely to incur financial loss due to pandemic-related shutdowns and job layoffs. Consequentially, many families grappled with housing insecurity and evictions as they were less likely to have the financial reserves to compensate for the missed paychecks. Although there were moratoriums on evictions during the COVID-19 shutdown, those moratoriums were set to expire within a specified timeframe. Those individuals would then become housing insecure or end up in substandard housing. The quality of affordable housing matters, since housing has significant health implications.

Housing Instability and Race and Ethnicity

This risk of housing displacement or eviction is highest among renters of color; people of color experience more unstable housing than their White peers. For example, Black households were 54% rent burdened compared with 42.7% of White households (Joint Center for Housing Studies, 2021). Predominantly Black and racially segregated neighborhoods are associated with economic disinvestment, fewer community resources, less green space for

exercise or play, higher violence and crime rates, air pollution, overcrowded housing, pest infestations, and mold (Benfer et al., 2020). Housing stability, quality, safety, and affordability all affect health, as do the environmental and social characteristics of neighborhoods (Benfer et al., 2020).

The relationship between housing and health has many facets. The immediate housing environment includes neighborhood characteristics such as walkability, safety, and the psychosocial effects of stress associated with financial instability and the fear of foreclosure.

Foreclosure is associated with depression, anxiety, increased alcoholic intake, psychological stress, and suicide (Taylor, 2018). People who cannot afford their rent or mortgage are less likely to have sufficient food intake, have a source of regular healthcare, or be able to seek healthcare when the need arises. People who are persistently homeless have higher rates of physical and mental illness and are at risk for increased mortality. Homeless individuals often experience trauma while living on the streets or staying in shelters, and both have long-term adverse effects on psychological well-being (Taylor, 2018). Housing instability among youth is associated with increased risks of teen pregnancy, early drug use, and depression. Lack of stable and safe housing disrupts employment, community networks, and the education process for children, and contributes to food insecurity, leading to poor health.

Health equity in housing could involve subsidies to expand affordable housing to individuals in a wide range of income levels and the positioning of affordable housing in high-opportunity neighborhoods (Swope & Hernández, 2019). The Moving to Opportunity (MTO) program is one example of the difference housing makes for individuals and families.

Moving to Opportunity Program

The MTO program was a 10-year demonstration project (randomized control study) that compared families who moved from public housing in high-poverty neighborhoods to less impoverished areas with those who remained in public housing. The moved families were provided rental assistance and counseling and relocated to neighborhoods with better housing, educational districts, employment prospects, and more social order, though still categorized as poor neighborhoods. Evidence supporting the demonstration project revealed that persons in highly impoverished areas fared worse than those who lived in less disadvantaged communities on a range of economic, health, and educational outcomes (Chetty et al., 2016a). Schmidt and colleagues (2020) found that changes in the social context of neighborhoods improved girls' mental health and mitigated some behavioral risk challenges for boys. Antonakos and colleagues (2020) found that housing environments impact health through environmental exposures. The demonstration project further showed that children who moved by the age of 13 had higher college attendance rates, higher incomes, and were less likely to become single parents than those who moved after the age of 13 (Chetty et al., 2016b). This finding suggests the duration of exposure to better environments is an influencer of health and is associated with better health outcomes (Chetty et al., 2016a). This 10-year demonstration project produced evidence that housing policies related to health-promoting environments are an upstream measure to promote health equity.

FOOD SECURITY

According to the USDA, food security means having consistent access to enough food to maintain an active, healthy life (USDA, 2022). In 2021, 89.8% of US households were food secure. The remaining 10.2% of households had low or very low food security and lacked access to adequate food due to limitations of money or other resources. The USDA measures food security on four levels. Food security is the ready availability of nutritious, wholesome foods and the ability to acquire foods without resorting to emergency food supplies, scavenging, stealing, or other socially undesirable strategies. Examples of food insecurity include skipping meals or going hungry because the individual lacks the finances to buy or gain access to food. The experience of not having enough food can have harmful consequences on health. The USDA describes households with high or marginal food security as food secure and those with low or very low food security as food insecure (Table 2.4).

A family's position on this continuum is determined by the household's responses to survey questions about behaviors and experiences associated with difficulty meeting their basic food needs. The questions on the survey cover a wide range of severity of food insecurity, are targeted to the household rather than the individual, and range from least severe (e.g., "We worried whether we would run out of food before we got money to go

TABLE 2.4   **Levels of Food Security**

Level of Food Security	Description
High food security	The household did not have difficulty or worries about consistently accessing nutritious foods in adequate amounts.
Marginal food security	At times, the household had worries or anxieties about accessing food, but the quality, variety, and quantity of their food intake was not substantially reduced or changed.
Low food security	Households reduced the quality, variety, and desirability of their diets, but the amount they ate and the frequency of their eating patterns were not disrupted.
Very low food security	At least one or more individuals' eating patterns were disrupted during the year, and food intake was reduced due to a lack of money or other resources to obtain food.

From: USDA, Economic Research Service (2022).

to the store and buy more food") to most severe (e.g., "In the last 12 months, did you ever not eat for a whole day because there wasn't enough money for food?") (Coleman-Jensen et al., 2021, p. 5). Fig. 2.8 highlights the characteristics of households with very low food security and Box 2.2 details survey questions.

Food insecurity varies by state and is more prevalent in some states than others. The prevalence of food insecurity is alarming as access to nutritious food is necessary for health. Not having healthy foods leads to poor health outcomes including psychological distress, diet-sensitive chronic diseases (e.g., hypertension, hyperlipidemia, diabetes), malnutrition, and obesity (Myers & Painter II, 2017). Notably, food insecurity is higher in racial and ethnic minority populations.

Food Safety Net Programs

Food safety net programs are designed to increase access to food, reduce food insecurity, and provide financial avenues for households to purchase sufficient food to meet their daily needs. The federal government's food assistance programs were designed to increase food security for low-income families and individuals by providing food or resources for a health-promoting diet.

Percentage of households reporting indicators of adult food insecurity, by food security status, 2020

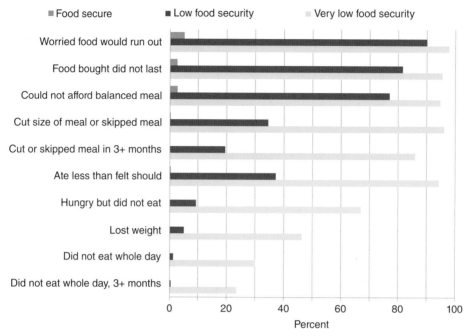

Fig. 2.8 Characteristics of households with very low food security. (USDA, Economic Research Service, using data from the December 2020 Current Population Survey Food Security Supplement, US Census Bureau.)

BOX 2.2   Food Security Survey Questions Used to Assess Households

Survey Questions

1. "We worried whether our food would run out before we got money to buy more." Was that often, sometimes, or never true for you in the last 12 months?
2. "The food that we bought just didn't last, and we didn't have money to get more." Was that often, sometimes, or never true for you in the last 12 months?
3. "We couldn't afford to eat balanced meals." Was that often, sometimes, or never true for you in the last 12 months?
4. In the last 12 months, did you or other adults in the household ever cut the size of your meals or skip meals because there wasn't enough money for food? (Yes/No)
5. (If yes to question 4) How often did this happen—almost every month, some months but not every month, or in only 1 or 2 months?
6. In the last 12 months, did you ever eat less than you felt you should because there wasn't enough money for food? (Yes/No)
7. In the last 12 months, were you ever hungry, but didn't eat, because there wasn't enough money for food? (Yes/No)
8. In the last 12 months did you lose weight because there wasn't enough money for food? (Yes/No)
9. In the last 12 months did you or other adults in your household ever not eat for a whole day because there wasn't enough money for food? (Yes/No)
10. (If yes to question 9) How often did this happen—almost every month, some months but not every month, or in only 1 or 2 months?

BOX 2.2   Food Security Survey Questions Used to Assess Households—cont'd

Questions 11–18 Were Asked Only if the Household Included Children Ages 0–17

11. "We relied on only a few kinds of low-cost food to feed our children because we were running out of money to buy food." Was that often, sometimes, or never true for you in the last 12 months?
12. "We couldn't feed our children a balanced meal, because we couldn't afford that." Was that often, sometimes, or never true for you in the last 12 months?
13. "The children were not eating enough because we just couldn't afford enough food." Was that often, sometimes, or never true for you in the last 12 months?
14. In the last 12 months, did you ever cut the size of any of the children's meals because there wasn't enough money for food? (Yes/No)
15. In the last 12 months, were the children ever hungry but you just couldn't afford more food? (Yes/No)
16. In the last 12 months, did any of the children ever skip a meal because there wasn't enough money for food? (Yes/No)
17. (If yes to question 16) How often did this happen—almost every month, some months but not every month, or in only 1 or 2 months?
18. In the last 12 months, did any of the children ever not eat for a whole day because there wasn't enough money for food? (Yes/No)

Coding of Responses
Questions 1–3 and 11–13 are coded as affirmative (i.e., possibly indicating food insecurity) if the response is "often" or "sometimes." Questions 5, 10, and 17 are coded as affirmative if the response is "almost every month" or "some months but not every month." The remaining questions are coded as affirmative if the response is "yes."

Assessing Food Security Status in Households Without Children
Households without children are classified as food insecure if they report 3 or more indications of food insecurity in response to the first 10 questions; they are classified as having very low food security if they report 6 or more food-insecure conditions out of the first 10 questions.

Assessing food Security Status in Households With Children Ages 0–17
Households with children are classified as food insecure if they report 3 or more indications of food insecurity in response to the entire 18 questions; they are classified as having very low food security if they report 8 or more food-insecure conditions in response to the set of 18 questions.
The food security status of children in the household is assessed by responses to the child-referenced questions (11–18). Households reporting two or more of these conditions are classified as having food insecurity among children. Households reporting five or more are classified as having very low food security among children.

From: Coleman-Jensen, A., Rabbitt, M. P., Gregory, C. A., & Singh, A. (2021). *Household food security in the United States in 2020, ERR-289. U.S.* Department of Agriculture, Economic Research Service. https://www.ers.usda.gov/webdocs/publications/102076/err-298.pdf.

The standard US food assistance programs can be found in Table 2.5.

Food Banks and Pantries

Food banks and pantries are community-based food resources designed to relieve hunger (Fig. 2.9). A food bank is a nonprofit organization that collects and distributes food to smaller frontline nonprofit organizations. The food bank stores and distributes food to food pantries, soup kitchens, homeless shelters, and group homes. In contrast, food pantries are also involved in food storage, preparation, and distribution but reach out directly to individuals and families who are food insecure. Food pantries rely heavily on food

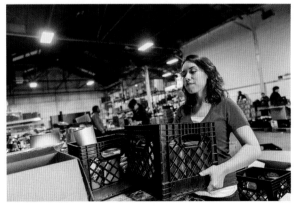

Fig. 2.9 Community-based food resources (From: iStock.com/SDIProductions.)

TABLE 2.5   US Food Assistance Programs and Food and Nutrition Services*

US Food Assistance Programs	Description
Supplemental Nutrition Assistance Program (SNAP), formerly known as the Food Stamp Program*	SNAP, formerly the Food Stamp Program, is the Nation's most prominent domestic food and nutrition assistance program for low-income Americans. It provides nutrition benefits to supplement the food budgets of needy families.
Special Supplemental Nutrition Program for Women, Infants, and Children (WIC)*	WIC safeguards the health of low-income pregnant, postpartum, and breastfeeding women, infants, and children up to age 5 who are at nutritional risk.
Summer Food Service Program (SFSP)*	This program ensures that children have access to nutritious meals and snacks during the summer when school is not in session by providing free meals to kids and teens in low-income areas.
National School Breakfast Program (SBP)*	The SBP is a federally assisted meal program operating in nonprofit public or private schools.
National School Lunch Program (NSLP)*	The NSLP operates in nonprofit public or private schools. It provides nutritionally balanced, low-cost, or free lunches to qualifying children daily.
Commodity Supplemental Food Program (CSFP)*	The CSFP works to improve the health of low-income older adults, beginning at age 60, by supplementing their diets with nutritious foods.
Meals on Wheels	Meals on Wheels is a nationwide network of community-based, nonprofit programs dedicated to providing older adults in their communities with nutritional support to allow them to remain in their homes. Meals on Wheels provides a nutritious meal and safety check to homebound older adults.

*These programs are administered federally and operated through state agencies.
From: https://www.fns.usda.gov/programs. https://www.mealsonwheelsamerica.org/americaletsdolunch/faqs.

banks to provide a steady food supply. Food banks may obtain food from food drives as the food often received can be used immediately or stored for later use. In addition, food banks receive food products from businesses, restaurants, bakeries, and individuals and monetary donations to purchase food products. Food pantries provide nonperishable foods such as canned goods, dried goods, and baked goods, although some may provide perishable goods such as dairy products, meats, and fresh produce directly to individuals on site. Additionally, some food pantries are mobile and deliver prepacked food boxes to individuals in communities that lack a food pantry.

COVID-19 and Food Insecurity

The economic crisis created by the COVID-19 pandemic led to one of the most unprecedented levels of food insecurity in recent decades. Historically, rates of food insecurity hovered around 11% to 12% but during early 2020, it was estimated that 38% of the US population was food insecure (USDA, 2020). The pandemic also created hardships for marginalized and vulnerable people who were already at disproportionally high risk for food insecurity (Wolfson & Leung, 2020). For example, households with children were more likely to experience food insecurity than those without children. In addition, Black Americans were 3.2 times more likely than White Americans to be food insecure, while Hispanic Americans were 2.5 times more likely to be food insecure than White Americans.

CONCLUSION

This chapter focused on the relationship between income and health, demonstrating the social gradient between higher- and lower-income individuals. Insufficient income to meet basic needs is a powerful influencer of health. The chapter points out how SES, whether determined by income, education, or employment, has a significant impact on health over the life course. Income is a driving force behind the disparities in health-related access to care, housing, and food. Income determines where one resides, and the residential neighborhood is where one is born, grows, lives, plays, works, and ages. Poverty can lead to unsafe housing, poor personal hygiene, unhealthy eating habits, poor neighborhood water and air quality, and many other issues surrounding economic and social disadvantage.

Communities can either enhance health or create health risks. A low income contributes to poor health but poor health can also cause a low income. Health is inextricably linked to income, and much of income is related to public policy, as with minimum wage laws, employment insurance, and access to healthcare.

Upstream measures—macrolevel factors—have the potential to impact society at large. Upstream approaches address factors that influence health, and those approaches have societal value. Upstream approaches are policies that benefit everyone and can create societal conditions to keep everyone healthy. For example, upstream interventions related to income and health are addressed through health policy and broad-based initiatives such as minimum wage laws to ensure that everyone earns livable wages or has access to employer-based health insurance. Minimum wage laws that allow individuals to make a livable salary enable the individual to afford housing and food, thereby reducing the potential to become housing or food insecure. Broad-based policy decisions related to neighborhood stability are an example of an upstream intervention. For example, ensuring that neighborhoods have appropriate lighting, walking paths, green spaces, and transportation routes prevents populations from being trapped in food deserts and provides spaces for exercise. Upstream interventions address educational systems, employment, community and residential housing, neighborhood safety and violence, and environmental toxins. Upstream interventions improve health disparities caused by inequities such as the lack of affordable, safe quality housing and food, and the ability to live in healthy built and natural environments, including access to safe and efficient transportation, quality education, livable wages, and access to health and human services.

These interventions are directed at the structural causes of health inequities. Nurses often see the downstream effects of upstream policy decisions that significantly impact health. Upstream measures can ultimately reduce health disparities commonly seen due to societal inequities. To adequately address broader societal issues requires upstream interventions that extend beyond what any healthcare provider or nurse can achieve alone. The key is for nurses to realize how upstream decisions have impacted the lives of the individuals often seen in emergency rooms, hospitals, or urgent care centers. The question becomes, how can nurses develop the habit of looking upstream? What can you do? First, challenge assumptions about the causes of health and illness. Think in terms of the big picture rather than at the individual level. Think about the conditions that create the economic and social circumstances and the built and physical environment of neighborhoods (National Collaborating Centre for Determinants of Health [NCCDH], 2014). Nurses can become civically involved by attending town hall and environmental zoning meetings and then reflecting on how proposed policies might impact health. Find interprofessional and community partners interested in taking action to reduce income inequality and poverty, unsafe working and living conditions, and systemic racism (NCCDH, 2014). With community partners, nurses can advocate for policy changes, meet with politicians, initiate letter-writing campaigns, and participate in committees in professional organizations advocating for change. Nurses should seek additional professional development opportunities for partnership building, political advocacy, public speaking, consensus building, community organizing, team building, and interprofessional collaboration (NCCDH, 2014). The key to advancing health equity is that nurses and other healthcare providers begin to examine how social factors impact health and look beyond providing downstream clinical care.

Midstream interventions are when nurses make referrals to assist in meeting an individual's nonclinical care needs. These actions may be based on the social needs assessment done when a person is admitted to a healthcare organization or goes to a clinic. Examples of midstream interventions include referrals to social workers or social service agencies for supplemental nutrition assistance programs such as Women, Infants, and Children or housing assistance. These midstream interventions assist patients with the challenges of living in poverty but do not address the root causes of poverty, which can be accomplished primarily through upstream interventions.

Downstream interventions related to income and health are when nurses provide clinical care to persons seeking healthcare. The provision of direct care can occur in an emergency room, acute care center, or community-based site. The care may be for a condition resulting from housing and food insecurity. If health inequities are linked to social injustices, then focusing on individual behaviors cannot adequately address the disparities that result from these inequities.

Nurses must understand poverty. Simulation exercises and games can provide students and nurses with a greater awareness of poverty. For example, Kuehn and colleagues (2020) found that poverty simulation tools gave students a greater understanding of the relationship between poverty and health. Simulation can also be effective in helping students learn about the structural aspects of poverty. For the most part, the impoverished are viewed as individuals who failed in life or did not "pull themselves up by the bootstraps." The US culture accepts poverty openly and tolerates income inequality and expressions of wealth and privilege while marginalized populations go without the necessities for life. Accepting poverty and income inequality in the United States is a social injustice. It feeds into the myth of meritocracy without considering the social inequities that impact marginalized and minoritized populations.

Drevdahl (2013) refers to social justice as having to do with fairness, especially concerning how people are treated, decisions are made, and resources are distributed, all of which apply to health and healthcare. Embedded within the American Nurses Association's *Code of Ethics*

is the acclamation that nurses should be advocates for social justice. Social justice is the active examination of, critique, and advocacy for change in the social structures, policies, laws, customs, power, and privilege that disadvantage marginalized groups (Fawcett, 2019). Nurses have a long history of advocacy for justice. For example, the American Academy of Nursing president stated, "The nursing profession advocates for social justice in the pursuit of optimal health.... This must extend to our understanding of the systems and structures that block this vision from becoming a reality" (American Nurses Association (ANA), 2020, paragraph 7). Health equity in the context of income and health means individuals have full access to opportunities, power, and resources necessary to achieve their full potential and optimal health. Given the mounds of evidence on the relationship between economic advantage, economic disadvantage, and health, any obstacle to having economic advantage harms health.

STUDENT REFLECTION QUESTIONS

1. Have you had clinical experiences where you provided care for individuals at the lower rungs of the socioeconomic ladder? Did you look at the person's situation as an individual, societal, or structural problem?
2. How would families near or below the poverty threshold benefit from a UBI program?
3. How can nurses become involved in multisectoral opportunities outside healthcare to improve the economic and social conditions that contribute to poverty?
4. Go to the website http://playspent.org. Play the online tool that allows you to experience what it is like to live on a lower-level income and meet the basic needs of yourself and your family (Urban Ministries of Durham. (n.d.)).

REFERENCES

American Academy of Family Physicians. (2021). Poverty and health—The family medicine perspective (position paper). https://www.aafp.org/about/policies/all/poverty-health.html.

American Nurses Association (ANA). (2020). The American Academy of Nursing and the American Nurses Association call for social justice to address racism and health equity in communities of color. https://www.nursingworld.org/news/news-releases/2020/the-american-academy-of-nursing-and-the-american-nurses-association-call-for-social-justice-to-address-racism-and-health-equity-in-communities-of-color/.

Antonakos, C. L., Coulton, C. J., Kaestner, R., Lauria, M., Porter, D. E., & Colabianchi, N. (2020). Built environment exposures of adults in the moving to opportunity experiment. *Housing Studies, 35*(4), 703–719. https://doi.org/10.1080/02673037.2019.1630560.

Bailey, Z. D., Feldman, J. M., & Bassett, M. T. (2021). How structural racism works—Racist policies as a root cause of U.S. racial health inequities. *The New England Journal of Medicine, 384*(8), 768–773. https://doi.org/10.1056/NEJMms2025396.

Beech, B. M., Ford, C., Thorpe, J., Bruce, M., & Norris, K. (2021). Poverty, racism, and the public health crisis in America. *Frontiers in Public Health, 9,* 699049, 1–9. https://doi.org/10.3389/fpubh.2021.699049.

Benfer, E. A., Mohapatra, S., Wiley, L. F., & Yearby, R. (2020). Health justice strategies to combat the pandemic: Eliminating discrimination, poverty, and health disparities during and after COVID-19. *Yale Journal of Health Policy, Law, and Ethics, 19*(3), 123–171.

Board of Governors of the Federal Reserve System. (2020). Disparities in wealth by race and ethnicity in the 2019 survey of consumer finances. https://www.federalreserve.gov/econres/notes/feds-notes/disparities-in-wealth-by-race-and-ethnicity-in-the-2019-survey-of-consumer-finances-20200928.htm.

Bor, J., Cohen, G. H., & Galea, S. (2017). Population health in an era of rising income inequality: USA, 1980–2015. *Lancet, 389*(10077), 1475–1490. https://doi-org.ezp.slu.edu/10.1016/S0140-6736(17)30571-8.

Braveman, P. A., Arkin, E., Proctor, D., Kauh, T., & Holm, N. (2022). Systemic and structural racism: Definitions, examples, health damages, and approaches to dismantling. *Health Affairs, 41*(2), 171–178.

Burtle, A., & Bezruchka, S. (2016). Population health and paid parental leave: What the United States can learn from two decades of research. *Healthcare (Basel), 4*(2), 30. https://doi-org.ezp.slu.edu/10.3390/healthcare4020030.

Buszkiewicz, J. H., Hill, H. D., & Otten, J. J. (2021). Association of state minimum wage rates and health in working-age adults using the National Health Interview survey. *American Journal of Epidemiology, 190*(1), 21–30. https://doi.org/10.1093/aje/kwaa018.

Centers for Disease Control and Prevention. (2021). Violence prevention. What are adverse childhood experiences? https://www.cdc.gov/violenceprevention/aces/fastfact.html?CDC_AA_refVal=https%3A%2F%2Fwww.cdc.gov-%2Fviolenceprevention%2Facestudy%2Ffastfact.html.

Chattoo, C. B., Young, L., Conrad, D., & Coskuntuncel, A. (2021). The rent is too damn high: News portrayals of housing security and homelessness in the United States. *Mass Communication and Society, 24*(4), 533–575.

Cheng, T. L., Johnson, S. B., & Goodman, E. (2016). Breaking the intergenerational cycle of disadvantage: The three generation approach. *Pediatrics, 137*(6), e20152467. https://doi-org.ezp.slu.edu/10.1542/peds.2015-2467.

Chetty, R., Hendren, N., & Katz, L. F. (2016a). The effects of exposure to better neighborhoods on children: New evidence from the moving to opportunity experiment. *American Economic Review, 106*(4), 855–902.

Chetty, R., Stepner, B. A., Shelby, L., Scuderi, B., Turner, N., Bergeron, A., & Cutler, D. (2016b). The association between income and life expectancy in the United States, 2001–2014. *JAMA, 315*(16), 1750–1766.

Coleman-Jensen, A., Rabbitt, M. P., Gregory, C. A., & Singh, A. (2021). *Household food security in the United States in 2020, ERR-289*. U.S. Department of Agriculture, Economic Research Service. https://www.ers.usda.gov/webdocs/publications/102076/err-298.pdf.

Commonwealth of Australia. (2012). *Allostatic load: A review of the literature*. Department of Veteran Affairs.

Donahoe, J. T., & McGuire, T. G. (2020). The vexing relationship between socioeconomic status and health. *Israel Journal of Health Policy Research, 9*, 68.

Drevdahl, D. J. (2013). Injustice, suffering, difference: How can community health nursing address the suffering of others? *Journal of Community Health Nursing, 30*(1), 49–58. https://doi.org/10.1080/07370016.2013.750212.

Fawcett, J. (2019). Thoughts about social justice. *Nursing Science Quarterly, 32*(3), 250–253. https://doi.org/10.1177/0894318419845385.

Glymour, M. M., Avendano, M., & Kawachi, I. (2014). Socioeconomic status and health. In Berkman, L. F., Kawachi, I., & Glymour, M. M. (Eds.), *Social epidemiology*. Oxford University Press.

Healthcare.gov. (n.d.). Federal poverty level. https://www.healthcare.gov/glossary/federal-poverty-level-fpl/

Howard, M. W. (2023). The U.S. could help solve its poverty problem with a universal basic income. In: *Scientific American*. https://www.scientificamerican.com/article/the-u-s-could-help-solve-its-poverty-problem-with-a-universal-basic-income/.

Howard, M. W. & Carter, V. J. (n. d). *Income inequality. Britannica Money*. https://www.britannica.com/money/income-inequality.

Joint Center for Housing Studies. (2021). Renter cost burdens by race and ethnicity. https://www.jchs.harvard.edu/ARH_2017_cost_burdens_by_race.

Khullar, D., & Chokshi, D. A. (2018). Health, income, & poverty: Where we are & what could help. *Health Affairs Health Policy Brief*. https://www.healthaffairs.org/do/10.1377/hpb20180817.901935/full/.

Kochhar, R. (2020). Unemployment rose higher in three months of COVID-19 than it did in two years of the great recession. *Pew Research Center*. https://www.pewresearch.org/fact-tank/2020/06/11/unemployment-rose-higher-in-three-months-of-covid-19-than-it-did-in-two-years-of-the-great-recession/.

Krisberg, K. (2016). Income inequality: When wealth determines health: Earnings influential as lifelong social determinant of health. *The Nation's Health, 46*(8), 1–17.

Kuehn, M. B., Grosch Mendes, C. M., Fukunaga Luna Victoria, G. M., Nemetz, E., & Rigos, Z. (2020). A poverty simulation's impact on nursing and social work students' attitudes towards poverty and health. *Creative Nursing, 26*(4), 256–262. https://doi.org/10.1891/CRNR-D-20-00051.

Marmot, M. G., Smith, G. D., Stansfeld, S., Patel, C., North, F., Head, J., White, I., Brunner, E., & Feeney, A. (1991). Health inequalities among British civil servants: The Whitehall II study. *Lancet, 337*(8754), 1387–1393. https://doi.org/10.1016/0140-6736(91)93068-k.

Myers, A. M., & Painter, M. A., II (2017). Food insecurity in the United States of America: An examination of race/ethnicity and nativity. *Food Security, 9*, 1419–1432.

National Collaborating Centre for Determinants of Health (NCCDH). (2014). *Let's talk: Moving upstream*. National Collaborating Centre for Determinants of Health, St. Francis Xavier University.

National Low Income Housing Coalition. (2021). The gap: A shortage of affordable rental homes. https://reports.nlihc.org/gap/.

Organization for Economic Co-operation and Development (OECD). (2021). Income inequality (indicator). https://data.oecd.org/inequality/income-inequality.htm.

Price, J. H., Khubchandani, J., & Webb, F. J. (2018). Poverty and health disparities: What can health professionals do? *Health Promotion Practice, 19*(2), 170–174.

Robert Wood Johnson Foundation (RWJF). (2013). How does employment, or unemployment affect health? https://www.rwjf.org/en/library/research/2012/12/how-does-employment–or-unemployment–affect-health-.html.

Rosell, B. (2019). Gentrification & homelessness. *Communique, 47*(8), 23–26.

Schmidt, N. M., Nguyen, Q. C., Kehm, R., & Osypuk, T. L. (2020). Do changes in neighborhood social context mediate the effects of the moving to opportunity experiment on adolescent mental health? *Health & Place, 63*, 102331. https://doi.org/10.1016/j.healthplace.2020.102331.

South, E., Venkataramani, A., & Dalembert, G. (2022). Building Black wealth—The role of health systems in closing the gap. *New England Journal of Medicine, 38*(9), 844–849.

Substance Abuse and Mental Health Services Administration (SAMHSA) Soar Works TA Center. (n.d.). Definitions of homelessness. https://soarworks.samhsa.gov/article/definitions-homelessness.

Swope, C. B., & Hernández, D. (2019). Housing as a determinant of health equity: A conceptual model. *Social Science & Medicine, 243*, 112571. https://doi.org/10.1016/j.socscimed.2019.112571.

Taylor, L. A. (2018). Housing and health: An overview of the literature. *Health Affairs Policy Brief.* https://doi.org/10.1377/hpb20180313.396577.

The Brookings Institute. (2020). Examining the Black-White wealth gap. https://www.brookings.edu/blog/up-front/2020/02/27/examining-the-black-white-wealth-gap/.

The Sentencing Project. (2020). Criminal justice facts. https://www.sentencingproject.org/criminal-justice-facts/.

The Urban Institute & Center on Society and Health. (2015). How are income and wealth linked to health and longevity? https://www.urban.org/research/publication/how-are-income-and-wealth-linked-health-and-longevity/view/full_report; food security measurement: https://www.ers.usda.gov/topics/food-nutrition-assistance/food-security-in-the-us/measurement.aspx#measurement. https://www.ers.usda.gov/topics/food-nutrition-assistance/food-security-in-the-us/key-statistics-graphics/#foodsecure.

Urban Ministries of Durham. (n.d.). Spent. https://playspent.org/html/.

US Census Bureau. (2021). Income and poverty in the United States: 2019. census.gov.

US Department of Agriculture, Economic Research Service. (2020). Data shows U.S. poverty rates in 2019 higher in rural areas than in urban for racial/ethnic groups. https://www.ers.usda.gov/data-products/chart-gallery/gallery/chart-detail/?chartId=101903.

US Department of Agriculture (USDA), Economic Research Service. (2022). Measurement. https://www.ers.usda.gov/topics/food-nutrition-assistance/food-security-in-the-us/measurement.aspx#measurement.

US Department of Health and Human Services (USDHHS), Office of Disease Prevention and Health Promotion (ODPHP). (n.d.). Healthy People 2030: Social determinants of health. https://health.gov/healthypeople/objectives-and-data/social-determinants-health.

US Department of Labor, Bureau of Labor Statistics. (2019). The employment situation—May 2019. https://www.bls.gov/news.release/archives/empsit_06072019.pdf.

US Department of Labor, Bureau of Labor Statistics. (2021). The employment situation—August 2021. https://www.bls.gov/news.release/archives/empsit_04022021.pdf.

Wagmiller, R. L., & Adelman, R. M. (2009). Childhood and intergenerational poverty: The long-term consequences of growing up poor. https://www.nccp.org/publication/childhood-and-intergenerational-poverty.

Wang, J., & Geng, L. (2019). Effects of socioeconomic status on physical and psychological health: Lifestyle as a mediator. *International Journal of Environmental Research and Public Health, 16*(2), 281. https://doi.org/10.3390/ijerph16020281.

Wolfson, J. A., & Leung, C. W. (2020). Food insecurity during COVID-19: An acute crisis with long-term health implications. *American Journal of Public Health, 110*(12), 1763–1765. https://doi-org.ezp.slu.edu/10.2105/AJPH.2020.305953.

Yearby, R., Clark, B., & Figueroa, J. (2022). Structural racism in historical and modern US health care policy. *Health Affairs, 2*, 187–194. https://doi.org/10.1037/hlthaff.2021.01466.

Education, Educational Access, and Educational Quality

Sabita Persaud

Education creates the voice through which human rights can be claimed and protected.
—*Universal Declaration of Human Rights*

CHAPTER OUTLINE

LEARNING OBJECTIVES

1. Evaluate education and educational attainment as social determinants of health.
2. Analyze the bidirectional relationship between education and educational attainment and health.
3. Articulate the pathways by which literacy, early childhood education (ECE), the school-to-prison pipeline (STPP), and limited English proficiency (LEP) impact the health of individuals and communities.
4. Describe nursing-led strategies that address the health-related inequities that result from educational access, quality, and attainment.

SOCIAL GRADIENT OF EDUCATION AND HEALTH

Over the life course, education serves many purposes, including the acquisition of knowledge, development of healthy supportive relationships that contribute to a sense of well-being, and development of problem-solving skills and self-efficacy. It also provides the ability to earn a living, evaluate information, and seek alternative solutions (Raghupathi & Raghupathi, 2020). At the community level, education impacts the level of social engagement, which contributes to maintaining cohesive, safe, and healthy communities. Notably, there is a bidirectional association between education and health—just as education impacts health outcomes, educational outcomes are affected by health. Understanding the relationship between education and health allows nurses to plan, implement, and evaluate appropriate and effective interventions for individuals, families, and communities.

To fully explore the relationship between education and health, one must do so in the context of the social gradient. The social gradient in health refers to the relationship between health status and social status. Health is not experienced equally by all, and there is a distinct social gradient that exists among socioeconomic groups.

Health outcomes can reflect persistent inequities in opportunities, access, and use of services. While poverty is a primary cause of social exclusion and inequity, it is exacerbated by racial and gender discrimination. In essence, the lower a person's socioeconomic status, the worse their health. When examining death rates among children under the age of 5 years by household income, for example, the link between socioeconomic status and health is marked, with those in the lowest income groups affected most.

Education and Health

A person's life course is affected by several factors, including social, political, and cultural structures. As these processes contribute to the systematically unequal distribution of power and resources among different groups, health inequities emerge (WHO, 2018). Health inequities result from social status through differential exposure to health hazards, differential vulnerabilities to health conditions, the availability of material resources, and differential consequences of poor health based on socioeconomic status (Pan American Health Organization, 2017). The socioeconomic circumstances of a person clearly affect their health throughout their life span. A focus on educational outcomes for the most disadvantaged groups can have a positive influence on health disparities. This disadvantage may be in the form of a lack of access to health services or quality education, impacting the same groups with accumulated effects felt throughout their lives and from generation to generation. In recent decades, the gradient in health outcomes owing to educational achievement has broadened in the United States, resulting in a wider gap in health status (Montez & Berkman, 2014; Zimmerman & Woolf, 2014). Focusing on improving educational outcomes for the most disadvantaged groups can positively impact health inequalities.

EDUCATIONAL GRADIENT

Educational attainment is the highest level of formal education completed. Between 2000 and 2019, educational attainment rates among 25- to 29-year-olds rose at all levels. Higher levels of education are linked to higher earnings and employment rates (National Center for Education Statistics [NCES], 2022). More-educated people have more job security and higher incomes; greater access to health-promoting activities; access to higher-quality healthcare, health benefits, food, and living conditions; and are more likely to be part of social networks that promote healthy behaviors (Raghupathi & Raghupathi, 2020; Zajacova & Lawrence, 2018). They also face reduced exposure to conditions that undermine health, such as work-related stress and unsafe working environments. In addition, education provides skills needed for individuals to apply health-related information to their lives. Conversely, those with less education self-report worse overall health, more chronic conditions, and have a shorter life expectancy and shorter survival rates when sick (Raghupathi & Raghupathi, 2020; Zajacova & Lawrence, 2018).

Education gradients are present across gender, race, ethnicity, household composition, and socioeconomic status. Among females, there has been a significant rise in educational attainment in recent decades. Among those who are employed full time, women are more likely to have a bachelor's degree than males. Despite these gains in educational attainment, there continues to be a wage gap between males and females (Day, 2019).

Disparities

When analyzing the educational gradient in gaps seen throughout childhood, family conditions contribute significantly (Jackson et al., 2017). Children who live in a home without a parent who has finished high school, in a single-parent home, or in poverty are all at risk for poorer educational outcomes (NCES, 2022). Parental educational attainment can have an impact on children's and families' health-related behaviors; the education level of the mother is more likely to have an impact than that of the father. Living in a household where neither parent had completed high school was most common among Hispanic children under age 18 while living in households where either parent completed a bachelor's or higher degree was most common among Asians (NCES, 2022). Children from divorced or single-parent families are more likely to have emotional, behavioral, physical, and academic problems compared with children from a father–mother family (Yu, 2015). Except for Black and American Indian/Alaska Native children, most children under the age of 18 live with married parents across racial/ethnic groups (NCES, 2022). According to the NCES, a higher percentage of children live in married-couple households than in mother- or father-only households across all groups, except for Black children. In 2018, over half of Black children lived in mother-only households compared with approximately one-third living in married-couple households (NCES, 2019). Family structures are becoming more diverse, and living arrangements are increasingly complex, making it difficult to draw clear connections to education. However, the research is clear that family structure may contribute to instability, limited resources, and lack of parental involvement, which are among the primary drivers of the stratification seen in education (Pribesh et al., 2020).

Economic Status

Poverty rates for Black and American Indian/Alaska Native children were highest in 2020, followed by Hispanic and Pacific Islander children. In 2019, it was reported that 16% of children lived in poverty (NCES, 2022). In recent years the poverty rate for children has decreased among all racial and ethnic groups, except for Pacific Islanders. The NCES (2019) reports that the poverty rate for children was highest in households where neither parent had completed high school and lowest in households where both parents had a bachelor's degree or higher. In 2020, Black and Hispanic students attended schools designated as high poverty at a rate higher than other racial/ethnic groups (NCES, 2022). High-poverty schools provide disproportionately fewer math, science, and college-preparatory classes than other schools, and have higher rates of students suspended or expelled (Government Accountability Office [GAO], 2016).

Education provides the knowledge, skills, and experience needed to navigate the world, and it is this understanding that empowers individuals to make informed, effective, and sustainable changes. The lack of access to quality education that provides opportunities to acquire these skills and knowledge can negatively impact the ability of individuals to achieve optimal health. Additionally, the most vulnerable individuals must overcome multiple risk factors to reach high levels of educational attainment. Education influences health throughout the life span and can mitigate the long-term impact of early life conditions on health. It is well established that educational attainment correlates with health indicators such as life expectancy, obesity, disease morbidity, smoking status, and use of preventive services (Campbell et al., 2014). There are also strong positive correlations between education and health outcomes in terms of mortality, morbidity,

and health-related behaviors. Declining mortality rates have been seen in males of all races and levels of education, with those with the highest levels of education experiencing the greatest declines (Hickey et al., 2018; Montez & Berkman, 2014). Among non-Hispanic White and Black females, there has been a decrease in life expectancy among those with more education and an increase in mortality among those with less education (Hickey et al., 2018; Montez & Berkman, 2014). This points to the confounding impacts that race and gender have on education and health.

As previously discussed, poverty negatively impacts both the academic achievement and overall health of young children. Children from more socioeconomically advantaged communities experience safer and more supportive environments and higher-quality education programs. Children from disadvantaged communities are more likely to need special education services, repeat grades, and drop out of school (Office of Disease Prevention and Health Promotion, n.d.).

Income

Income and wealth are key predictors of health status (Braveman et al., 2010; Zimmerman & Woolf, 2014). Education has become a primary path to financial stability, leading to stable employment that provides families with the means to achieve optimal health (Zajacova & Lawrence, 2018). Individuals with a higher level of education have a greater ability to access socioeconomic resources that contribute to a healthy lifestyle, and to live and work in environments that provide the resources required for healthy living (Zajacova & Lawrence, 2018).

In 2019, approximately 3.9% of people with a bachelor's degree or higher lived in poverty in the United States, compared with 23.7% of those without a high school diploma (NCES, 2019). The median earnings of 25- to 34-year-olds with a master's degree or higher are greater than for those with a bachelor's degree, and the median earnings for those with a bachelor's degree are more than 50% higher than for those with a high school diploma. Similarly, people with higher educational attainment have substantially higher employment rates than those with lower educational attainment (NCES, 2019). Those with a bachelor's degree earn roughly twice as much as those without a college education, but the wage gap between males and females widens as education levels increase (Day, 2019). For every dollar males with a bachelor's degree earn, females earn only 74 cents, compared with 78 cents for workers without a college degree. This pay disparity has been linked to higher levels of stress and poorer health behaviors such as alcoholism and medication nonadherence. It also contributes to poor sleep, diet, and exercise habits, and poor mental health (Treadwell, 2019). Individuals with advanced degrees have a better chance of obtaining rewarding jobs that pay more, provide more job satisfaction, and provide important health-related benefits such as health insurance coverage.

Compared with uninsured or inconsistently insured adults, adults with consistent health insurance coverage have access to more provider services and opportunities for help with disease management (Zimmerman & Woolf, 2014). People with lower incomes are more likely to be uninsured and are more vulnerable to rising healthcare costs due to higher copayments, deductibles, and premiums.

Economic vulnerability can negatively impact health by reducing one's ability to obtain essential resources such as food, transportation, stable and safe housing, and healthcare (Braveman et al., 2010). Braveman et al. (2010) also suggest that individuals with higher incomes have more resources to purchase healthy foods, more time to participate in regular exercise programs, and increased access to healthcare facilities.

Influence of Education on Health-Related Behaviors

Risk Behaviors

Those with a higher level of education are more likely to engage in healthy behaviors and less likely to develop unhealthy habits. Adults with less education are more likely to smoke and have unhealthy practices related to diet and exercise (Zajacova & Lawrence, 2018), whereas adults with a higher level of education are less likely to engage in risky behaviors and more likely to have a healthy diet and consistent exercise regimen. Education helps individuals develop cognitive skills, problem-solving abilities, and personal control, all needed to make thoughtful healthcare-related decisions (Raghupathi & Raghupathi, 2020). The ability to analyze and solve problems enhances one's ability to affect events and outcomes in one's life. These skills can have an indirect impact on health outcomes by improving socioeconomic circumstances, or they can have a direct impact by increasing understanding of complex content. Formal education offers opportunities to learn more about health and health risks through well-designed health education curricula and focus on health-promoting behaviors needed to prevent or manage diseases. As a result, those with more education are better equipped to recognize symptoms and seek care promptly (Raghupathi & Raghupathi, 2020). People with a higher level of education are also more aware of health risks and, as a result, may be more receptive to health education campaigns. Adults with a higher level of education are less likely to engage in risky behaviors and more likely to engage in health promotion related to nutrition and exercise habits (Zimmerman & Woolf, 2014). Quality education is essential to navigating healthcare as well as making lifestyle and personal health decisions.

Stress

Stress has different effects depending on whether it occurs in genetic makeup, experiences, coping mechanisms, or in response to various threats.

Under increasing stress, biological effects and mental consequences are apparent. The combination of high perceived stress and risky health behaviors has been linked to an increase in mortality among individuals of low socioeconomic status (Krueger et al., 2011). Individuals with a low level of education are also more likely to lack the coping skills and strategies required to mitigate the negative effects of stress (Raghupathi & Raghupathi, 2020). Negative health consequences may then worsen, affecting other aspects of life and accumulating over a lifetime.

Self-Efficacy

By developing skills that promote self-efficacy and self-empowerment, education may promote an internal locus of control, the belief that the life course is determined by one's own actions (Ross & Mirowsky, 2013). The highly educated have higher levels of perceived control. Those with low education may feel less in control, not only because they have fewer resources but also because they are more likely to experience a discrepancy between culturally desirable goals and the means to attain them (Ross & Mirowsky, 2013).

Social Networks

Education also promotes skills that help individuals form and maintain social relationships that are beneficial for health by providing social support and promoting healthier behaviors. Individuals with less education are more at risk for chronic occupational or economic stress and tend to have fewer coping capacities, making them less able to deal with these pressures (Krueger et al., 2011).

Individuals in a social network can relay information, establish behavioral norms, and serve as role models. The more educated a person is, the more likely they are to have the social support needed to mitigate the negative impacts of stressful events, and they are also less likely to experience these stressful events. Individuals with higher levels of education may also have larger social networks and be more involved in community-based organizations. On the other hand, a lack of social support is associated with higher mortality rates and poor mental health. Social support and networks are often established in the communities where people live, work, and play.

Impact on Society

Community characteristics such as food access, green space, and economic resources have all been linked to health outcomes. Unhealthy eating habits have been linked to health problems such as diabetes, hypertension, obesity, and heart disease, but access to healthier foods is often limited in communities with lower median incomes and lower levels of educational attainment. These communities often have an oversupply of outlets that sell little fresh produce and offer inexpensive calorie-dense foods and beverages. Adults with a higher level of education and income are more likely to live in communities with green space and access to outdoor places where community members can safely exercise. Green space in urban environments promotes positive social interactions that foster social cohesion and improve health and well-being. Positive health behaviors and outcomes, such as increased physical activity and social engagement, have also been linked to urban green spaces (Jennings & Bamkole, 2019). Green spaces, along with other important health-related resources, are lacking in low-income communities.

Exemplar

Education assists individuals in accessing and using available resources more efficiently, protecting against negative life events that can lead to unhealthy coping strategies. The relationship between education and smoking serves as an example. Differences in cigarette smoking by education represent one of the deadliest inequalities resulting from the social gradient. Approximately 15.5% of all adults in the United States currently smoke, and cigarette smoking is cited as the cause of 480,000 deaths per year, with smokers dying 10 years earlier on average than nonsmokers (CDC, 2020). The total economic cost of smoking in the United States is more than $300 billion a year, including $170 billion in direct medical care and more than $100 billion in lost productivity due to premature death (Assari & Mistry, 2018).

People living in poverty and those with lower levels of educational attainment in the United States have higher rates of cigarette smoking than the general population (US Department of Health and Human Services, 2020). Smoking is more prevalent among males, American Indians/Alaska Natives, people with behavioral health conditions, LGBTQ+ people, and people with lower incomes and education levels (CDC, 2020).

Educational inequalities related to smoking are an important concern for nurses, and an example of the many disadvantages experienced by those with less education (Maralani, 2013). Smoking-related causes of death are key contributors to widening educational gradients in mortality. Widening disparities in mortality for smoking-related causes of death, such as heart disease, lung cancer, chronic lower respiratory disease, and cerebrovascular disease have been observed. Additionally, people with less than a high school education have higher lung cancer incidence rates than those with a college education.

Compared with the less educated, the more educated are less likely to ever smoke, smoke fewer cigarettes per day, are more likely to successfully quit smoking, and are more likely to quit earlier in life (Maralani, 2013). People with a high school education smoke cigarettes for more than twice as many years as people with at least a bachelor's degree (CDC, 2019a). From 1966 to 2015, cigarette smoking declined by 83% among people in the United States with college degrees. However, the decline was less than half that among individuals who did not have a high school diploma (Assari & Mistry, 2018). Following the diagnosis of a chronic condition, more educated individuals are more likely to quit smoking and adhere to smoking cessation over time (Margolis, 2013). Adults with less than a high school education have less success quitting than those with a college education or greater (CDC, 2019a). Education is positively linked to attempts to quit smoking and the likelihood of success (Maralani, 2013). More educated individuals are more informed about healthcare issues, have the financial means to afford smoking cessation aids, can better translate information about the risks of smoking into quitting, and are more likely to use effective quitting methods (Maralani, 2014).

Education promotes skills such as knowledge acquisition, decision-making, coping skills, and self-efficacy, all of which contribute to a higher likelihood of attempting to quit smoking. Less-educated individuals may experience high levels of stress resulting from economic inequality, poor working conditions, discrimination, and poor conditions in the community that may trigger people to begin, escalate, and continue smoking (Hickey et al., 2018; Maralani, 2014). In addition, individuals with lower levels of education may also lack the skills and resources needed to successfully create and carry out a smoking cessation plan.

Cigarettes are commonly marketed as stress relieving, and nicotine dependence becomes both a source of stress and a deterrent to quitting. There is more exposure to cigarette advertising in low-income communities, since tobacco companies target these communities (CDC, 2019a). Because low-income neighborhoods have a higher concentration of tobacco retailers, they are more vulnerable to point-of-sale marketing. Individuals living in low-income communities have the least knowledge about the health risks of smoking, the fewest resources and social supports, and often the least access to services to help them quit (CDC, 2020). Education, as a social determinant, interacts with many other factors to dictate the impact of smoking on individuals and communities. Smoking serves as an example of the bidirectional relationship between education and health.

Education improves literacy, aids in the formation of good habits, and enhances cognitive ability. Educational attainment can help improve health by increasing access to better jobs, which in turn increases financial security through higher incomes. Education can help people navigate complex healthcare-related issues.

EARLY CHILDHOOD EDUCATION

Long-term health is heavily influenced by educational attainment. It is critical that children have the opportunity to grow socially and cognitively so they can thrive and succeed academically, which is critical for their overall well-being and future success. There is immense physical, cognitive, socioemotional, and language development in the early years of childhood. Every child should have an equal early education that lays the groundwork for learning, healthy growth and development, and long-term success. Many children, however, do not have access to high-quality programs and related support services, and as a result, ECE continues to face challenges in terms of achieving equity, access, and excellence. Inequities that occur in early childhood are especially concerning because of the long-term consequences. Positive experiences promote cognitive, social, emotional, and physical development in children, whereas negative experiences can stifle them. Adult diseases such as coronary artery disease, chronic lung disease, and cancer have been linked to less-than-optimal early childhood experiences. Children from low-income families are more likely to have negative experiences in early childhood, which can delay their development and impede school readiness.

Health-Related Benefits

ECE programs seek to provide opportunities and exposures that can mitigate the impacts of adverse childhood experiences and positively impact children's lives, as well as the lives of their caregivers (Campbell et al., 2014; Smith, 2020). There is a wealth of research that supports that ECE is a key factor in child development and well-being and a protective factor against future disease and disability (Black et al., 2017). ECE programs strengthen the foundation for educational attainment by enhancing social and educational skills before children enter the K-12 system.

High-quality ECE programs have been shown to be precursors to maintaining a positive life trajectory. These programs provide direct and indirect benefits to the child, family, and community and are delivered in various ways and settings to meet the needs of diverse populations. Classroom-based ECE programs result in lower special education placement, higher grade retention, and higher graduation rates (McCoy et al., 2017). This is especially important for children from disadvantaged backgrounds, as these programs not only provide education but also support programs that serve as buffers and strengthen the caregiver's ability to meet their children's needs (Bakken et al., 2017; Smith, 2020). The needs of disadvantaged children may be served by participation in ECE programs, since these programs strive to prevent or minimize gaps in school readiness between low-income and more economically advantaged children. High-quality ECE programs that are intentionally designed to meet the needs of low-income and racial and ethnic minority children improve long-term educational and health outcomes and reduce disparities (Black et al., 2017).

ECE programs continue to address changing work roles and family compositions, helping equalize opportunities for children from low-income families and enhance child development and well-being (Kamerman & Gatenio-Gabel, 2015). In the United States, programs such as Head Start are designed to provide all children with enriched experiences and learning opportunities that can improve school readiness.

Educational Quality

ECE programs include a range of part-day, full-school-day, and full-work-day programs and are funded and delivered in various ways in both the public and private sectors. Preschools and nursery schools include the range of programs offered under public and private education auspices or provide compensatory education under special legislation and are largely half-day or cover the typical school day. Center-based childcare typically refers to full-day programs or free-standing and independent programs that offer care corresponding to traditional working hours. Family childcare refers to care for several children in the caregiver's home.

While access to ECE programs is a priority, attention must also be paid to the quality of programs. The quality of these programs is an important factor due to the potential impact on the long-term educational attainment and health of children (Black et al., 2017). High-quality programs address academic, social-emotional, and physical domains and seek to ensure children are developing in ways that enable them to be healthy and ready for school. Comprehensive child assessments, staff with professional knowledge and skill, ongoing support for teachers, support for diverse learners, meaningful family engagement, low teacher-to-student ratio, and comprehensive program assessment are all characteristics of high-quality programs (Weshcler et al., 2016). Children enrolled in low-quality programs with limited resources, safety concerns, and low teacher support have poorer physical and mental health (Office of Disease Prevention & Health Promotion [ODPHP], n.d.).

Disparities

Children from families at all income levels can benefit from high-quality ECE, though economically disadvantaged children benefit more. Children from low-income families have less access to high-quality ECE than children from middle-income families, placing them at further disadvantage. ECE can provide disadvantaged children with opportunities to achieve school readiness and lifelong employment, and bolster long-term health outcomes (ODPHP, n.d.). Children who participate in ECE programs are less likely to be involved in the child welfare system, have better language development, and have more positive health outcomes than those who do not (Smith, 2020). This is in part because participation in ECE programs can open access to preventative services for children and their families. Primary prevention interventions, such as requiring up-to-date immunizations, enrolling participants in children's health insurance programs, and providing nutritious meals, are all part of quality programs. Secondary prevention services include vision and hearing screenings and home visit programs. Intensive therapy and trauma interventions are examples of tertiary services afforded to those who attend quality programs. These types of preventive and early intervention programs target children's and families' education, relationships, health behaviors, and well-being.

Growth and Development

Healthy eating is essential in early childhood, not only for the obvious health benefits but also for the numerous associated academic benefits. Children experiencing poverty, food insecurity, and inadequate dietary intake are at risk for poor health and development in the short and long term (Black et al., 2017). Low-income preschoolers who attend a center-based program are less likely to be food insecure than those who are cared for solely by their parents or by an unrelated adult at home (Gundersen & Ziliak, 2016). Children typically spend 6 hours a day in school and consume half of their daily calories during that time, providing an opportunity for ECE programs to intervene.

ECE programs can positively impact healthy growth and development through the provision of meal services. Programs such as the federally funded Supplemental Nutrition Assistance Program (SNAP) and Child and Adult Food Program are designed to alleviate problems related to nutrition in early childhood, with the goal of improving overall health and well-being. Access to and participation in these programs support physical health, development, and nutrition. Under the US Department of Agriculture's (USDA) Child and Adult Food Program, participating centers receive federal support to provide nutritious meals and snacks for eligible children, providing meals for over 4 million children in 2018 (USDA, 2019). SNAP is the largest federal nutrition assistance program. Participation in SNAP during childhood decreases the likelihood of obesity, hypertension, heart disease, and heart attack in young adults. Women who participated in the program as children have increased educational attainment, higher earnings and income, and decreased rates of poverty and reliance on public assistance programs (Keith-Jennings et al., 2019).

Support

High-quality ECE programs also promote positive developmental outcomes, stability, predictability, and support. Early childhood settings offer supportive and healthy environments that can help children cope with stressful events and develop resilience. Relationships with teachers, staff, and peers complement the role of parents and caregivers in helping children build positive social interactions. Access to teachers and trained staff increases the likelihood of early identification of social, health, and cognitive challenges in individual children, enabling early referral for intervention. Furthermore, parental interactions with teachers strengthens parents' capacities, including their ability to reinforce the education and socialization of their children (Ramon et al., 2018). Programs that promote supportive and nurturing relationships between caregivers and children influence parental and child outcomes by increasing positive parent–child interactions and strengthening parents' social support (Morris et al., 2017). These connections are especially important for disadvantaged children, who are at a higher risk of poor health outcomes and developmental delays (Bitsko et al., 2016). Parental support and involvement benefits children, parents, and programs in ways that extend beyond academic achievement. ECE programs that provide parental support, such as home visits and parent groups, have several additional benefits, including increased trust and decreased stress, which can improve the family's overall health and well-being (Black et al., 2017). Accessible and affordable high-quality childcare can lead to a significant increase in parental employment and income levels, which can lead to improved child outcomes and set the foundation for educational attainment (Zajacova & Lawrence, 2018). Parents who have access to childcare are more likely to work and do so for longer periods. This increased workforce participation and job experience ultimately translate into long-term financial benefits for families with children attending preschool.

Long-Term Benefits

Not only does ECE benefit children while they are enrolled, but there are also significant long-term benefits. Participating in an intensive ECE program from preschool to third grade is linked to higher educational attainment through adulthood. Starting with a high-quality ECE program, a seamless continuum of high-quality education means that early investments can be improved and expanded upon in later years. For example, participants in early Head Start have been found to have a lower risk for cardiovascular disease and associated risk factors such as obesity, hypertension, hyperglycemia, and hypercholesterolemia, delaying or avoiding the occurrence of chronic disease as adults (Campbell et al., 2014).

Impact on Society

The benefits of early childhood education (ECE) extend to the community through lower expenditures, such as reduced spending for special education and involvement in child protection and welfare systems. Investing in ECE also reduces involvement with the criminal justice system, lowering the societal costs of the criminal justice system and incarceration.

Because educational attainment is positively correlated with health outcomes, investment in ECE is critical to the reduction of health disparities. Innovative partnerships between healthcare and ECE delivery systems are imperative to address the root causes of health disparities and reduce access barriers to social supports that can help improve health equity. Children entering ECE who do not possess the foundational skills, knowledge, and attitudes necessary for success in school are at risk of long-term academic, social, and behavioral difficulties. Children who attend high-quality ECE programs are more likely to complete high school and continue their education. Additionally, children who do not possess the foundational skills are more likely to drop out before finishing high school, engage in criminal behavior, become pregnant as teenagers, and become addicted to tobacco, alcohol, and other drugs (McCoy et al., 2017). The combination of behavioral issues and academic failure is also linked to poor physical and mental health in adulthood. While ECE programs are not directly intended to improve child health, there are clear indications that they may lead to short- and long-term improvements in health-related outcomes for those who participate. More emphasis must be placed on ensuring that all children have access to ECE opportunities.

FORMAL SCHOOLING (K-12)

Health risk behaviors are generally higher among those with less than 9 years of formal education, begin to decline among those with 9 to 12 years of formal education, and continue to decline with additional years of education (Ramon et al., 2018). This emphasizes the significance of educational attainment for future health. Academic achievement in adolescents is a predictor and determinant of adult health outcomes (CDC, 2019b). When academic success is measured in terms of grades, there is a link between high school student grades and risk behaviors, with higher grades being associated with lower rates of risk behavior. Early sexual initiation, violence, and substance use have all been linked to lower educational attainment and poor grades and test scores. Students with higher grades are more physically active and are less likely to use marijuana (CDC, 2019b).

Schools can play an important role in promoting young people's health and safety and assisting them in developing lifelong healthy habits. Students spend a significant portion of their day in the school setting, allowing for increased access to health services and opportunities for health-related interventions. Unfortunately, those who attend less-resourced schools are not afforded the same experiences and access as those who attend more-resourced schools. For example, students at less-resourced schools are at least three times more likely than those who attend more-resourced schools to have stressors, including unstable housing, hunger, and lack of medical and dental care, that could interfere with learning (Kelleher, 2015). Moreover, teachers at underresourced schools spend significantly more time dealing with class interruptions, counseling students, and discussing community problems and societal inequities than their peers in adequately resourced schools (Kelleher, 2015). Low-income children do not have the same access to resources and enrichment opportunities as those from higher-income communities. However, when presented with opportunities such as gifted-and-talented programs, students who attend high-poverty schools are half as likely as those who attend underresourced schools to participate in these enrichment activities. This is most likely due to socioeconomic factors that take precedence. Despite multiple interventions such as targeted funding, innovative enrichment programs, and new school governance models, a significant improvement in overall outcomes for low-income children has not yet been seen (US Department of Education, n.d.). Until this is comprehensively addressed, these children will be disadvantaged not only in education but also in health.

SCHOOL-TO-PRISON PIPELINE

The STPP refers to policies that directly and indirectly push students out of school and onto a pathway into the criminal justice system, disproportionately impacting the most vulnerable students (Berlowitz et al., 2017; Heitzeg, 2009). These policies and practices include zero-tolerance policies related to suspension and expulsion, policing and surveillance, and referrals to law enforcement (Heitzeg, 2009). More recently, the STPP has come under increased scrutiny, and the country's reliance on law enforcement to address issues related to mental health, substance use, and poverty has been highlighted (Aronowitz et al., 2021). Zero-tolerance policies are applied to minor violations of school rules and penalize students for actions that could be handled within schools. Zero-tolerance policies "mandate the application of predetermined consequences, most often severe and punitive in nature, that are intended to be applied regardless of the gravity of the behavior, mitigating circumstances, or situational context" (American Psychological Association Zero Tolerance Task Force, 2008, p. 852). The application of these policies varies from district to district, but infractions range from possession of tobacco, alcohol, and drugs to threatening behavior, dress code violations, truancy, bullying, and tardiness (Curran, 2019). Students who are victims of these policies are denied educational access and the associated benefits.

DISPARITIES

Zero-tolerance policies negatively impact educational attainment by increasing suspensions and expulsions and referrals to alternative educational settings and programs. Those expelled or suspended are more likely to be left behind, stop going to school, use social welfare programs, and be incarcerated (McElrath et al., 2020).

While zero-tolerance policies are widely enacted, students with disabilities, those belonging to racial and ethnic minorities, those who speak English as a second language, those who identify as LGBTQ+, and those who have experienced trauma have significantly higher rates of suspension than other students (Mallett, 2016). In 2018, Black students represent 39% of school suspensions yet comprise only 15.5% of all public school students (GAO, 2018). Preschool-aged Black males are excessively disciplined compared with students from other ethnic groups, with a likelihood of being suspended that is nearly three times as great as that of White students. LGBTQ+ youth are particularly at risk for suspension and expulsion due to the bullying and harassment they experience and are often punished for their attempts to defend themselves (Himmelstein & Brückner, 2011). Students with disabilities are also suspended more than their nondisabled peers. Black boys with disabilities are referred to law enforcement, arrested for school-related accidents, or expelled from school at an even higher rate (GAO, 2018). These inequalities exist regardless of the type of disciplinary action, school poverty level, or type of school attended.

Impact on Education and Health

Students who miss instruction due to suspension or expulsion are less likely to perform well academically and receive lower scores on standardized and statewide exams (National Council on Disability [NCD], 2016). Suspension puts students at greater risk for subsequent disciplinary action, repeating a grade, and being involved with the criminal justice system (Noltemeyer et al., 2015). Those who have been suspended multiple times are more likely to be arrested or convicted (Monahan et al., 2014). In addition, students who have been incarcerated as a juvenile are more likely to be incarcerated as adults and less likely to graduate from high school (Aizer & Doyle, 2015).

Students with disabilities who receive special education services in school have poorer outcomes and are suspended and expelled more often than their peers without disabilities (NCD, 2016). Students with disabilities face significant nonacademic consequences of zero-tolerance policies, as they are more likely than their nondisabled peers to rely on school services such as academic support, mental health counseling, occupational therapy, and physical therapy. The inability to attend school impedes access to much-needed treatment, which may result in poor health, low self-esteem, physical problems, substance abuse, lower academic achievement, and difficulties with peer interactions. Students with emotional disturbances are substantially more likely to be suspended or expelled in a single school year or over the course of their academic careers than students with other disabilities. Racial and ethnic minority students with disabilities are disproportionately classified as having emotional disturbances, placing them at even higher risk for suspension or expulsion (Mallett, 2016). It is estimated that 20% of children in the United States suffer from a mental disorder, and most schools lack sufficient therapy facilities to assist them (NCD, 2016). In fact, zero-tolerance disciplinary measures often result in students with mental health issues being suspended, expelled, or jailed.

Long-Term Impact

Zero-tolerance policies are a conduit for vulnerable children to be funneled into the criminal justice system. Incarceration is associated with significant mental and physical health effects during adolescence and young adulthood. Being imprisoned *amplifies* the mental, emotional, and behavioral problems that these youth face (Barnert et al., 2018). It is estimated that about two-thirds of children and adolescents in the juvenile justice system have at least one diagnosable mental health problem, compared with less than 20% of the general population (Development Services Group, Inc. & Office of Juvenile Justice and Delinquency Prevention, 2017).

Children and adolescents who stay in the justice system as adults face poorer health outcomes, including physical limitations, mental illness, and increased risk for suicidal thoughts and attempts, than those never incarcerated or incarcerated at an older age (Barnert et al., 2018). Individuals who have been imprisoned not only have substantial healthcare needs but also face many obstacles to receiving health benefits and accessing care.

Even after release, those who have been incarcerated find themselves at high risk for continued poor health outcomes. The process of reentering society after incarceration can be stressful for individuals, their families, and communities. People who have been incarcerated have higher morbidity and mortality rates than the general population. Additionally, rates of hospitalization increase and utilization of mental health and substance abuse treatment decreases after release (American Academy of Family Physicians Foundation, 2017). In addition to health risks, former prisoners face stigma that can lead to disruptions in their social networks, higher risks of fatal drug overdoses, suicide, and economic disadvantage. These challenges affect not only formerly incarcerated individuals but also their families and communities, many of which face inequities resulting from complex social determinants of health.

Impact on Society

Communities whose schools have high rates of suspension and expulsion are impacted when community youth are unable to complete their education and/or become incarcerated. The high rates of arrest and imprisonment in neighborhoods served by schools that use these disciplinary methods are also cause for concern, as they have a range of negative health effects for communities by leading to ill mental and physical health in previously incarcerated people, their families, and community members (Wang & Wildeman, 2017). Furthermore, these discipline policies have indirect adverse effects on nonsuspended students in schools with high suspension rates. Schools with high suspension use have shown lower mean scores on state achievement tests than schools with lower suspension use, even among those students who were not suspended (Noltemeyer et al., 2015).

Role of the Nurse

Nurses and other providers have an opportunity to improve children's long-term health outcomes by advocating that unnecessary and potentially harmful exposures to incarceration are minimized. There is also an additional responsibility to prevent detrimental health effects for those who are exposed to the criminal justice system (Barnert et al., 2017). Nurses working in schools must take an active role in the assessment and screening process with a keen eye for hidden disabilities and exposure to trauma (National Association of School Nurses, 2018). As part of the interdisciplinary team, nurses should collaborate and coordinate to create plans to support children with disability-related diagnoses (e.g., anxiety) who are at risk for disciplinary action.

HEALTH LITERACY AND NUMERACY

Proficiency in literacy and numeracy is necessary to access economic and social opportunities and resources needed to reach optimal health and wellness. Development of these skills is a lifelong process, with those who struggle with basic skills frequently excluded from resources and opportunities needed for optimal health.

Health Literacy

Health literacy is an asset that increases a person's capacity for health action through language proficiency, reading, and numeracy skills (Wittenberg et al., 2018). This concept, as defined by the CDC (2021), is comprised of two components: personal and organizational. Personal health literacy is "the degree to which individuals have the ability to find, understand, and use information and services to inform health-related decisions and actions for themselves and others" (CDC, 2021, paragraph 1). Organizational health literacy is the degree to which organizations equitably enable individuals to make informed health-related decisions (CDC, 2021). The definition of health literacy has evolved over time with increased emphasis on a person's ability to make well-informed health-related decisions based on the information obtained (Loan et al., 2018). The addition of organizations to the definition encourages a commitment to health literacy at the systems level.

A separate but related concept, health information literacy refers to "the set of abilities needed to: recognize a health information need; identify likely information sources and use them to retrieve relevant information; assess the quality of the information and its applicability to a specific situation; and analyze, understand, and use the information to make good health decisions" (Schardt, 2011, p. 1). Health information literacy focuses on information-related practices and capabilities, whereas health literacy emphasizes communication between health professionals and patients (Lawless et al., 2016). Both are equally important concepts for nursing to address.

Health Numeracy

Numeracy is the "ability to access, use, interpret, and communicate mathematical information and ideas, to engage in and manage mathematical demands of a range of situations in adult life" (CDC, 2021, paragraph 3). Health numeracy refers to the extent to which people access, comprehend, and interact with numerical health information to make health decisions (Peters et al., 2019). Numeracy-related healthcare tasks include reading a growth chart, interpreting nutrition and medication labels, and understanding laboratory results. The current evidence related to the impact of numeracy on health outcomes is not conclusive but still important to consider.

Influence on Health Outcomes

Multiple social determinants, such as economic status, education, and neighborhood and built environment, influence and are influenced by health literacy and numeracy. Low health literacy (LHL) can be viewed as the result of a combination of life circumstances, such as limited access to or poor education, LEP, learning differences and disabilities, and cognitive impairment (Mantwill et al., 2015). Research suggests that individuals who face the most social disparities are the most likely to have lower levels of health literacy (Mantwill et al., 2015).

Individuals with lower health literacy and numeracy may face challenges as they access, navigate, and understand the healthcare system. The complexity of the healthcare environment requires individuals to take on an expanded role that includes seeking information, advocating for rights and understanding responsibilities, measuring and monitoring one's own health, and making informed health-related decisions (Institute of Medicine, 2004). Individuals must have a sufficient level of health literacy and numeracy to successfully engage in health-related activities such as:

- Accessing health care services
- Providing informed consent
- Calculating medication dosages
- Communicating with healthcare providers
- Evaluating health-related information
- Interpreting test results

Health literacy and numeracy skills are dependent on the context of the health-related situation, individual skills and experiences, or changes to the larger healthcare system. At some point, a person may need assistance with understanding important health information or navigating a complex health system. Even those with higher levels of education may encounter complex health situations that are difficult to understand. However, individuals with cognitive decline associated with age and disability, lower education levels and socioeconomic status, and LEP are at the highest risk.

Cost of Low Literacy

There are significant personal and economic costs associated with limited health literacy, including increased chronic illness and disability, increased hospitalization, greater emergency room utilization, and lower quality of life (Dodson et al., 2015; Loan et al., 2018; McDonald & Shenkman, 2018). Annually, low health literacy costs between $105 billion and $238 billion in direct healthcare costs, with indirect costs between $1.6 trillion and $3.6 trillion (Hudson et al., 2017). On average, health payers and employers spend $26 more on patients with low health literacy, totaling $4.8 billion across the healthcare industry each year (Accenture, 2017). Moreover, patients with LHL are more likely to have less knowledge of disease processes and more difficulty managing their disease, thus increasing the need for healthcare services and associated costs. Low health literacy can also have a negative effect on provider–patient communication as patients with LHL tend to be passive in their communication with providers, less likely to engage in shared decision-making, and more likely to be unsatisfied with provider interactions (Muscat et al., 2019). The advantages of higher levels of health literacy include increased patient safety, decreased hospitalizations, and increased savings for the healthcare system.

Role of the Nurse

Gathering, comprehending, and applying the information needed to make informed decisions and change health behaviors can be challenging for those with low health literacy and numeracy. Nurses can serve as advocates for improved health literacy through prioritizing health literacy and numeracy assessment, implementing effective and creative interpersonal communication strategies, and developing accessible and understandable health education materials (Nesari et al., 2019). If nursing fails to join in the responsibility, health inequities faced by the most vulnerable populations will be magnified.

Assessment

Assessing health literacy allows nurses and other providers to gain insight into a patient's knowledge, behaviors, attitudes, and skills. As the largest segment of the healthcare workforce, nurses are ideally positioned to screen and document patients' health literacy skills. Nurses have the responsibility of facilitating health education activities and thus should have the knowledge and skills needed to assess health literacy, identify those at risk, and implement appropriate interventions (Nesari et al., 2019; Wittenberg et al., 2018).

Despite this responsibility, the impact of health literacy on access to care and adherence to plans of care is often omitted from nursing assessments (Dickens et al., 2013). Nurses often rely on their personal judgment or patient's educational level to assess health literacy, which could lead to an overestimation and a nurse communicating in a manner that the patient does not comprehend (Dickens et al., 2013; Wittenberg et al., 2018). Because health literacy includes a patient's ability to read as well as how they understand and utilize health information, nurses should assess the health literacy levels of all patients, taking the universal precautions approach that all patients are at risk for not understanding health information (Brega et al., 2015; Loan et al., 2018).

Notably, individuals with low literacy skills may already feel marginalized and fear being exposed (Muscat et al., 2019). For this reason, nurses must prioritize promoting shame-free environments (Loan et al., 2018), which may involve the inclusion of a formal literacy test as part of an encounter. In situations where this may occur, it is best for the nurse to use general assessment questions and behavioral clues to assess health literacy. It is common for individuals with low health literacy to mask the issue; however, a thorough nursing assessment may uncover a barrier to understanding.

Nurses must make use of established tools to assess and communicate with patients who have limited health literacy. The Newest Vital Sign (NVS) and Short Assessment of Health Literacy (SAHL) are widely used tools to assess health literacy. The NVS, which is available in 10 languages, is a 3-minute functional literacy assessment where individuals are assessed for low literacy levels. The SAHL, a 2.5-minute tool available in Spanish and English, tests the patient's comprehension and pronunciation of 18 terms (Agency for Healthcare Research and Quality, 2019). Health numeracy has not gained as much attention in research and healthcare, making assessment more difficult. Nurses must be innovative in using interpersonal communication strategies to assess health numeracy levels.

Interpersonal Communication Strategies

After patients have been identified as having limited health literacy and/or numeracy, this information should be included in their treatment plans so that appropriate nursing actions and follow-up care are implemented (Loan et al., 2018). The universal precautions approach to reduce miscommunication includes nursing interventions that focus on simplifying communication and confirming comprehension for all patients (Brega et al., 2015). Interpersonal communication strategies such as the teach-back method can be used. This method, recommended by the Agency for Healthcare Research and Quality (2019), is a communication strategy that verifies patients' understanding of health information to improve adherence to treatment plans and protect patient safety. The teach-back method involves the nurse providing information and then asking the patient to repeat the key points in their own words. This communication cycle continues until the patient has received and understands key points (Badaczewski et al., 2017). The teach-back method allows nurses to assess an individual's understanding and reteach or modify teaching as needed while empowering individuals through greater understanding.

Verbal instruction should be reinforced with printed or digital materials that are easy to read and include photos, infographics, and illustrations. Nurses must join the interdisciplinary team in assessing, selecting, and creating easy-to-understand forms and health information materials. There are several tools available to assess health information. The CDC Clear Communication Index, a 20-item evidenced-based index, is one widely used tool that can be applied to assess health education materials. The index places emphasis on information clarity and comprehension for diverse groups. Use of this tool increased the likelihood that diverse users could identify the intended message and understand the words and numbers in the materials (Baur & Prue, 2014).

Although ideal, it may not be feasible for nurses to assess health education materials prior to dissemination, as these are often distributed at the system level. In these cases, nurses may need to rely on interpersonal communication skills and strategies. One of the most common strategies is to use plain language to simplify verbal or written health information. Health education materials should be developed with specific audiences and literacy levels in mind. Plain language strategies are designed to help users find, understand, and use materials to meet their needs (Table 3.1). Use of plain language helps ensure that patients with low educational attainment and low health literacy and numeracy can be actively engaged in their own health (Table 3.1).

TABLE 3.1   Plain Language Strategies
Plain Language Strategies
• Use simple words and/or phrases
• Avoid medical and nursing jargon
• Reduce abbreviations and acronyms
• Use active voice
• Place the main message first

Nurses are poised to be the most important advocates for individuals with low health literacy and should have the knowledge and skills needed to implement strategies that not only meet the needs of those with low health literacy but also improve overall health literacy. The ability to assess patients' health literacy is essential to identify patients who most need help obtaining, processing, and applying health-related information. Furthermore, nurses should take the lead in ensuring that disseminated health information meets the literacy needs of the intended audience.

DIGITAL LITERACY

E-health is the "use of information and communication technologies (ICT) for health and health-related fields, including telehealth, telemedicine, mobile health (mHealth), electronic medical or health records, big data, wearables, and even artificial intelligence" (WHO, paragraph 1, n.d.). Digital health literacy (DHL), or e-health literacy, refers to the ability to utilize health information from electronic sources and apply that knowledge to address a health issue (Norman & Skinner, 2006). DHL allows people to take a more active role in achieving optimal health outcomes, thus having a positive impact on the overall healthcare system. DHL can lead to improved prevention, increased awareness of health-promoting activities, and overall improvement in health outcomes. However, the use of technology to engage in healthcare is dependent on access to the Internet and being skilled in its use. E-health literacy is influenced by a person's health status, education, and motivation, and the availability of technology (Norman & Skinner, 2006). E-health literacy is dynamic, evolving over time as new technologies are introduced and the personal, social, and environmental contexts transform.

As the healthcare system continues to integrate the digital health ecosystem (Fig. 3.1), the ability to navigate digital health tools and services is increasingly important. Though the future of healthcare is digital, the lack of access to digital technologies continues to be a barrier to healthcare in the United States. Patient-oriented health tools such as health apps, patient portals, and online patient records, which are rapidly increasing in supply and demand, are designed to empower patients to monitor their health and take initiative with their care.

Disparities

Poverty, a lack of access to the Internet and digital health technologies, low involvement with digital health, and

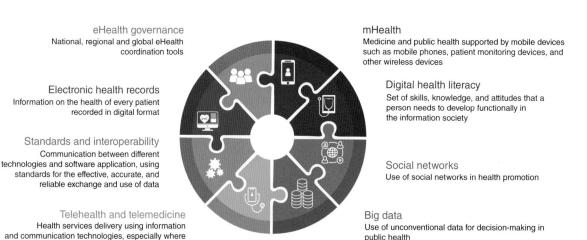

eHealth governance
National, regional and global eHealth coordination tools

Electronic health records
Information on the health of every patient recorded in digital format

Standards and interoperability
Communication between different technologies and software application, using standards for the effective, accurate, and reliable exchange and use of data

Telehealth and telemedicine
Health services delivery using information and communication technologies, especially where distances is a barrier to receiving healthcare

mHealth
Medicine and public health supported by mobile devices such as mobile phones, patient monitoring devices, and other wireless devices

Digital health literacy
Set of skills, knowledge, and attitudes that a person needs to develop functionally in the information society

Social networks
Use of social networks in health promotion

Big data
Use of unconventional data for decision-making in public health

Fig. 3.1 Digital health ecosystem.

low DHL are all factors that can lead to poor health outcomes. Individuals along the lowest social gradients are also the most vulnerable regarding access to and understanding of health information (Liobikienė & Bernatonienė, 2018). In addition to experiencing digital exclusion, they are also likely to be less aware of issues of privacy, health data use, and data protection. Internet access and related skills are closely linked to inequalities involving income, education, race and ethnicity, age, and geography, adding another barrier to the ability to benefit from technological innovations (Harris et al., 2019). Adults who are not digitally literate are less educated, older, and more likely to be Black, Hispanic, or a non-US native. They have lower labor force participation rates and work in lower-skilled jobs than digitally literate adults (Mamedova & Pawlowski, 2018). As a result of evolving digital technologies, traditionally underserved groups may gain access to previously unattainable services. However, the growing reliance on technology to access health information and services can widen health disparities for those who lack access or the skills to use these technologies.

Disparities in broadband access can exacerbate disparities in other social determinants of health that have an impact on health outcomes. For example, for those in digitally isolated communities, a lack of broadband can limit educational and economic opportunities. The digital divide—the gap between those who have access to information and communication technologies and those who do not—encompasses access to broadband Internet connection, devices, and health information (Hall et al., 2015). This divide diminishes a person's ability to communicate with providers, research health-related topics, connect with medical resources, and participate in telehealth. Today, there is an additional need to focus on how individuals use digital health information to make healthcare decisions, engage in health behaviors, and navigate the health system (Box 3.1).

Access and Availability

Greater reliance on technology in healthcare creates a barrier to care for those who have limited digital literacy. Approximately 21 million Americans (6.5%) do not have broadband Internet access (Federal Communications Commission [FCC], 2019). Broadband encompasses high-speed, reliable Internet delivered through fiber, wireless, satellite, digital subscriber line, or cable (FCC, 2019). The most vulnerable members of society

---

BOX 3.1 Exemplar

During the COVID-19 pandemic, there was a significant increase in the use of digital health services to provide healthcare in a safe manner. Telehealth became a widely used vehicle to provide clinical services through remote telecommunication technologies. Telehealth also allows for improved access and quality of care for vulnerable patients who need health services for acute or chronic conditions. A successful telehealth visit requires access to smartphones, tablets, or computers and a reliable Internet connection. In addition to equipment, individuals must also be able to navigate online platforms and patient portals. Due to acute shortages of healthcare providers and geographic barriers to care, rural communities, in particular, face healthcare access challenges. Remote delivery of healthcare services via telehealth has the potential to improve access to care in these communities but is dependent on fast and reliable broadband access.

---

are most likely to be without stable broadband Internet access. This includes those of low socioeconomic status, those with lower levels of education, ethnic and racial minorities, rural populations, and the elderly (Anderson, 2020). Older, low-income African Americans with less than a high school diploma who live in rural areas are the most likely not to use the Internet (Anderson & Perrin, 2017).

The availability of broadband Internet must continue to be prioritized, as should access to affordable and usable digital devices. Individuals from ethnic minorities or lower socioeconomic groups are more likely to rely on a smartphone for Internet service, decreasing the stability of the Internet connection. Those with lower levels of education are also more likely to rely solely on a smartphone for Internet access. Of those aged 65 or older, over one-third do not have a desktop or laptop, and more than half do not have a smartphone (Anderson, 2020). This will become increasingly important as the development and use of health-related apps continue to grow. Unaddressed, these disparities will further decrease access to health services for those that are most in need.

Knowledge and Skills

The adoption of new knowledge and skills needed to use technology can be a challenge, particularly for older adults. Due to a general lack of access to digital technologies and relevant skills to use them, low-income older adults face greater challenges in this area (Hargittai & Dobransky, 2017). Compared with those younger, older adults have lower rates of Internet and social media use (Anderson & Perrin, 2017). Higher-income older adults have higher levels of digital literacy than lower-income older adults and are more likely to engage in a variety of online activities (Hargittai & Dobransky, 2017). Although older adults have shown an interest in digital technologies, many, particularly those from marginalized groups, are unsure how to use them. Approximately two-thirds of adults over the age of 65 use the Internet (Anderson & Perrin, 2017). Internet usage among older adults varies by age group, with more "young-old" adults (65–69) using the Internet than "oldest-old" adults (80 and older), and the more affluent have higher levels of Internet social media use (Hargittai et al., 2018).

The increased availability of online health information and services poses a challenge to those with limited literacy skills or Internet experience. Many describe the Internet as stressful, overwhelming, and even inaccessible. Contributing to the plethora of available health-related information are social media and networking platforms such as Facebook, Twitter, Instagram, Snapchat, YouTube, and WhatsApp.

Social Media

Social media is a platform that enables people to communicate and interact with one another and share opinions and content in digital and online spaces, and it represents a source of health information for people across the world. Social media empowers both providers and patients to share experiences and opinions about health issues with a wide range of audiences. Social media is also used to seek and share health-related information. As more people obtain health-related information online, it is critical to ensure that content delivered through online resources is accessible to a wide range of target audiences, especially the most vulnerable.

Differences in access to technology combined with sociodemographic factors may affect the use of social media health interventions, potentially resulting in health inequities. It is estimated that 72% of Americans use social media; however, sociodemographic differences are seen among users based on specific platforms. Overall, 64% percent of those with a high school education or less use social media compared with 79% of college graduates (Pew Research Center, 2020). Moreover, those who reside in suburban and urban areas report higher levels of social media use than those who reside in rural areas. One criticism leveled at the use of social media for health is the difficulty in reaching older populations who may require more medical attention but may also have less access. According to the Pew Research Center (2020), only 40% of those aged 65 or older report using at least one social media site compared with 82% of those aged 30–49. However, adults aged 65 and up are becoming more active on social media, with rates steadily increasing in recent years. This method of accessing health-related information and services will only become more common, emphasizing the importance of providing accurate information online.

Misinformation is incorrect information whereas disinformation is misinformation spread with the intent of deceiving the audience. Misinformation and disinformation have created needless uncertainty, anxiety, fear, and anger in society, all of which have detrimental effects. The digital literacy required to evaluate online information necessitates cognitive skills, particularly the ability to fact-check the information obtained. While social media allows for rapid information dissemination, misinformation and disinformation infiltrate and spread on health-related social media.

Social media has the potential to significantly improve health outcomes but must be used with care and consideration. Again, the skills obtained through educational attainment are needed to maximize the positive impacts of social media and lessen the likelihood that mis/disinformation influences health behaviors.

Role of the Nurse

As the use of digital technologies to deliver health information and engage people in interventions becomes more common, there will be a greater need to understand the best methods and channels for disseminating information in the most accessible and understandable way. Nurses can advocate for access to and accessibility of digital health services for all using a holistic approach that addresses the factors that impact the health and quality of life of individuals, families, and communities. Digital health interacts with social determinants of health in a way that indirectly contributes to health inequities. There is a great risk that health disparities may widen as access to healthcare continues to be difficult for the most vulnerable segments of the population.

Healthcare professionals must work to ensure that momentum in closing all levels of the digital divide does not wane.

LIMITED ENGLISH PROFICIENCY

Low health literacy and LEP are distinct but related barriers to health communication. LEP describes those who do not speak English as their primary language and have limited spoken and written English fluency, hindering access and communication, interfering with the patient–provider relationship, and leading to disparities in health (Price et al., 2012).

The US Census Bureau (2019) reported that individuals with LEP accounted for approximately 9% (25.2 million) of the US population over age 5. Approximately 21% of the population report speaking a language other than English at home. The top three languages reported were Spanish, Chinese, and Tagalog (US Census Bureau, 2019). As immigration and migration continue to expand, the healthcare system must be equipped to handle potential issues in communication.

Language barriers exacerbate the impact of other social determinants of health, deepening disparities in healthcare access and outcomes. Language barriers make it more difficult for vulnerable patients to speak for themselves, ask questions, and navigate healthcare systems. The language of healthcare, in itself, is difficult to understand but is especially challenging for those with language barriers (Feinberg et al., 2020). Individuals with LEP experience language-related barriers that adversely affect health outcomes and interfere with the process of accessing and utilizing care and services.

Disparities

Language-related barriers to care exist in both primary and acute care settings. Compared with English-proficient patients, patients with language barriers experience delays in preventative services, longer wait times, and missed office visits in primary care settings (Feinberg et al., 2020). Individuals with LEP may not understand their diagnosis and treatment plans, which can result in decreased service utilization and adherence to treatments, missed office visits, and delayed disease management. In acute care settings, individuals with LEP experience higher rates of adverse events such as falls and surgical infections, worse postoperative pain management,

and lower-quality healthcare experiences (Kenison et al., 2017). Disparities among hospitalized children of parents with LEP include decreased quality care, poorer health status, and increased risk of adverse events (Zurca et al., 2017). Reducing language barriers is critical to improving care quality, lowering the risk of medical errors, and increasing access to services. The negative health outcomes patients with language barriers face when interacting with healthcare providers, accessing interpreters, and addressing medical concerns are numerous. These are further exacerbated by a lack of knowledge related to the right to have qualified interpreters and other language access provisions at no extra cost. Many patients with LEP have trouble communicating and comprehending medical details, which is both limiting and stressful (Kenison et al., 2017). This stress is amplified in healthcare settings, and these limitations impact patient safety, health outcomes, and health equity.

Role of the Nurse
Communication

When caring for patients with LEP, the communication process is often impaired. Providers may be faced with diagnostic uncertainty, which can lead to increased rates of diagnostic testing and hospital admission (Schulson et al., 2018). Communication issues have also been cited as the primary cause of serious adverse events, with patients with LEP being more likely than English-speaking patients to experience serious harm (Wasserman et al., 2014). Therefore improving communication with those who have LEP must be a priority for nurses. When communicating with a patient with LEP, nurses and other providers must gauge their own limitations and know when to engage language services. The Standards for Culturally and Linguistically Appropriate Services (CLAS) clearly direct that language assistance programs, including bilingual personnel and interpreter services, must be offered and provided at no cost to each patient/consumer with minimal English proficiency at all points of communication, in a timely manner, during all hours of operation in healthcare organizations receiving federal funds (Office of Minority Health [OMH], 2018). A lack of language services results in poor communication and limits the necessary exchange of important information between the provider and patient.

Nurses working in community-based settings should engage with community health workers (CHWs) to conduct health education and skill-building initiatives to empower community members with LEP. CHWs are front-line public health outreach professionals with a deep connection to the communities they serve, and an in-depth awareness of the experiences, culture, language, and needs of its members. Serving as an outreach worker, patient navigator, peer counselor, health adviser, and/or health educator, they can bridge the gap between healthcare practitioners and communities. CHWs can help ensure that health education is provided to the community in a health-literate and culturally appropriate way. They are also positioned to advocate for the use of medical interpreters.

The CLAS standards also recommend that services include the provision of bilingual workers, such as CHW's that can interact directly with patients/consumers in their chosen language, as a first priority. When such staff members are unavailable, the next best choice is the face-to-face interpretation given by qualified staff, contract, or volunteer interpreters. If an in-person interpreter is unavailable, telephone interpreter services can be used (OMH, 2018). Although federal regulations mandate that healthcare providers provide qualified interpreters for patients with LEP, there are significant inconsistency and noncompliance with these regulations resulting in healthcare inequity (Diamond et al., 2019).

Interpretive Services and Language Concordance

Medical interpretive services can close gaps in communication by interpreting important information between patients and providers. The use of professional interpreters decreases communication errors, improves utilization of services and clinical outcomes, and increases patient satisfaction among those with LEP (Price et al., 2012). Often, "unofficial" and untrained interpreters are used to translate in healthcare settings, leading to errors and omissions that result in clinical consequences. This is especially true when bilingual staff and patient family members are used. When informal and untrained interpreters are used, providers tend to avoid sensitive issues such as sexual health, domestic abuse, drug and alcohol use, and end-of-life care (Diamond et al., 2012). To ensure high-quality, equitable care for patients with LEP, healthcare systems must develop and implement effective systems for medical interpretation or connect patients with healthcare professionals who speak their preferred language.

Language concordance, the provider's use of the patient's preferred language, enhances healthcare encounters. Language-concordant providers are often able to ask more in-depth and personal questions than providers who use an interpreter. Patients who have language-concordant providers have greater trust and medication compliance, higher satisfaction and engagement, and fewer emergency room visits (Diamond et al., 2012). Patients who do not speak the same language as their providers have been shown to have higher service utilization rates, longer lengths of stay, higher readmission rates, and increased diagnostic testing (Diamond et al., 2019). Among Spanish-speaking patients, the use of language-concordant physicians has been shown to significantly improve health outcomes, for example, greater medication adherence and better glycemic control (Diamond et al., 2019; Parker et al., 2017).

To provide high-quality care, effective communication is important. This can be challenging when caring for patients with LEP. However, failure to overcome language barriers can have unintended negative effects on health outcomes. All members of the interdisciplinary team are responsible for providing coordinated treatment that meets the needs of those with LEP. While communication barriers are a major contributor to health inequalities, inequities faced by those with limited English literacy, cultural differences, stigma, and systemic barriers should also be considered. Developing a plan of care that addresses language-related barriers, updating health information for languages most commonly encountered, using interpreters, recruiting and checking the language proficiency of bilingual workers, and training staff on cultural sensitivity are all techniques that can be used to provide the best care for patients with LEP. Individuals with LEP often have overlapping vulnerabilities. Nurses should be mindful of these overlaps and advocate for the requisite services and support to address the needs of patients with LEP.

CONCLUSION

To influence health outcomes effectively, nurses at all levels and in all environments must be trained to recognize and address the social determinants of health. Evidence-based strategies that maximize both early childhood development and education must be prioritized to enhance the health of the whole community. Failure to act in this manner contributes to expanded health disparities through perpetuating intergenerational and socioeconomic disadvantage. A multifaceted, multidisciplinary approach is required, and nurses are positioned to advocate for a health-literate society at all levels.

Upstream Interventions

As a profession, nursing must recognize that treating the consequences of inequity through tertiary programs and services alone will not eliminate health inequities. The underlying and multifaceted causes of these inequities must be addressed. Nursing must respond to the call to create a health-literate society by actively participating in research, education, and action. Regardless of the practice setting, nurses have a professional and ethical duty to act in a consistent, purposeful manner that meets each patient's particular information needs. Integrating evidence-based strategies related to health literacy must become the standard of practice.

This begins with involvement in upstream interventions that include the development of a policy agenda for equity in education and educational access with strategic activities specific to nursing. Nurses at all levels are encouraged to develop their capacity and fully participate in advocacy, action, and political processes. Nurses should take the same policy-related actions to address educational gaps as they would if campaigning for medically focused issues. Policies aimed at making the experience of seeking health information easier, more useful, and more positive in general, especially for those with lower health literacy, can help mitigate the effects of negative long-term health outcomes associated with LEP and lower health literacy.

As the most trusted professionals, nurses must make use of their collective voice in policy to represent the vulnerable and marginalized. This requires collaborating with other sectors to support system-level policies that improve both education and health. Interventions that work in isolation to improve education equity have not been completely effective, pointing to a need for policies that tackle the issue with a multidisciplinary approach. Collaboration with other sectors and community-based organizations is critical to developing policies that address these inequities.

Nurses must take the lead in creating health-literate organizations, ensuring the integration of evidenced-based strategies, policies, and procedures designed to maximize patients' abilities to navigate, understand, and use health information and services. Additional research is also needed for the strategic and ongoing development and evaluation of novel methods that address education and its impacts on health outcomes.

To improve awareness and knowledge, all nurses should engage in professional development activities related to education and educational attainment as a social determinant of health. This should include the multiple pathways by which educational quality and access impact health throughout the life span. Nurses involved in health education should consider sharing content on strategies that create a patient-centered, stigma-free environment that enhances health literacy with peers and other members of the interdisciplinary team.

Midstream

Generally, the healthcare sector is responsible for direct clinical care, the public health sector is responsible for population health and disease control, and social service agencies are responsible for access to resources and services. Improving the health of all requires collaboration, coalition building, and partnerships among healthcare, public health, and social services professionals. The social determinants of health, particularly education, are complex and intertwined; no single entity can adequately address the issue in a silo.

The creation and growth of intersectional partnerships between the health and early education sectors are core to paving a new way forward. Partnerships allow for more family-centered approaches that are needed to successfully meet the housing, nutrition, employment, and health and wellness needs of parents and young children. Collaborative efforts that target individuals at higher risk for negative health outcomes due to low educational attainment should also be developed.

The diverse needs of those who are more vulnerable due to the STPP, low educational achievement, reduced English proficiency, and low health literacy necessitate cooperation with a wide variety of agencies, organizations, and individuals. Attempting to address the negative consequences of the STPP will require collaboration and coalition building. Not only must nursing, education, mental health, and other healthcare professionals, law enforcement, and the criminal justice system be involved in a meaningful way, but they must all share a vision and understanding of the work. Nurses, particularly in school health, have a unique opportunity to decrease the impact of the STPP by educating those in the education and criminal justice systems on alternative responses, as well as behavioral and substance use disorders, trauma, and crisis management.

Understanding how to connect with resources, form partnerships, build coalitions, and work effectively in a multidisciplinary team requires skill, guidance, and training. This may require additional education and training for nurses serving as advocates for these vulnerable groups. Delivery of programs that encourage life-long learning may improve the knowledge and skills of nurses, positively influencing the health of those they care for.

Downstream

Downstream efforts prevent, minimize, and manage the impacts of disease, but they cannot alter the underlying conditions at the core of an individual's health problems. However, their impact cannot be dismissed. Nurses must address health literacy at each encounter, from diagnosis to discharge.

All nurses should view health literacy as a priority and strive to maintain competency. This begins with the assessment of one's own level of knowledge and skills relevant to the impacts of educational quality and access on health outcomes, making sure to fill in any gaps. Nurses should share their knowledge with one another and other members of the multidisciplinary team.

As a member of the team that has a significant amount of direct contact with clients, nurses should act as role models for other members of the interprofessional team, including CHWs, social workers, nutritionists, and case managers. This includes the incorporation of a thorough health literacy assessment and the distribution of appropriate health-related knowledge and materials.

There are many opportunities to create spaces where nurses can provide an appropriate level of health education. For example, nurses can plan health fairs or health education sessions with interactive materials that are appealing and appropriate for various learners, such as parents, siblings, and grandparents.

Targeted interventions, such as weight management, that focus on healthy behaviors specifically designed for those with lower levels of education and literacy also have the potential to make a significant impact. However, care must be taken that interventions targeting individuals with low educational levels are not perceived to have stigmatizing effects.

Improvements in patient–provider interactions may also help reduce disparities. Nurses can take the lead by using and sharing the health literacy universal precautions approach. This approach ensures that patients of all education levels have access to health information that is understandable. Strategies such as plain language communication can be modeled to make health information accessible, useful, and understandable to diverse groups.

Nursing has an opportunity to significantly influence the relationship between education and health. Higher levels of educational attainment lead to improved job prospects and higher incomes resulting in health benefits, increased social growth and enhanced social skills, and increased skills required for improving awareness, attitudes, and behaviors necessary for optimal health. A lack of quality or accessible education can also lead to increased health disparities by perpetuating intergenerational and socioeconomic disadvantage cycles. To avoid this, nurses must strategically engage with those working in education, understand the connections between education and health, and advocate for the role of education in creating and maintaining healthy communities.

■ CASE STUDY

Student Case Study 1

Part I: S.G. is a 68-year-old Spanish-speaking female new to your clinic. She is being seen today to follow up on previous lab work. S.G. has had diabetes for over 20 years and has a history of elevated cholesterol. She has taken Metformin and Glipizide for the past 10 years. However, although S.G. reports "good" fasting blood glucose levels, her most recent labs show that her diabetes is uncontrolled. Based on S.G.'s hemoglobin A1C (7.4%), the provider prescribes Lantus 10u with a titration of 2 units every 3 days until fasting blood glucose is >130. S.G. appears to understand English, nodding appropriately when asked questions. However, she often responds in a mix of Spanish and English.

1. How might the nurse assess S.G.'s level of health literacy in English and/or Spanish? What strategies might

the nurse employ to ensure S.G. is able to obtain, interpret, and apply the information? What concerns, if any, should the nurse have about using either a formal or informal interpreter?

Part II: During a teaching session, the nurse notices that when S.G. was asked to draw 10 units of insulin, she draws 1 unit instead. The nurse also notes that the patient had difficulty understanding the acceptable range for her fasting blood glucose levels. However, S.G. tells the nurse that she is confident in her ability to properly administer her insulin.

2. What is the most likely cause of S.G.'s confusion? How might the nurse address this? What strategies should the nurse use to facilitate S.G.'s understanding of injection techniques? What are some of the potential consequences of S.G. not understanding the information presented by the nurse? What follow-up should the nurse plan for S.G.?

Student Case Study 2

Mr. Husseni is a 52-year-old male living with his elderly father and three children. Mr. Husseni appears to have limited comprehension of English, although it is not his native language. The family lives in a two-bedroom apartment in a socioeconomically disadvantaged urban neighborhood. His community has limited health resources, and the closest hospital is 15 minutes away by car. During the COVID-19 pandemic, Mr. Husseni continued to work as a rideshare and food delivery driver, placing all household members at higher risk of COVID-19 infection. However, he is unable to stop working because the family needs his income. Mr. Husseni is a smoker and has poorly controlled diabetes, placing him at risk for worse health outcomes from COVID-19 infection.

Mr. Husseni tends to minimize risk and has limited trust in the healthcare system. The nurse for an extensive primary care practice contacts Mr. Husseni to schedule a telehealth visit with his provider, to allow Mr. Husseni to receive care while avoiding exposure to the community. Mr. Husseni refuses that visit and states that he will wait until he can come into the office.

1. What are some of the issues reflected in this case study?
2. What are some of the potential barriers that may have caused Mr. Husseni to refuse the telehealth visit?
3. What are the nurse's priority interventions/actions?
4. What factors should the nurse consider to ensure that Mr. Husseni receives maximum benefit from the telehealth visit?
5. What strategies to address health literacy might the nurse include in Mr. Husseni's care plan?
6. How might Mr. Husseni's outcome from the telehealth visit vary compared with that of a male of the same age living in more economically advantaged circumstances?

STUDENT REFLECTION QUESTIONS

1. Children living in highly impoverished areas often attend schools with fewer qualified teachers, fewer academic resources and enrichment opportunities, and high teacher turnover. How might these circumstances impact students' quality of education and long-term academic success? What impact, if any, could their educational experiences have on their socioeconomic status in later life?
2. Since education is a social determinant of health, how might attending underresourced schools influence an individual's life trajectory?

3. Going back to school to get needed education is not an option for most adults. What can you do as a nurse for patients who come into the healthcare system at any point (e.g., clinic, emergency room, urgent care center, or hospital) with LEP and limited literacy to ensure the patient's understanding of the prescribed healthcare treatment plans?

STUDENT LEARNING ACTIVITY 1: HEALTH LITERACY

Locate a piece of written health communication (webpage, brochure, poster, infographic, etc.). Use the CDC Clear Communication User's Guide and Index Scoring Sheet to critique the health literacy level of the material.

The CDC's Clear Communication Index Website, Widget, and Score Sheet are located at: https://www.cdc.gov/ccindex/ and https://www.cdc.gov/healthcommunication/pdf/clearcommunicationindex/fillableformmay2013.pdf

- Provide a synopsis of the CDC's Clear Communication Index results, including the final score.
- Outline areas where the piece scored well and areas that were missed.
- Describe how the missed areas might adversely affect the target audience.

- Provide suggestions for how the piece could be modified to improve its health literacy and increase the index score.

■ STUDENT LEARNING ACTIVITY 2: PLAIN LANGUAGE

Word List

Choose 15 technical words related to a specific health topic, such as diabetes, carcinoma, or hypertension.

For each word, create a minidictionary with easy-to-read definitions and phonetic spellings to clarify pronunciation.

Example:

Hypertension (Hi-per-ten-shun): Blood pressure that is too high.

REFERENCES

Accenture. (2017). *The hidden cost of healthcare system complexity.* https://www.accenture.com/_acnmedia/pdf-104/accenture-health-hidden-cost-of-healthcare-system-complexity.pdf.

Agency for Healthcare Research and Quality. (2019). *Health Literacy Measurement Tools (Revised).* https://www.ahrq.gov/health-literacy/research/tools/index.html.

Aizer, A., & Doyle, J. (2015). Juvenile incarceration, human capital and future crime: Evidence from randomly-assigned judges. *The Quarterly Journal of Economics.* https://doi.org/10.3386/w19102.

American Academy of Family Physicians Foundation. (2017). *Incarceration and health: A family medicine perspective.* https://www.aafp.org/about/policies/all/incarceration.html.

American Psychological Association Zero Tolerance Task Force. (2008). Are zero tolerance policies effective in the schools? An evidentiary review and recommendations. *American Psychologist, 63*(9), 852–862. doi:10.1037/0003-066X.63.9.852.

Anderson, M. (2020). *Mobile technology and home broadband 2019.* Pew Research Center. Retrieved from https://www.pewresearch.org/internet/2019/06/13/mobile-technology-and-home-broadband-2019/.

Anderson, M., & Perrin, A. (2017). *Technology use among seniors.* Pew Research Center: Internet, Science & Tech. https://www.pewresearch.org/internet/2017/05/17/technology-use-among-seniors/.

Aronowitz, S. V., Kim, B., & Aronowitz, T. (2021). A mixed-studies review of the school-to-prison pipeline and a call to action for school nurses. *Journal of School Nursing, 37*(1), 51–60. https://doi.org.ezproxy.snhu.edu/10.1177/1059840520972003.

Assari, S., & Mistry, R. (2018). Educational attainment and smoking status in a national sample of American adults: Evidence for the Blacks' diminished return. *International Journal of Environmental Research and Public Health, 15*(4a), 763. https://doi.org/10.3390/ijerph15040763.

Badaczewski, A., Bauman, L. J., Blank, A. E., Dreyer, B., Abrams, M. A., Stein, R., Roter, D. L., Hossain, J., Byck, H., & Sharif, I. (2017). Relationship between teach-back and patient-centered communication in primary care pediatric encounters. *Patient Education and Counseling, 100*(7), 1345–1352. https://doi.org/10.1016/j.pec.2017.02.022.

Bakken, L., Brown, N., & Downing, B. (2017). Early childhood education: The long-term benefits. *Journal of Research in Childhood Education, 31*(2), 255–269. https://doi.org/10.1080/02568543.2016.1273285.

Barnert, E. S., Abrams, L. S., Tesema, L., Dudovitz, R., Nelson, B. B., Coker, T., Bath, E., Biely, C., Li, N., & Chung, P. J. (2018). Child incarceration and long-term adult health outcomes: A longitudinal study. *International Journal of Prisoner Health, 14*(1), 26–33. https://doi.org/10.1108/IJPH-09-2016-0052.

Barnert, E. S., Dudovitz, R., Nelson, B. B., Coker, T. R., Biely, C., Li, N., & Chung, P. J. (2017). How does incarcerating young people affect their adult health outcomes? *Pediatrics, 139*(2), e20162624. https://doi.org/10.1542/peds.2016-2624.

Baur, C., & Prue, C. (2014). The CDC Clear Communication Index is a new evidence-based tool to prepare and review health information. *Health Promotion Practice, 15*(5), 629–637. https://doi.org/10.1177/1524839914538969.

Berlowitz, M. J., Frye, R., & Jette, K. M. (2017). Bullying and zero-tolerance policies: The school to prison pipeline. *Multicultural Learning and Teaching, 12*(1). https://doi.org/10.1515/mlt-2014-0004.

Bitsko, R. H., Holbrook, J. R., Robinson, L. R., Kaminski, J. W., Ghandour, R., Smith, C., & Peacock, G. (2016). Health care, family, and community factors associated with mental, behavioral, and developmental disorders in early childhood—United States, 2011–2012. *Morbidity and Mortality Weekly Report, 65*(9), 221–226. https://doi.org/10.15585/mmwr.mm6509a1.

Black, M. M., Walker, S. P., Fernald, L., Andersen, C. T., DiGirolamo, A. M., Lu, C., McCoy, D. C., Fink, G., Shawar, Y. R., Shiffman, J., Devercelli, A. E., Wodon, Q. T., Vargas-Barón, E., Grantham-McGregor, S. & Lancet Early Childhood Development Series Steering Committee. (2017). Early childhood development coming of age: Science through the life course. *Lancet, 389*(10064), 77–90. https://doi.org/10.1016/S0140-6736(16).

Braveman, P. A., Cubbin, C., Egerter, S., Williams, D. R., & Pamuk, E. (2010). Socioeconomic disparities in health in the United States: What the patterns tell us. *American Journal of Public Health, 100*(Suppl. 1), S186–S196. https://doi.org/10.2105/AJPH.2009.166082.

Brega, A. G., Barnard, J., Mabachi, N. M., Weiss, B. D., De-Walt, D. A., Brach, C., & West, D. R. (2015). *AHRQ Health Literacy Universal Precautions Toolkit* (2nd ed.). Agency for Healthcare Research and Quality. Retrieved from http://www.ahrq.gov/professionals/quality-patient-safety/quality-resources/tools/literacy-toolkit/.

Campbell, F., Conti, G., Heckman, J. J., Moon, S. H., Pinto, R., Pungello, E., & Pan, Y. (2014). Early childhood investments substantially boost adult health. *Science, 343*(6178), 1478–1485. https://doi.org/10.1126/science.1248429.

CDC. (2019a). *Current cigarette smoking among adults in the United States.* https://www.cdc.gov/tobacco/data_statistics/fact_sheets/adult_data/cig_smoking/index.htm.

CDC. (2019b). *Health and academics.* https://www.cdc.gov/healthyyouth/health_and_academics/index.htm.

CDC. (2020). *Tobacco-related disparities.* https://www.cdc.gov/tobacco/disparities/index.htm.

CDC. (2021). *Understanding literacy and numeracy.* https://www.cdc.gov/healthliteracy/learn/UnderstandingLiteracy.html.

Curran, F. C. (2019). The law, policy, and portrayal of zero tolerance school discipline: Examining prevalence and characteristics across levels of governance and school districts. *Educational Policy, 33*(2), 319–349. https://doi.org/10.1177/0895904817691840.

Day, J. (2019). *College degree widens gender earnings gap.* https://www.census.gov/library/stories/2019/05/college-degree-widens-gender-earnings-gap.html.

Development Services Group, Inc. & Office of Juvenile Justice and Delinquency Prevention. (2017). *Intersection between mental health and the juvenile justice system.* https://www.ojjdp.gov/mpg/litreviews/Intersection-Mental-Health-Juvenile-Justice.pdf.

Diamond, L., Izquierdo, K., Canfield, D., Matsoukas, K., & Gany, F. (2019). A systematic review of the impact of patient-physician non-English language concordance on quality of care and outcomes. *Journal of General Internal Medicine, 34*(8), 1591–1606. https://doi.org/10.1007/s11606-019-04847-5.

Diamond, L. C., Luft, H. S., Chung, S., & Jacobs, E. A. (2012). "Does this doctor speak my language?" Improving the characterization of physician non-English language skills. *Health Services Research, 47*(1 Pt. 2), 556–569. https://doi.org/10.1111/j.1475-6773.2011.01338.x.

Dickens, C., Lambert, B. L., Cromwell, T., & Piano, M. R. (2013). Nurse overestimation of patients' health literacy. *Journal of Health Communication, 18*(Suppl. 1), 62–69. https://doi.org/10.1080/10810730.2013.825670.

Dodson, S., Beauchamp, A., Batterham, R., & Osborne, R. (2015). Health literacy, inequity, and health outcomes. *Belges De Santé Publique, 72*(1), 11.

Federal Communications Commission. (2019). *Broadband deployment report (Report No. FC 19-44).* Retrieved from https://docs.fcc.gov/public/attachments/FCC-19-44A1.pdf.

Feinberg, I., O'Connor, M. H., Owen-Smith, A., Ogrodnick, M. M., & Rothenberg, R. (2020). The relationship between refugee health status and language, literacy, and time spent in the United States. *Health Literacy Research and Practice, 4*(4), e230–e236. https://doi.org/10.3928/24748307-20201109-01.

Government Accountability Office. (2016). *K–12 education. Better use of information could help agencies identify disparities and address racial discrimination (GAO Publication No.16-345).* Retrieved from https://www.gao.gov/assets/gao-16-345.pdf.

Government Accountability Office. (2018). *K–12 education. Discipline disparities for Black students, boys, and students with disabilities (GAO Publication No. 18-258).* Retrieved from https://www.gao.gov/assets/gao-18-258.pdf.

Gundersen, C., & Ziliak, J. (2016). Food insecurity among children in the United States. *Southern Economic Journal, 82*(4), 1059–1061. https://doi.org/10.2307/26632306.

Hall, A. K., Bernhardt, J. M., Dodd, V., & Vollrath, M. W. (2015). The digital health divide: Evaluating online health information access and use among older adults. *Health Education & Behavior, 42*(2), 202–209.

Harris, K., Jacobs, G., & Reeder, J. (2019). Health systems and adult basic education: A critical partnership in supporting digital health literacy. *Health Literacy Research and Practice, 3*(Suppl. 3), S33–S36. https://doi.org/10.3928/24748307-20190325-02.

Hargittai, E., & Dobransky, K. (2017). Old dogs, new clicks: Digital inequality in skills and uses among older adults. *Canadian Journal of Communication, 42*(2), 195–212. https://doi.org/10.22230/cjc.2017v42n2a3176.

Hargittai, E., Piper, A. M., & Morris, M. R. (2018). From internet access to internet skills: Digital inequality among older adults. *Universal Access in the Information Society, 18*(4), 881–890. https://doi.org/10.1007/s10209-018-0617-5.

Heitzeg, N. A. (2009). Education or incarceration: Zero tolerance policies and the school to prison pipeline. *Forum on Public Policy, 2*, 1–21.

Hickey, K. T., Masterson Creber, R. M., Reading, M., Sciacca, R. R., Riga, T. C., Frulla, A. P., & Casida, J. M. (2018). Low health literacy: Implications for managing cardiac patients in practice. *The Nurse Practitioner, 43*(8), 49–55. doi:10.1097/01.NPR.0000541468.54290.49.

Himmelstein, K. E., & Brückner, H. (2011). Criminal-justice and school sanctions against nonheterosexual youth: A national longitudinal study. *Pediatrics, 127*(1), 49–57. https://doi.org/10.1542/peds.2009-2306.

Hudson, S., Rikard, R. V., Staiculescu, I., & Edison, K. (2017). *Improving health and the bottom line: The case for health literacy. Appendix C.* In *Building the case for health literacy: Proceedings of a workshop.* The National Academies Press.

Institute of Medicine. (2004). *Health literacy: A prescription to end confusion.* The National Academies Press.

Jackson, M., Kiernan, K., & McLanahan, S. (2017). Maternal education, changing family circumstances, and children's skill development in the United States and UK. *The Annals of the American Academy of Political and Social Science, 674*(1), 59–84. https://doi.org/10.1177/0002716217729471.

Jennings, V., & Bamkole, O. (2019). The relationship between social cohesion and urban green space: An avenue for health promotion. *International Journal of Environmental Research and Public Health, 16*(3), 452. https://doi.org/10.3390/ijerph16030452.

Kamerman, S. B., & Gatenio-Gabel, S. (2015). Early childhood education and care in the United States: An overview of the current policy picture. *International Journal of Child Care and Education Policy, 1*(1), 23–34. https://doi.org/10.1007/2288-6729-1-1-23.

Keith-Jennings, B., Llobrera, J., & Dean, S. (2019). Links of the Supplemental Nutrition Assistance Program with food insecurity, poverty, and health: Evidence and potential. *American Journal of Public Health, 109*(12), 1636–1640. https://doi.org/10.2105/AJPH.2019.305325.

Kelleher, K. (2015). *Unequal schools, generations of poverty.* UCLA Blueprint. https://blueprint.ucla.edu/feature/unequal-schools-generations-of-poverty/.

Kenison, T. C., Madu, A., Krupat, E., Ticona, L., Vargas, I. M., & Green, A. R. (2017). Through the veil of language: Exploring the hidden curriculum for the care of patients with limited English proficiency. *Academic Medicine, 92*(1), 92–100. https://doi.org/10.1097/ACM.0000000000001211.

Krueger, P. M., Saint Onge, J. M., & Chang, V. W. (2011). Race/ethnic differences in adult mortality: The role of perceived stress and health behaviors. *Social Science & Medicine, 73*(9), 1312–1322. https://doi.org/10.1016/j.socscimed.2011.08.007.

Lawless, J., Toronto, C. E., & Grammatica, G. L. (2016). Health literacy and information literacy: A concept comparison. *Reference Services Review, 44*(2), 144–162. https://doi.org/10.1108/rsr-02-2016-0013.

Loan, L. A., Parnell, T. A., Stichler, J. F., Boyle, D. K., Allen, P., VanFosson, C. A., & Barton, A. J. (2018). Call for action: Nurses must play a critical role to enhance health literacy. *Nursing Outlook, 66*(1), 97–100. https://doi.org/10.1016/j.outlook.2017.11.003.

Liobikienė, G., & Bernatonienė, J. (2018). The determinants of access to information on the Internet and knowledge of health related topics in European countries. *Health Policy, 122*(12), 1348–1355.

Mallett, C. A. (2016). The school-to-prison pipeline: From school punishment to rehabilitative inclusion. *Preventing School Failure: Alternative Education for Children and Youth, 60*(4), 296–304. https://doi.org/10.1080/1045988x.2016.1144554.

Mamedova, S., & Pawlowski, E. (2018). *A description of US adults who are not digitally literate (NCES 2018-161).* US Department of Education. National Center for Education Statistics, Institute of Education Sciences. https://nces.ed.gov/pubs2018/2018161.pdf.

Mantwill, S., Monestel-Umaña, S., & Schulz, P. J. (2015). The relationship between health literacy and health disparities: A systematic review. *PLoS One, 10*(12), e0145455. https://doi.org/10.1371/journal.pone.0145455.

Maralani, V. (2013). Educational inequalities in smoking: The role of initiation versus quitting. *Social Science & Medicine, 84*, 129–137. https://doi.org/10.1016/j.socscimed.2013.01.007.

Maralani, V. (2014). Understanding the links between education and smoking. *Social Science Research, 48*, 20–34. https://doi.org/10.1016/j.ssresearch.2014.05.007.

Margolis, R. (2013). Educational differences in healthy behavior changes and adherence among middle-aged Americans. *Journal of Health and Social Behavior, 54*(3), 353–368. https://doi.org/10.1177/0022146513489312.

McCoy, D. C., Yoshikawa, H., Ziol-Guest, K. M., Duncan, G., Schindler, H., Magnuson, R., Yang, R., Koepp, A., & Shonkoff, J. (2017). Impacts of early childhood education on medium- and long-term educational outcomes. *Educational Researcher, 46*(8), 474–487. https://doi.org/10.3102/0013189x17737739.

McDonald, M., & Shenkman, L. J. (2018). Health literacy and health outcomes of adults in the United States: Implications for providers. *The Internet Journal of Allied Health Sciences and Practice, 16*(4), article 2.

McElrath, K., Guevara, L., Shekarkhar, Z., & Brown, J. M. (2020). Out-of-school suspensions: Counter-narratives from the student perspective. *Journal of Qualitative Criminal Justice & Criminology, 8*(3). https://doi.org/10.21428/88de04a1.ee4217b2.

Monahan, K., VanDerhei, S., Bechtold, J., & Cauffman, E. (2014). From the school yard to the squad car: School discipline, truancy, and arrest. *Journal of Youth & Adolescence, 43*, 1110–1122.

Montez, J. K., & Berkman, L. F. (2014). Trends in the educational gradient of mortality among US adults aged 45–84 years: Bringing regional context into the explanation. *American Journal of Public Health, 104*(1), e82–e90. https://doi.org/10.2105/ajph.2013.301526.

Morris, A. S., Robinson, L. R., Hays-Grudo, J., Claussen, A. H., Hartwig, S. A., & Treat, A. E. (2017). Targeting parenting in early childhood: A public health approach to improve outcomes for children living in poverty. *Child Development, 88*(2), 388–397. https://doi.org/10.1111/cdev.12743.

Muscat, D. M., Morony, S., Trevena, L., Hayen, A., Shepherd, H. L., Smith, S. K., Dhillon, H. M., Luxford, K., Nutbeam, D., & McCaffery, K. J. (2019). Skills for shared decision-making: Evaluation of a health literacy program for consumers with lower literacy levels. *Health Literacy Research and Practice, 3*(Suppl. 3), S58–S74. https://doi.org/10.3928/24748307-20190408-02.

National Association of School Nurses. (2018). *The school nurse's role in behavioral/mental health of students.* Position statements. https://www.nasn.org/advocacy/professional-practice-documents/position-statements/ps-behavioral-health.

National Center for Education Statistics. (2019). *Indicator 27: Educational attainment.* https://nces.ed.gov/programs/raceindicators/indicator_rfa.asp.

National Center for Education Statistics. (2022). *Report on the condition of education 2022 (NCES 2022-144).*

National Council on Disability. (2016). *Breaking the school-to-prison pipeline for students with disabilities.* https://ncd.gov/publications/2015/06182015/.

Nesari, M., Olson, J. K., Nasrabadi, A. N., & Norris, C. (2019). Registered nurses' knowledge of and experience with health literacy. *Health Literacy Research and Practice, 3*(4), e268–e279. https://doi.org/10.3928/24748307-20191021-01.

Noltemeyer, A. L., Ward, R. M., & Mcloughlin, C. (2015). Relationship between school suspension and student outcomes: A meta-analysis. *School Psychology Review, 44*(2), 224–240. https://doi.org/10.17105/spr-14-0008.

Norman, C. D., & Skinner, H. A. (2006). eHealth literacy: Essential skills for consumer health in a networked world. *Journal of Medical Internet Research, 8*(2), e9. https://doi.org/10.2196/jmir.8.2.e9.

Office of Disease Prevention and Health Promotion. (n.d.). *Early childhood development and education. Healthy People 2020.* https://www.healthypeople.gov/2020/topics-objectives/topic/social-determinants-health/interventions-resources/early-childhood-development-and-education.

Office of Minority Health. (2018). *The National CLAS Standards.* https://minorityhealth.hhs.gov/omh/browse.aspx?lvl=2&lvlid=53.

Pan American Health Organization. (2017). *Social determinants of health in the Americas. Health in the Americas 2017.* https://www.paho.org/salud-en-las-americas-2017/?p=45.

Parker, M., Fernandez, A., & Moffet, H. (2017). Association of patient-physician language concordance and glycemic control for limited–English proficiency Latinos with type 2 diabetes. *JAMA Internal Medicine, 177*(3), 380–387. https://doi.org/10.15760/honors.252.

Peters, E., Tompkins, M. K., Knoll, M. A., Ardoin, S. P., Shoots-Reinhard, B., & Meara, A. S. (2019). Despite high objective numeracy, lower numeric confidence relates to worse financial and medical outcomes. *Proceedings of the National Academy of Sciences, 116*(39), 19386–19391. https://doi.org/10.1073/pnas.1903126116.

Pew Research Center. (2020). *Demographics of social media users and adoption in the United States.* https://www.pewresearch.org/internet/fact-sheet/social-media/#who-uses-social-media.

Pribesh, S. L., Carson, J. S., Dufur, M. J., Yue, Y., & Morgan, K. (2020). Family structure stability and transitions, parental involvement, and educational outcomes. *Social Sciences, 9*(12), 229.

Price, E. L., Pérez-Stable, E. J., Nickleach, D., López, M., & Karliner, L. S. (2012). Interpreter perspectives of in-person, telephonic, and videoconferencing medical interpretation in clinical encounters. *Patient Education and Counseling, 87*(2), 226–232. https://doi.org/10.1016/j.pec.2011.08.006.

Raghupathi, V., & Raghupathi, W. (2020). The influence of education on health: An empirical assessment of OECD countries for the period 1995–2015. *Archives of Public Health, 78*(1). https://doi.org/10.1186/s13690-020-00402-5.

Ramon, I., Chattopadhyay, S. K., Barnett, W. S., Hahn, R. A., & Community Preventive Services Task Force. (2018). Early childhood education to promote health equity: A community guide economic review. *Journal of Public Health Management and Practice, 24*(1), e8–e15. https://doi.org/10.1097/PHH.0000000000000557.

Ross, C. E., & Mirowsky, J. (2013). The sense of personal control: Social structural causes and emotional consequences. In C. S. Aneshensel, J. C. Phelan, & A. Bierman (Eds.), *Handbooks of sociology and social research. Handbook of the sociology of mental health* (pp. 379–402). Springer Science+Business Media. https://doi.org/10.1007/978-94-007-4276-5_19.

Schardt, C. (2011). Health information literacy meets evidence-based practice. *Journal of the Medical Library Association, 99*(1), 1–2. https://doi.org/10.3163/1536-5050.99.1.001.

Schulson, L., Novack, V., Smulowitz, P. B., Dechen, T., & Landon, B. E. (2018). Emergency department care for patients with limited English proficiency: A retrospective cohort study. *Journal of General Internal Medicine, 33*(12), 2113–2119. https://doi.org/10.1007/s11606-018-4493-8.

Smith, J. M. (2020). Early childhood education programs as protective experiences for low-income Latino children and their families. *Adversity and Resilience Science, 1*(3), 191–204. https://doi.org/10.1007/s42844-020-00013-7.

Treadwell, H. M. (2019). Wages and women in health care: The race and gender gap. *American Journal of Public Health, 109*(2), 208–209. https://doi.org/10.2105/AJPH.2018.304866.

Truth Initiative. (2017). *Tobacco is a social justice issue: Low-income communities.* https://truthinitiative.org/research-resources/targeted-communities/tobacco-social-justice-issue-low-income-communities.

US Census Bureau. (2019). *2019: ACS 5-year estimates data profiles.* https://data.census.gov/cedsci/profile?q=&g=0100000US&table=DP02&tid=ACSDP1Y2018.DP02&hidePreview=true&vintage=2018.

US Department of Agriculture. (2019). *FNS 01: Child and adult care food program.* https://www.fns.usda.gov/fns-101-cacfp.

US Department of Education. (n.d.). *Equity of opportunity.* https://www.ed.gov/equity.

US Department of Health and Human Services. (2020). Smoking cessation: A report of the surgeon general – key findings. Retrieved from https://www.hhs.gov/surgeon-general/reports-and-publications/tobacco/2020-cessation-sgr-factsheet-key-findings/index.html.

Wang, E. A., & Wildeman, C. (2017). Mass incarceration, public health, and widening inequality in the USA. *Lancet, 389*(10077), 1464–1474. https://doi.org/10.1016/S0140-6736(17)30259-3.

Wasserman, M., Renfrew, M. R., Green, A. R., Lopez, L., Tan-McGrory, A., Brach, C., & Betancourt, J. R. (2014). Identifying and preventing medical errors in patients with limited English proficiency: Key findings and tools for the field. *Journal for Healthcare Quality, 36*(3), 5–16. https://doi.org/10.1111/jhq.12065.

Weshcler, M., Melnick, H., Maier, A., & Bishop, J. (2016). *The building blocks of high-quality early childhood education programs.* https://learningpolicyinstitute.org/product/building-blocks-high-quality-early-childhood-education-programs.

Wittenberg, E., Ferrell, B., Kanter, E., & Buller, H. (2018). Health literacy: Exploring nursing challenges to providing support and understanding. *Clinical Journal of Oncology Nursing, 22*(1), 53–61. https://doi.org/10.1188/18.CJON.53-61.

WHO. (n.d.). *Using e-health and information technology to improve health.* https://www.who.int/westernpacific/activities/using-e-health-and-information-technology-to-improve-health.

WHO. (2018). *Health inequities and their causes.* https://www.who.int/news-room/facts-in-pictures/detail/health-inequities-and-their-causes.

Yu, J. (2015). Parental education matters for adolescent health: The importance of parental education in the US. *Journal of Studies in Social Sciences, 11*(2), 160–195.

Zajacova, A., & Lawrence, E. M. (2018). The relationship between education and health: Reducing disparities through a contextual approach. *Annual Review of Public Health, 39*(1), 273–289. https://doi.org/10.1146/annurev-publhealth-031816-044628.

Zimmerman, E., & Woolf, S. H. (2014). *Understanding the relationship between education and health.* NAM Perspectives. Discussion Paper, National Academy of Medicine, Washington, DC. https://doi.org/10.31478/201406a.

Zurca, A. D., Fisher, K. R., Flor, R. J., Gonzalez-Marques, C. D., Wang, J., Cheng, Y. I., & October, T. W. (2017). Communication with limited English-proficient families in the PICU. *Hospital Pediatrics, 7*(1), 9–15. https://doi.org/10.1542/hpeds.2016-0071.

The Physical, Natural, and Built Environment

Diana Ruiz

> *Health is about much more than genetics and medical care.*
> —*Robert Wood Johnson Foundation (RWJF, n.d.)*

CHAPTER OUTLINE

LEARNING OBJECTIVES

1. Examine the concept of the physical, natural, and built environment at the local and national levels.
2. Describe the impact of the physical, natural, and built environment on health and well-being.
3. Evaluate challenges and opportunities in the physical, natural, and built environment related to health in one's community.
4. Formulate a plan to assess and evaluate the built environment using a systematic and collaborative approach.
5. Describe the nurse's role in advocating for a stronger and healthier physical, natural, and built environment.

THE ENVIRONMENT AND HEALTH

Health can be defined in many ways. Historically, health has been described as a "state of complete physical, mental and social well-being, and not merely the absence of disease or infirmity" (WHO, 1946, para 1). The traditional medical model implies that health exists as a state free of illness or disease. Patients are generally considered to be in "good health" when they lack acute illness and are in a state of balance and homeostasis. However, physiologic and physical health are the tip of the iceberg when it comes to achieving a broader definition of health. Can an individual be healthy if he or she lives in an unsafe neighborhood with violence and poor sanitation? Does health exist despite the absence of positive social interactions and relationships? Can a person be healthy and still lack safe places to learn, work, worship, and play? Can physical and physiologic health be completely separated from other vital aspects of life, such as social determinants of health?

Take a moment to reflect on current clinical experiences and/or professional nursing practice. During the provision of care for patients in an acute care or community clinic setting, are social determinants considered when assessing the patient's health status, behavior, and choices? Do nurses have a general understanding of the environment in which patients live and how it may impact their well-being? Can nurses effectively assess social determinants during a routine interview, assessment, or other interaction with patients? Is this type of assessment within the scope of a nursing student's or registered nurse's responsibilities? The answer, of course, should be yes to all these questions. It is the professional nurse's responsibility to assess and understand a patient's status in terms of health, environment, and general well-being. In other words, nurses must engage patients in deeper conversations to better appreciate how to support their health journey and reduce barriers to achieving health equity. This includes moving from a superficial nurse–patient relationship to a bidirectional partnership with open dialogue that includes social determinants that impact health.

Achieving health at the individual level and, more importantly, health equity at the population level goes far beyond the traditional definition of health. Health encompasses an amalgamation of one's life, including but not limited to physical, emotional, and psychological health; spirituality; religion; food security; safety; a clean environment; education; and positive social bonds. The WHO continues in its commitment to achieving health globally, reiterating in 2017 a list of key issues that pertain to human rights and health. More specifically, the WHO advocates the need to evaluate and address social determinants of health, including water, food, gender equality, housing, and education, to fully achieve health (2017). Therefore it is globally understood that health is not independent of one's environment and the associated social determinants of health.

The environment in which individuals live, work, play, and learn can have a significant impact on overall health and well-being (CDC, 2018). The environment is of such significance to health that the recently published "Healthy People 2030" framework focuses on strategic initiatives to improve overall living conditions with a broader goal of improving health outcomes. A fundamental component of the 2030 framework is a goal to promote healthier environments to improve health. To achieve this goal, numerous environmental health objectives have been identified, such as reducing exposure to harmful toxins, improving safe drinking water, reducing air pollution, and increasing public transportation options (US Department of Health and Human Services, 2020a).

ORIGINS OF HEALTH

Where does health begin? Does it begin in the encoding of DNA upon conception, or is it defined much later and based on health behaviors and choices? Does it stem from the family household in which an individual is raised? Or is it perhaps influenced by the neighborhoods in which people live and the schools they attend? If one believes that health is solely defined by genetics and subsequent health patterns and behaviors, this is partially correct. Independent of everyone's unique genetic makeup, one's overall health status is significantly influenced by the physical, natural, and built environment in which the individual lives, works, learns, and plays. The built environment includes the physical structural components and environmental elements that influence day-to-day life. Much like genetic markers code and predict an individual's future health, morbidity, and mortality, the physical and built environment have the potential to code and define future success, survival, and illness patterns. For example, individuals are much more likely to develop pulmonary symptoms and conditions if they live in areas with documented poor air quality related to manufacturing facilities and transportation in the built environment. Conversely, if one lives in a community with clean air, land, and water, all of which meet the US Environmental Protection Agency (EPA) standards, the person is less likely to develop health conditions directly related to pollutants in the environment. The EPA works diligently to ensure that the health of individuals is protected and laws are enforced to meet national standards. The EPA (2022) set forth seven key goals in the most recent fiscal year 2022–26 Strategic Plan, including to:
1. Tackle the climate crisis.
2. Take decisive action to advance environmental justice and civil rights.
3. Enforce environmental laws and ensure compliance.
4. Ensure clean and healthy air for all communities.
5. Ensure clean and safe water for communities.
6. Safeguard and revitalize communities.
7. Ensure the safety of chemicals for people and the environment.

In its fiscal year 2022–26 Strategic Plan, the EPA addresses climate change and advancing environmental justice and civil rights as core to its mission. The impacts of climate change threaten the lives and livelihoods of all. Global air temperature has warmed by 1.8°F in the last century (US EPA, 2022). As a result, several climate-related changes, such as droughts, wildfires, melting glaciers, and flooding, frequently occur. The Strategic Plan outlines several strategies to reduce the deleterious effects of climate change. To advance environmental and civic justice, the plan identifies mitigation strategies that focus on clean air, clean water, and safe land throughout communities nationwide, including those that have been historically disenfranchised (US EPA, 2022). Additionally, the EPA regularly monitors and enforces compliance with environmental laws to ensure clean and healthy air and water for communities.

These extensive goals reflect the impact the environment has on health. In an even broader sense, health is defined by the foods consumed, the quality of drinking water, the cleanliness of the air, and the environment in which one lives, works, learns, worships, and plays. Some of these environmental attributes occur by choice—such as choosing where to live—but some do not. Children do not have the autonomy to choose where they live or what school they attend. Instead, they are at the mercy of the decisions of their caregiver(s) or guardian(s). As adults, people have free will and the ability to choose where to live, work, and attend school, but many important decisions are ultimately determined by financial constraints. A lack of financial means to live in a clean and safe environment can negatively impact health, despite a desire to live in a more favorable environment.

If an individual lacks a solid foundation of health in their environment, the remaining aspects of physical health can be inconsequential in the present and future. Overcoming an unhealthy environment, regardless of circumstances, can be challenging and insurmountable for some. This chapter delves deeper into the social determinants of health as they relate to the physical, natural, and built environment.

CREATING A CULTURE OF HEALTH TO PROMOTE EQUITY

Everyone deserves to live the healthiest life possible.
—*RWJF, 2021a*

The RWJF is internationally recognized as a leader in health, equity, and social justice. The Foundation supports a plethora of community-based initiatives and programs to advance health equity in the United States. RWJF is well known for innovative, cross-sector collaboration and grassroots efforts to lead national change.

The RWJF, alongside the RAND Corporation and many other stakeholders, currently leads a sustainable, extensive, and robust national movement to promote health and equity through the creation and implementation of the Culture of Health (COH) framework. Embedded within the framework are the "10 Principles for a Culture of Health." As shown in Box 4.1, each principle provides direction and a call to action. The principles focus on achieving equity across sectors and supporting collaboration to improve health and create a broad sense of unity to improve living conditions for all (RWJF, 2021c).

The importance of the physical, natural, and built environment in terms of health underlies many of the COH principles and should not be underemphasized. Specifically, the principles call for health promotion across geographic, demographic, and social sectors,

> **BOX 4.1 10 Principles for a Culture of Health**
> 1. Good health flourishes across geographic, demographic, and social sectors.
> 2. Attaining the best health possible is valued by our entire society.
> 3. Individuals and families have the means and the opportunity to make choices that lead to the healthiest lives possible.
> 4. Business, government, individuals, and organizations work together to build healthy communities and lifestyles.
> 5. No one is excluded.
> 6. Everyone has access to affordable, quality healthcare because it is essential to maintain, or reclaim, health.
> 7. Healthcare is efficient and equitable.
> 8. The economy is less burdened by excessive and unwarranted healthcare spending.
> 9. Keeping everyone as healthy as possible guides public and private decision-making.
> 10. Americans understand that we are all in this together.
>
> From: Robert Wood Johnson Foundation. (2021). *How we got here.* https://www.rwjf.org/en/cultureofhealth/about/how-we-got-here.html#ten-underlying-principles.

again emphasizing the importance of environmental factors for health. The COH framework postulates that all individuals have equal opportunities to make choices that lead to healthy lives.

The initial 2015 "From Vision to Action" report set forth a comprehensive road map and framework for all sectors in society to collaborate to create a COH (RWJF, 2015). The updated COH framework continues to promote four key action areas, with a focus on the unique impact of the environment:

1. Making health a shared value
2. Fostering cross-sector collaboration
3. Creating healthier, more equitable communities
4. Strengthening the integration of health services and systems (RWJF, 2021b)

Each of the four action areas contributes to the central goals of improved population health, well-being, and equity. To determine action area program effectiveness, the following specific outcomes are measured: enhanced individual and community well-being, managed chronic disease and reduced toxic stress, and reduced healthcare costs (RWJF, 2021b). The framework concepts reflect that health does not exist solely within the traditional healthcare definition and structure and thus warrants a systemic, broader approach through cross-sector collaboration with a focus on the impact of the environment.

Under the umbrella of the third action area focus, creating healthier, more equitable communities, the RWJF framework further explains that the built environment, social and economic environment, and policy and governance all drive the creation of healthier communities. The perception of safety and security inside and outside of one's home, the walkability of a neighborhood, and access to learning and social resources such as libraries are all tangible physical environment characteristics that can contribute positively to population health. The attributes of the social and economic environment also directly correlate with health and include residential segregation, housing affordability, and the availability of early childhood education. For example, one might question how racial segregation can impact health. The segregation of low-income racial groups can lead to reduced educational and economic opportunities, along with barriers to accessing vital social and health resources. This further expands the existing health equity gap between various racial groups.

IMPACT OF THE BUILT ENVIRONMENT ACROSS THE LIFE SPAN

The built environment can impact individuals across the life span in different ways. As a young child, play is vital for healthy growth and development. Outdoor play in a safe environment has the added benefits of fresh air, exposure to sunlight, and the development of gross motor skills while running, climbing, and jumping. However, a parent or guardian is unlikely to allow a child to play outdoors if there is no safe area in which to do so. The child becomes limited in play and remains constrained in the internal built environment.

The built environment moderates and either enables or disables human action (Matthews & Lippman, 2020). The design of buildings for school-aged children can have a profound impact on student success. Crowded, outdated, and unsafe schools create negative learning environments that may predispose children to unnecessary stress and illness. Conversely, well-designed, clean, safe schools provide a solid educational and social foundation for children to grow and excel.

Many schools, businesses, and organizations have partnered with agencies such as the US Green Building Council (USGBC) to enhance and improve the overall built environment. As part of its key mission, the USGBC strives to transform the design of communities and buildings to enable a socially responsible and healthy environment that improves the quality of human lives (USGBC, 2017). The USGBC provides strategies and resources for school administrators and teachers to create sustainable, green classrooms that enable learning and student success. The USGBC framework also has a significant impact on the work environment, which is discussed later in this chapter.

As an adolescent, socialization with peers is essential for healthy development. Socialization outside the school setting is common in the teenage years and often includes visiting each other's homes. However, an unsafe neighborhood, lack of walkability, or unsafe and inadequate transportation can create social isolation for adolescents. Worse yet, living in an unsafe neighborhood with high crime rates can either increase the likelihood of an adolescent becoming a victim or wrongfully engaging in unhealthy behaviors. The broad availability of illegal drugs and substances, along with the presence of criminal activity in high-crime neighborhoods, can further increase adolescents' risk for harm and injury. Risky behaviors in adolescence can negatively impact academic success and future career opportunities.

As a young to middle-aged adult, one's environment can impact stress levels, physical activity opportunities, and work/school commute times. Community design and transportation infrastructure can increase risk and stress if they create stressful driving conditions like heavy traffic. Long commute times can add unnecessary stress and transportation costs and can limit family/social bonding times if prolonged. Excessive automobile use without the potential to carpool and share rides can further contribute to negative air quality.

The built environment can have a significant impact on the quality of life of the aging American population. The concept of aging in place, remaining in one's adulthood home as age increases, is not feasible or realistic for many. Limited income, poor health, and disability can lead to difficulties in maintaining one's home and thus create barriers to health. Environmental change, neighborhood redesign, and the natural degradation of older buildings can create unsafe living conditions in one's home. Thus it is important to consider alternative housing options, when necessary, with elderly patients to promote health and security. Healthcare providers cannot simply assume that elderly patients are safer and likely to be healthier by remaining at home. Nurses must include a discussion of the patient's built environment and housing conditions in the routine patient interview process.

SHORT-TERM IMPACTS OF THE BUILT ENVIRONMENT

Researchers continue to focus on the short- and long-term impacts on health of the physical, natural, and built environment. Some impacts can be seen immediately as a direct result of an environmental failure, such as the case of the Flint water crisis discussed later in this chapter. However, long-term effects may be more subtle and can span current and future generations.

The short-term impacts of a negative built environment can be straightforward. Living in a neighborhood with a high crime rate immediately increases the likelihood of being a crime victim or participant in criminal activity. Living in a community with high air pollution can lead to daily respiratory symptoms or other ailments. The inability to routinely access healthy foods can lead to poor eating habits, obesity, and other health conditions with more long-term consequences. The inability to access safe walking paths can lead to decreased daily physical activity. These are just a few examples of how the physical, natural, and built environment can directly impact day-to-day activities in the short-term.

LONG-TERM IMPACTS

The long-term impacts of the environment in which people live, work, learn, and play remain an ongoing topic of research. Many reputable national and global organizations have strategic plans to measure the long-term impacts of the environment on health outcomes. Examples include the Office of Disease Prevention and Health Promotion, the RWJF, and the EPA.

The long-term impacts of an unhealthy environment can take years, if not decades, to be identified and measured. Not all impacts are "visible" and can therefore be difficult to measure objectively. For example, if an individual lives in a community with limited access to safe housing, they may grow up lacking a sense of security, thus limiting their ability to succeed as a productive adult. If schools have insufficient funding for technology and extracurricular activities, outdated buildings and supplies, and teacher shortages, students are less likely to perform well academically. Receiving a poor or substandard education may impact one's future success in attaining a college degree and/or obtaining a job with a higher income. However, these outcomes can be challenging to quantify and measure over the long term.

The concept that a relationship exists between the environment and health is generally accepted. However, one may question how this occurs. How strong is this association, and can it be measured objectively? Is it conclusive? In a systematic literature review conducted by Smith et al. (2017), researchers sought to establish interrelationships between various environmental attributes and health. The review of 28 studies found positive impacts on health when there is improved walkability, access to parks and playgrounds, and adequate transportation infrastructure.

Furthermore, one may question what specifically within the built environment impacts health and long-term outcomes. What attributes have the greatest impact? In a 2020 study conducted by Phan et al. (2020), researchers used Google Street View images to pinpoint which specific elements in the built environment had greater associations with morbidity and mortality. Interestingly, they found that aspects such as crosswalks had a marked impact on health. A higher number of crosswalks led to a reduction in obesity rates for adults and adolescents and, interestingly, also led to a reduction in premature mortality. Of equal significance, researchers found various associations, although not statistically significant, between more visible structural wire presence in the environment and higher rates of obesity, premature mortality, and decreased overall physical activity. One can assume that visible wire presence implies more buildings, more congested living areas, and perhaps fewer green areas.

Ongoing research is warranted in this area to further ascertain the direct correlations between the physical, natural, and built environment and overall health. Community design and infrastructure can improve health and overall quality of life when planned strategically. Future generations will continue to benefit from informed community design, environmental protection regulations, careful consideration of the built environment, and ongoing health policy development to achieve equity.

HEALTH-PROMOTING GOODS AND SERVICES

Access to Healthcare Services

Geographical location directly impacts access to safe, effective, and affordable healthcare. Medically underserved areas (MUAs) exist across the country in rural and urban communities and pose significant challenges to healthcare access. The Health Resources and Services Administration (HRSA, 2021) designates areas such as counties, neighboring counties, and census tract groups as MUAs when there is insufficient access to primary care. Medically underserved populations (MUPs) are designated based on a shortage of primary care providers in a subpopulation that may be vulnerable as a result. These subpopulations face additional challenges, such as economic, cultural, and language barriers to health (HRSA, 2021). In the case of MUPs, individuals are somewhat victims of their environment. The inability to access care due to a shortage of healthcare providers, coupled with unique subpopulation characteristics, makes achieving health an even greater feat.

Affordable access to care may be more predominant in states with Medicaid expansion or other state-funded health plans. In an effort to expand access for low-income individuals, the Patient Protection and Affordable Care Act of 2010 reduced the uninsured rate across the country. However, some states, such as Texas, still have a relatively high uninsured rate, making healthcare access difficult and possibly unaffordable. According to the 2021 RWJF "County Health Rankings & Roadmaps" summary for Texas, approximately 20% (or 1 in 5 Texans) still lack insurance. Accessing healthcare services becomes an even greater challenge when individuals lack insurance and/or personal means to pay for such services. This creates a domino effect of healthcare avoidance, delayed treatment, and the potential for poor outcomes.

Access to Food and Food Insecurity in the Built Environment

The built environment contributes to health patterns, behaviors, and day-to-day choices, even when it comes to food and nutrition. The built environment can impact cost, convenience, and access to healthy food. Individuals who lack transportation or safe walking paths to areas outside their immediate periphery easily become confined in the built environment and are forced to make decisions about food and nutrition based on geography. Barriers in the built environment can lead to individual choices that contradict the desire to consume healthy foods. For example, individuals living in remote, racially segregated, or unsafe neighborhoods may have decreased access to nutritious foods due to the poorly designed built environment and lack of public transportation and/or suitable walking paths.

Access to nearby built environment structures, such as local convenience/corner stores with limited healthy options versus grocery stores with a variety of nutritious foods, guides the immediate decision-making process. Convenience stores are well known to carry unhealthy foods, alcohol, and tobacco rather than healthy foods and fresh produce (Minkler et al., 2019). Living near convenience/corner stores where food is readily available, less costly, and easier to access can deter individuals from shopping at grocery stores and farmer's markets outside their neighborhood. The built environment in this circumstance heavily influences the ability and decision to purchase unhealthy foods.

As part of a cross-sector community initiative, the San Francisco Healthy Retail SF program was established in 2014 to incentivize local corner stores to offer healthier options. The program included incentives for corner store owners to redesign their store layout and offer a greater variety of fresh produce and healthy food options while also reducing the supply of tobacco and alcohol. A specific neighborhood in San Francisco was initially selected for the program due to the high food insecurity rates among its residents. The program was formally launched with the use of a three-legged stool framework including community engagement, redesign, physical environment, and business operation support (Minkler et al., 2019). Fortunately, the program met great success and led to a 12-month increase in produce sales of 35% in the model corner stores. The model also led to a ripple effect in other corner stores, including those not receiving incentives. This can be attributed to the power of strategic planning and cross-sector collaboration to promote health equity. The redesigned built environment in these corner stores contributed to healthier food options and thus healthier choices by individuals.

The ability to purchase healthy foods in one's neighborhood is a luxury that should not be taken for granted. Unfortunately, many neighborhoods across the country have not been strategically designed with walkability, safe paths, accessibility, and public transportation options in mind. Families with substantial socioeconomic burdens living in such poorly designed built environments must make difficult decisions daily regarding how to meet basic needs with limited income. According to the US Census Bureau, in 2019, 10.5% of Americans lived in poverty. While this is a favorable decline for the fifth consecutive year, there remain approximately 34 million people living in poverty (Semega et al., 2020). Organic and generally healthier food options typically come at a significantly higher cost, and socioeconomically challenged families have little choice but to purchase higher-density/higher-caloric, lower-cost foods. This may not be a decision, but rather the only option for families with lower incomes. A fixed income coupled with limited food-purchasing options in the immediate built environment collectively contribute to food insecurity and thus negatively impact health.

Food insecurity, as defined by the US Department of Agriculture (USDA), occurs when there is a lack of certainty regarding the ability to have or obtain food to meet the needs of all family members at any time point throughout the year due to insufficient funds or resources. This definition also includes households that have very low and low food security. According to a 2020 report by Coleman-Jensen et al., approximately 10.5% of American households experienced food insecurity at some point in 2019, as shown in Fig. 4.1. While this number was down from the previous year (11.1%), 35.2 million individuals were still living without secure

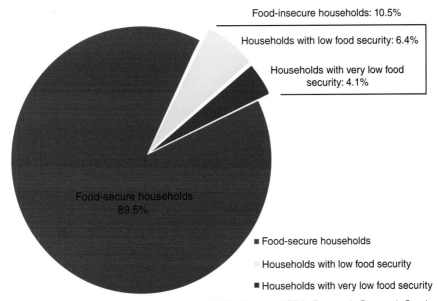

Fig. 4.1 US households by food security status, 2019. (Source: USDA, Economic Research Service, using data from the December 2019. Current Population Survey, Food Security Supplement.)

and consistent access to food to promote health. The built environment, unfortunately, can contribute to food insecurity simply by its design. A built environment that prohibits individuals from accessing food safely and consistently can negatively affect overall health. A lack of transportation or availability of nutritious food is an example of how the design of the built environment can negatively impact access to food.

Promoting Health in the Work Environment

Over 12 million people die globally each year because of unhealthy home or work environments (Prüss-Ustün et al., 2016). The importance of the work environment cannot be overemphasized when it comes to physical and mental health. Working full time requires that approximately 40 hours per week be spent within the construct of the built environment of the workplace. Most of an individual's day (or night) is typically spent in a workplace setting when working full-time hours. While American jobs vary vastly in schedules, skills required, duties, and industry, most occur within the constraints of a physical building. Therefore the work environment must support health by providing a positive environment in and around the built environment.

The USGBC prioritizes health promotion from a physical and design standpoint. The Council's main platform, Leadership in Energy and Environmental Design (LEED), includes objective ratings and a framework to share protocols, guidelines, and systems for ongoing green design and development in a variety of environments (USGBC, 2017). An analysis conducted by Worden et al. (2020) further explains the correlation between health and the built environment. The analysis supports much of the underlying message of this chapter, namely that health does not exist, and cannot be attained, solely within the construct of the health sector. On the contrary, the health sector needs substantial support from all social sectors, including the real estate industry, to truly promote health. The LEED framework from the USGBC can be applied in the workplace environment to address exterior building design and construction, interior design, operations and maintenance, and surrounding neighborhood development. These elements collectively have the potential to impact the overall "health status" of the work environment and thus the health of employees.

Two specific environmental aspects that can positively promote health and physical activity in the workplace include walkability and the greenness of the outdoor environment. Marquet and Hipp (2019) report that employees' perception of the walkability of the work environment can increase physical activity. If an employee perceives walking as accessible and safe in the context of the work environment (inside and outside the physical structure), the individual is more likely to engage in episodes of physical activity throughout the day. This can also include using stairs versus elevators to move throughout the workplace. Workplace walkability must include safety and ease of access for it to be of benefit in health promotion.

To promote employee satisfaction, workplace engagement, and employee retention, many employers strive to support their employee's overall health and well-being through a variety of workplace initiatives. Examples of workplace wellness programs are as diverse as the organizations themselves. Some organizations offer unique incentives for employees to reduce absenteeism and employee healthcare expenditures. Such programs include reduced healthcare insurance premium fees when biometric goals are met or with the avoidance of nicotine use. Other programs offer a more preventative approach by supporting physical activity breaks during work, providing on-site gymnasiums, and even offering community discount programs for recreational activities. Innovative and cutting-edge employers have begun to research the impact of a healthy work environment on productivity and employee retention. Newer efforts underway include the use of standing desks, walking meetings, and ergonomically designed work and meeting spaces. According to Kava et al. (2021), the work environment is an ideal place to implement evidence-based interventions to reduce chronic illness, including smoke-free campuses, access to healthy foods, and physical activity programs as the norm. The completion of a detailed workplace assessment can provide insight into areas for improvement in the physical and built environment.

HOUSING SECURITY AND QUALITY

Impact of Social Determinants on Health and Housing

Social determinants of health include the social/non-medical aspects of life that directly contribute to health and well-being. Social determinants such as accessible nutritious food, recreation and physical activity opportunities, neighborhood walkability, green space, transportation, quality of education, income earning potential, and racial disparities within the community all have significant impacts on health. Social determinants can impact overall quality of life and contribute to short-term and long-term health outcomes, both positively and negatively. Social determinants encompass all living conditions, including homelessness, substandard housing, and residential or racial segregation.

Existing structural racism in the housing and banking industries plays a role in the ongoing segregation and marginalization of vulnerable racial and ethnic groups. Multiple generations of families may continue to live in segregated neighborhoods with substandard housing due to the inability to access quality education and limited employment opportunities with reduced earning potential. The inability to purchase housing in more desirable neighborhoods is directly related to one's education, employment, and income potential. Residential and racial segregation are associated with poor health. Substandard living conditions can contribute to low birth weight in infants, preterm labor (Mehra et al., 2017), and unfavorable cancer survival rates (Landrine et al., 2017).

Population-Specific Considerations

Health disparities continue to prevail in the United States despite ongoing and widely disseminated efforts to achieve health equity. Some disparities are more prominent in certain neighborhoods and practically nonexistent in others. The segregation of certain vulnerable populations continues and leads to generations of poor living conditions and socioeconomic hardships. Strategic efforts to increase access to adequate housing and improved community design for socioeconomically challenged families can help reduce geographical disparities for vulnerable populations across generations.

The physical, natural, and built environment can look very different for individuals that live in the same city, county, or even zip code. As described in the student reflection activity, "A Tale of Two Families," not all neighborhoods are created alike, even when in close proximity. In other words, not all neighborhoods in the same community are homogenous in terms of safety, education, food security, economics, housing, employment, cleanliness, sanitation, and so on. Therefore when considering the impact of the overall environment on an individual, family, or subpopulation, it is vital to consider both the immediate and peripheral environmental factors and challenges patients face.

The perception that poor individuals live in isolated neighborhoods and thus have less exposure to positive contributors to health is a valid concept within the context of the built environment. In a study of over 400,000 individuals using publicly available data from Twitter across 50 of the largest population centers in the United States, Wang et al. (2018) assessed urban mobility and isolation among various populations. Researchers found that mobility out of lower-income neighborhoods is common; however, it remains limited when it comes to exposure to middle-class and predominantly White neighborhoods. This finding further supports the historical notion that underexposure to certain aspects of society still exists for lower-income families. Furthermore, researchers found that race had a greater impact on mobility and exposure to positive attributes than income, further indicating that segregation continues to exist across the country despite the widespread diversity of the population (Wang et al., 2018).

INFRASTRUCTURE, PUBLIC TRANSPORTATION, ZONING, AND HEALTH IMPACT ASSESSMENTS

The built environment, as defined by the US Department of Health and Human Services (2020b) as the physical aspects of where individuals live, learn, work, and play. It includes human-made physical structures and buildings that surround individuals, such as homes, schools, places of worship, social organizations, places of employment, and establishments frequently visited, such as grocery stores, retail stores, and restaurants. However, the built environment does not exist independently of the natural environment, which is heavily influenced by the overall climate and ongoing extreme climate changes.

One's geographic location offers a unique contribution to overall health. A well-designed, sustainably built environmental infrastructure promotes safety, security, physical activity opportunities, access to public transportation, food security, access to vital social resources, and social interactions. Paine and Thompson (2017) elaborate that key indicators for a favorable built environment should be established and utilized for community comparison and outcome measurement. Such indicators include access to utilitarian and physical activities, socialization and shared community spaces, crime prevention, and access to nutritious foods. These key indicators provide a solid base for future health research and public health policy regarding community design, infrastructure, and zoning.

According to Rider (2020), the transportation infrastructure of a community has a significant impact on climate change and public health outcomes. Communities with an abundance of single-driver vehicles tend to produce more environmental pollutants and noise. Isolation can occur when adequate public transportation does not exist. A lack of public transportation further reduces the likelihood of exposure to societal and financial resources outside of one's immediate environment. Interestingly, public transportation availability can contribute to an increase in physical activity when walking to and from transportation stations.

Windshield Survey and Health Impact Assessments

Are you familiar with the phrase "seeing is believing"? Does the phrase apply to the impact of the environment on an individual's health? Must one visualize poor living and environmental conditions to appreciate their potential impact on health? If so, completing a windshield survey can provide a beneficial and objective perspective.

It is easy to become accustomed to the subtle, and not so subtle, structures in the built environment. One can pass abandoned buildings while driving every day and easily overlook their dilapidated state. The environment can easily blur into the background of one's daily commute, walk, or other common activities. However, it is never truly "in the background" but rather at the forefront of people's decision-making. The routes driven, places visited, and walking paths taken are directly affected by the physical, natural, and built environment. Daily routine decisions may feel isolated from the built environment, but they are grounded in what the environment has to offer. A person is much more likely to take a walk in a park that is well lit, has maintained greenery and clean equipment, and is in a safe neighborhood. Most individuals are unlikely to dine at a restaurant that has poor structure, is near a high-traffic intersection, or lacks a well-lit parking lot. And yet, individuals may not verbalize these issues when deciding where to eat or which park to visit on a sunny day. Rarely do individuals pause and truly assess their environment with a clear and objective lens. The completion of a windshield survey offers us a unique ability to "see" one's community for what it truly is—a vastly complex compilation of education, religion, politics, healthcare, transportation, law enforcement, and the physical, natural, and built environment.

A windshield survey is an objective preliminary assessment of key components of a community. It can be completed as if one is viewing the community from the windshield of a vehicle, hence the name. Some individuals complete the assessment while driving through a community, while others choose to walk, looking through the same objective lens. The assessment can serve as the initial step toward conducting a formal, comprehensive community assessment and often leads to the creation of a plan to address community infrastructure deficiencies. This type of survey can be completed using a variety of templates or frameworks to ensure that all core components are at least minimally assessed.

One such template is the Social Factors and Safety/Cleanliness/Religion and Recreation/Education and Economics/Employment/Natural Environment and Nutritional Outlook (SCREEN) tool (Fig. 4.2). This windshield assessment tool focuses on six key components of the physical, natural, and built environment that impact health:

Societal factors and safety. Is there a sense of safety and security while driving or walking through the neighborhood? Are there easily accessible crosswalks throughout the area? Are law enforcement vehicles seen patrolling the area? Are police or fire stations in sight? Do the roads appear to be well maintained, well lit, and easily accessible? Is there evidence of social interactions among people? Is there evidence of social gathering locations and buildings? Are homelessness, illegal drug use, or other criminal activities evident in the community?

Cleanliness. What do streets, homes, and buildings generally look like? Are they clean and free of debris/clutter? Are the homes well maintained? Is there any evidence of illegal waste/dumping in the area? Are there abandoned properties or homes that appear unsafe due to visible structural issues?

Religion and recreation. Are there churches of different denominations in the area? Do they appear well kept and clean? Are there parks in the community? Do they appear to have operational equipment for children to play on? Are there areas that support physical activity? Do you see walking paths or bike lanes?

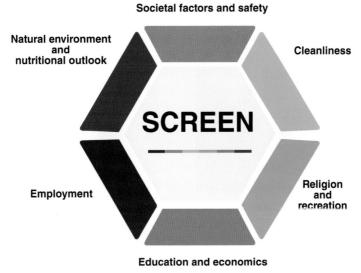

Fig. 4.2 The Social Factors and Safety/Cleanliness/Religion and Recreation/Education and Economics/ Employment/Natural Environment and Nutritional Outlook (SCREEN) tool. (Source: Developed and designed by Diana Ruiz.)

Education and economics. What is the overall impression of the local schools? Are they well kept? Are there children outside playing? Are the playgrounds securely fenced? What first impression do you get regarding the socioeconomic status of the area? Do you see evidence of poverty such as poor living structures, abandoned buildings, and homelessness? Are any homeless shelters identifiable? What other signs of wealth or poverty are visible?

Employment. Does the neighborhood appear to have diversity in terms of employment opportunities? Are there open businesses with evidence of customers? Do the businesses appear clean and in good structural standing? Is there a variety of open businesses?

Natural environment and nutritional outlook. What does the natural environment look like? Are there trees, grass, and sources of water? Are there notable signs of air pollution or indications of pollution? Are there any manufacturing plants, oil refineries, or other sources of pollution visible? From a nutritional outlook, are there many fast food and/or dine-in restaurants? Is there a variety of grocery and other stores? Were any food banks, mobile food pantries, or other food dispensaries identified in the area?

The utilization of a guided template such as the SCREEN tool can facilitate the objective assessment and documentation of a preliminary community assessment. The data

identified in a windshield survey can be invaluable in the process of completing a comprehensive community assessment. Moreover, the completion of a windshield survey offers insight into the daily challenges faced by individuals living in the community. It can be an eye-opening experience, particularly when completed in areas outside of one's immediate community. A windshield assessment can ultimately yield a deeper understanding of the unique challenges and disparities faced by the populations served. Individuals living in vulnerable and deficient neighborhoods may become accustomed to poor living conditions and may fail to see the abundant impact on behaviors, choices, and overall health outcomes. Figs. 4.3 and 4.4 show the windshield survey in action related to housing.

The RWJF "County Health Rankings & Roadmaps" program is an excellent resource for assessing health impacts, national disparities, challenges, and opportunities from traditional and nontraditional health perspectives. The county, state, and national rankings provide invaluable information regarding health outcomes and factors, including key components of the physical, natural, and built environment. Moreover, the "County Health Rankings & Roadmaps" model measures variable aspects of life that impact quality and length of life. They include broad categories covering:

- Health behaviors
- Clinical care

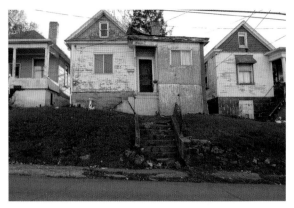

Fig. 4.3 Image of a House. (From iStock.com/LawrenceSawyer.)

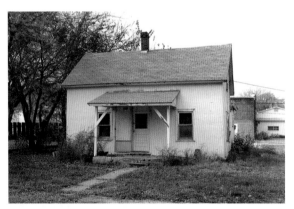

Fig. 4.4 Image of a House. (From iStock.com/lillisphotography.)

- Social and economic factors
- Physical environment (University of Wisconsin Population Health Institute, 2014).

Within each broad category, the model dives further into assessing community data and provides a "snapshot" of the overall health of the community. The county snapshot provides an excellent bird's eye view of various key factors impacting health. Community and county-level data can then be compared with the highest-performing national comparison for reference and guidance (University of Wisconsin Population Health Institute, 2014).

With regard to the physical, natural, and built environment, the RWJF "County Health Rankings & Roadmaps" annual report provides information specific to air pollution, drinking water violations, severe housing problems, driving alone to work, long commutes, traffic

volume, homeownership rates, severe housing cost burdens, and broadband access (County Health Rankings, 2021). Broadband access is discussed in detail later in this chapter. Each of these environmental factors can be further analyzed to determine trends, make comparisons, and identify barriers to health and opportunities for community collaboration and necessary improvement. It is essential to understand these factors in one's community to understand and meet increasingly complex patient needs across the continuum of care. It is no longer enough to understand the intricacies of health solely within the healthcare setting. Diverse and growingly complex patient populations warrant a fresh and innovative approach to achieving healthy equity, focusing on individual environments. For example, utilizing data directly from the Environmental Public Health Tracking Network and the Safe Drinking Water Information System, RWJF provides a comprehensive overview of the environmental stance of a particular county, offering nurses information about potential illness-causing factors. A county with a particularly high air pollution rating can be expected to have higher rates of respiratory illnesses as a result. Armed with this information, nurses can work toward improving population health by advocating for businesses to utilize clean air practices.

ENVIRONMENTAL JUSTICE: AIR, LAND, AND WATER

To gain a deeper appreciation of the environment, one must explore the immediate and proximal areas surrounding their home, work, and school. Individuals should assess and evaluate structures that can be seen when looking outside. What physical aspects of the environment immediately stand out? Is the neighborhood an urban area congested with people, vehicles, and buildings? Or does the neighborhood seem rural, remote, and quiet, with open land? Are there trees, natural vegetation, or perhaps bodies of water? What about concrete sidewalks, busy streets, and rushing traffic? Is the land lush and green or dry and desert-like? Is the open sky visible or obscured by human-made structures and electrical wire posts? Are the eyes drawn to the natural or built environment? What noises pervade when listening quietly? An individual's natural environment ties in directly with the physical and built environment and can easily become blurred. However, each component contributes differently to overall health and health behaviors.

Physical and natural environments encompass many aspects of an individual's day-to-day life. They include the geographical locations in which individuals live, work, learn, and play. They can include natural resources and land elements such as trees, mountains, bodies of water, and other aspects such as water quality, air pollution, community cleanliness and sanitation, housing status, and driving conditions in the immediate periphery and beyond.

Environmental health is a vast and complex science, independent of this discussion. There are a tremendous number of elements to study and understand about environmental health. Experts can spend a lifetime studying and researching characteristics of the environment and their impacts on health. For this chapter's purposes, the focus is specifically on the immediate impacts of the physical and natural environment on overall health and the ability to attain health equity. However, it is important to note that, ultimately, public health and climate change are intertwined at the national and global levels. Public health is impacted by transportation and its harmful effects, the use and misuse of essential land, and the presence of buildings, regardless of size and capacity (Rider, 2020). It is no surprise that Western modernization and industrialization come with a heavy environmental price tag.

The physical environment directly impacts access to clean water, clean air, and safe housing. Dating back to the days of Florence Nightingale, the importance of clean air, water, and housing for health has long been established. According to the WHO, premature morbidity and mortality can be prevented by living in a healthier environment. In fact, the environment's impact on health is so strong that the WHO reports approximately 1 in 4 deaths are preventable globally (24%) and attributable to the environment (WHO, 2016a). In the United States, 11% of deaths are attributed to the environment (WHO, 2016b). This statistic is a profound reminder that health is very much dependent upon the physical, natural, and built environment, as nearly 1 in every 10 deaths is related to the environment and associated risks.

Water Under Pressure: The Case of the Flint Water Crisis

We are, at times, victims or by-products of the environment in which we live. Some parts of our country are notorious for poor air and water quality. Let us explore the case of Flint, Michigan.

The Flint water crisis began in April 2014 when a significant financial decision was made by Flint officials to change the town's main water source. The change was made from purchasing water from the Detroit Water and Sewage Department, whose source was Lake Huron, to temporarily using water directly from the Flint River, which would be processed by its own Flint Water Service Center. The decision was only intended to be temporary until a long-term solution was finalized, which was to join the newly formed Karegnondi Water Authority. Despite forewarnings about the potential implications of using water with questionable quality, the Flint Water Service Center began delivering water to residents, and within a matter of weeks, individuals began to show vague symptoms of exposure to contaminated water. Residents soon reported a change in water color (reddish color), taste, and odor. Many residents also reported new-onset skin rashes, occurring particularly in young children. By late 2014, Flint received a Safe Drinking Water Act violation notice, and further extensive sampling and testing began. By September 2015, a local pediatrician, Dr. Hanna-Attisha, published an alarming report indicating that blood lead levels in local children had significantly increased since the 2014 transition to the Flint Water Service Center distribution. Shortly after this report, the decision was made to change the water source back to Lake Huron via the Detroit Water and Sewage Department, but the damage had already been done. Public trust was lost, and many residents experienced ongoing health conditions. Although difficult to directly correlate, numerous deaths also occurred in Flint because of Legionellosis during this time frame, which increased significantly when the water source changed (Masten et al., 2016).

Ultimately the Flint water crisis made national news and became one of the most significant American environmental health issues in the 21st century. It is a frightening example of how fragile our basic needs can be when they go unmet. It is also a reminder that basic needs such as clean water and air cannot be taken for granted, even in highly industrialized countries. As our population continues to grow across most areas in the United States, it is of great importance that proper city planning occurs to support the complex water needs of communities. Strategies such as community planning, strategic zoning, and municipal ordinances to reduce property lot size and vegetation can increase assurances that safe and clean drinking water will be available for future generations (Stoker et al., 2019).

PLANETARY HEALTH AND CLIMATE CHANGE

Every American is vulnerable to the health impacts associated with climate change.
—Crimmins et al., 2016

Climate change continues to be an area of concern across many sectors of society, from politics to healthcare. Although consensus is lacking as to the causes of climate change, the impacts are irrefutable. Climate change may result in an increased incidence of respiratory and heat-related illnesses as temperatures continue to rise globally. Additionally, climate and extreme temperatures have a direct impact on the ability to grow and produce vital foods and thus may contribute to food insecurity in the future. Vulnerable populations, including children, the elderly, the disabled, and those of lower socioeconomic status, may be impacted more severely (Crowley, 2016).

The EPA explains that climate changes associated with extreme weather patterns, such as record-high temperatures and heavy rainstorms, are attributed to rising levels of carbon dioxide and greenhouse emissions in the atmosphere due to human behaviors (EPA, 2021). In 2016, the US Global Change Research Program produced a comprehensive, evidence-based assessment of the impacts of climate change on human health in the United States. The assessment revealed that climate change is associated with temperature-related deaths, air quality concerns, extreme environmental events, vector-borne diseases, water-related illnesses, food safety/nutrition/distribution concerns, and mental health and well-being, and has a greater impact on vulnerable populations. In essence, all aspects of life are directly impacted by climate change patterns. The report conveys a clear message regarding the significantly negative impacts of climate change on health and health outcomes. Data from the report should be used as a guide for environmental reform and increased regulation of greenhouse emissions and other industrial hazards (Crimmins et al., 2016).

In January 2021, President Biden issued an Executive Order titled "Public Health and Environment and Restoring Science to Tackle the Climate Crisis." In Section 1, "Policy of the Executive Order," there is a call to:
- Empower workers and communities

- Promote and protect public health and the environment
- Conserve national treasures and monuments with symbolic meanings

Broadly speaking, the Executive Order requires a recommitment to the advancement of environmental justice by outlining necessary actions in eight key document sections. While all sections of President Biden's order are of interest and potential benefit, Section 5 focuses specifically on addressing the social cost and burden of detrimental environmental practices by accounting for the benefits of reducing climate pollution. The intent of this section is to provide tangible costs associated with greenhouse emissions in terms of impacts on human health, agricultural productivity, and property damage. The information is to be utilized by agencies to make socially responsible decisions regarding greenhouse emissions regulations (The White House, 2021).

A position statement from the American College of Physicians (ACP) calls for healthcare providers (physicians) to become well educated in climate change and to actively engage in advocacy for environmental protection strategies. Additionally, the ACP proposes that healthcare providers and administrators assess and act upon healthcare-related energy consumption. Due to excessive energy utilization in the healthcare sector, second only to the food industry, the ACP recommends establishing sustainable and energy-efficient practices in hospitals while preparing for the future healthcare needs of those impacted by extreme conditions resulting from climate change (Crowley, 2016). Addressing climate change threats and causes warrants a multifaceted, comprehensive, cross-sector, global approach. The future health of the planet will be shaped by the decisions made by all. Many nursing organizations have made public statements recognizing climate change as a public health concern. Additionally, the American Nurses Association's (ANA) policy agenda calls for preparing nurses to engage in conversations about the impact of climate change on health, especially in vulnerable populations (ANA, 2022).

As mentioned earlier, from the days of Florence Nightingale, nurses have made the connection between health and clean air, clean water, and a safe place to live and work. Butterfield and colleagues (2021) describe what nurses can do concerning climate change through activism and advocacy centered on equity, justice, and morality. Leffers et al. (2018) identified upstream climate strategies, such as mitigation through laws and policies, that can reduce sources of pollution that contribute to climate change. For example, the healthcare sector is thought to contribute approximately 10% of greenhouse gas emissions in the United States (Cook et al., 2019). Nurses often implement the downstream interventions necessary to care for those suffering from the harmful effects of climate change. For more information on what nurses can do about climate change, the Nurses Climate Challenge is a global initiative designed to educate nurses on the damaging effects of climate change and the necessary mobilization for action (Nurses Climate Challenge, 2021).

BROADBAND ACCESS, TECHNOLOGY, AND HEALTH

Access to reliable and fast broadband Internet service provides a wealth of benefits such as access to socialization with friends and family, education for individuals of all ages, diverse employment opportunities, healthcare services such as telemedicine, and social service resources. The ability to talk to a loved one, apply for a new job, and pursue a college degree using broadband has become the norm. As defined by the Federal Communications Commission, broadband has minimum download speeds of at least 25 megabits per seconds (Mbps) and upload speeds of at least 3 Mbps. Individuals of varied age groups have adapted to modern technology, with broadband as a key component. However, limited or inaccessible broadband can contribute negatively to an individual's overall health and quality of life. As explained by the Johns Hopkins University (JHU) Center for Applied Public Research, broadband is a critical aspect of life and yet can vary according to race, income, and geographical location. It can further contribute to social inequity and widen the gap when not readily available to all. Approximately one-third of households nationwide do not have Internet access (JHU Center for Applied Public Research, 2020).

Although broadband was made public over 30 years ago, it remains inaccessible and/or unaffordable to many. Internet reliability and speed are minimal expectations for some yet luxuries for others. From a geographical standpoint, access to the Internet can be almost nonexistent and a barrier to accessing essential health services, community resources, education, and employment.

TABLE 4.1 Broadband Access Based on Household Income

Household Income in Past 12 Months	Percent of Households Without Internet Subscription
$75,000 or more	4.3%
$20,000–$74,999	15.6%
Less than $20,000	35.6%

Data from: US Census Bureau. (2019). *American community survey-types of computers and Internet subscriptions.*https://data.census.gov/cedsci/table?q=S2801&tid=ACSST1Y2019.S2801&hidePreview=false.

Despite the perception that living in a rural area is the main contributor to limited broadband access, cost also remains a major prohibiting factor in the use of broadband in populations of lower socioeconomic status.

In 2019, the American Community Survey reported data indicating that 13.4% of households did not have any form of Internet subscription. Interestingly, this rate significantly increased as the annual income per household decreased. Table 4.1 shows the percentage of households without an Internet subscription according to average household income. Cost, remote living conditions, and technical inadequacies continue to create broadband accessibility issues for low-income groups. If no regulatory actions are taken at the national level, the absence of reliable broadband will continue to be a barrier to health, socialization, education, and employment opportunities.

HEALTHY ENVIRONMENT, HEALTHY FUTURE FOR ALL: IMPLICATIONS FOR NURSING PRACTICE

A safe and healthy environment in which to grow can have a profound impact on an individual's ability to overcome poverty, disparities, and other social determinants of health. For nurses, a holistic approach to providing care is the norm. However, it is not the norm for nurses to be intimately involved in aspects of the physical, natural, and built environment in which patients live. Understanding and appreciating the impact the environment has on the patients and populations served is an invaluable tool to promote comprehensive health. An individual cannot simply be well in the physiological realm. It is virtually impossible to maintain health while living in an unsafe or unhealthy physical, natural, and built environment.

In alignment with the ANA "Code of Ethics for Nurses with Interpretive Statements Provision 1.3," nurses support and empower individuals "to live with as much physical, emotional, social, and religious or spiritual well-being as possible" (ANA, 2015, para 2). Hence, assessing a patient's environment and acting upon detrimental elements is deeply embedded in professional nursing practice.

Unfortunately, the acuity and complexity of patients in the acute care hospital setting can limit students' and nurses' time to explore social determinants of health on a deeper level. Conflicting priorities may prevent deeper conversations surrounding social determinants of health. Thus these vital principles and concepts must be learned and assimilated into practice to meet the diverse and vast social and medical needs of patients. Nurses should be adequately prepared to identify and address social determinants of health with confidence. The inclusion of innovative population health education beyond the traditional classroom walls will ensure students are exposed to diverse populations during experiential community-based learning activities. Engaging in nontraditional clinical experiences supports the goal of providing compassionate and equitable care (Ruiz, 2020). Examples of such experiences include working at an animal shelter, serving homeless individuals in shelters, working with city code enforcement officers to promote neighborhood cleanliness, working with the parks and recreation department to increase green spaces and walkability, and working with community agencies focused on improving housing and living conditions. Moreover, unique clinical experiences in which students partner with local community agencies, government entities, and nonprofit agencies can enhance students' overall confidence when working in a diverse interprofessional team.

With the recent publication of "The Future of Nursing 2020–2030: Charting a Path to Achieve Health Equity" report, a greater emphasis now exists on exploring all aspects of health, including creating a COH, reducing health disparities, and improving the health and well-being of the US population (National Academies of Sciences, Engineering, & Medicine, 2021). The new report aligns well with the Healthy People 2030 goal of improving health and safety where individuals live, learn, work, and play (US Department of Health and Human Services, 2020a). While the Future

of Nursing report adamantly supports interprofessional and cross-sector collaboration, it will ultimately be the nursing profession that works to lead and align public health, healthcare, social services, and public policies to eliminate health disparities and achieve health equity for all (National Academies of Sciences, Engineering, & Medicine, 2021).

The utilization and incorporation of evidence-based population health tools and frameworks in the classroom represent an excellent way to translate such knowledge into professional nursing. The 10 Essential Public Health Services framework shown in Fig. 4.5 provides a solid foundation for nursing students to explore the three core functions of public health: assessment, policy development, and assurance (10 Essential Public Health Services Futures Initiative Task Force, 2020). Naturally, the concept of equity is the central focus of the Public Health Essentials framework. Of note, the framework includes key nursing aspects of assessing, diagnosing, planning, intervening, and evaluating collaborative interventions, all of which are also fundamental to nursing practice.

"Health equity means that everyone has a fair and just opportunity to be as healthy as possible. This requires removing obstacles to health such as poverty, discrimination, and their consequences, including powerlessness and lack of access to good jobs with fair pay, quality education and housing, safe environments, and health care" (Braveman et al., 2017, p. 1). Constraints and challenges in the physical, natural, and built environment can harm quality of life and overall health outcomes. Basic necessities such as employment, education, housing, healthcare, access to food, and overall safety and security may be limited within the constraints of a particular built environment.

Characteristics of the natural environment may further contribute negatively to health. For example, lower socioeconomic neighborhoods are less likely to have safe walking paths, parks, bicycle paths, and accessible public transportation options. This can limit physical activity, socialization, and access to resources outside the community. Therefore health equity cannot be attained by all when elements in the environment create barriers.

The use of the Public Health Services framework in the learning environment can provide students with a visual guide and road map for how to promote equity and work to remove barriers to health for individuals and populations. The framework empowers and challenges nurses to fully practice their education and

To protect and promote the health of all people in all communities

The 10 Essential Public Health Services provide a framework for public health to protect and promote the health of all people in all communities. To achieve optimal health for all, the Essential Public Health Services actively promote policies, systems, and services that enable good health and seek to remove obstacles and systemic and structural barriers, such as poverty, racism, sex discrimination, and other forms of oppression, that have resulted in health inequities. Everyone should have a fair and just opportunity to achieve good health and well-being.

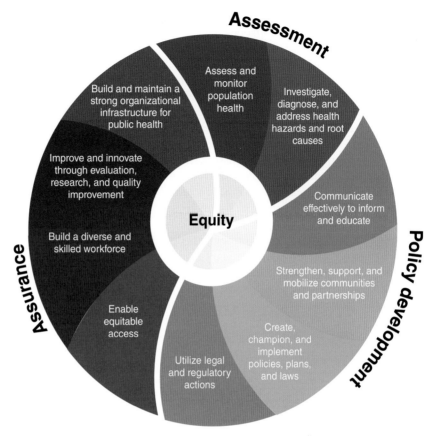

Fig. 4.5 The 10 Essential Public Health Services framework. (From: 10 Essential Public Health Services Futures Initiative Task Force. (2020). *10 Essential Public Health Services EPHS Toolkit.* https://spark.adobe.com/page/Qy1veOhGWyeu5/.)

degree through engagement in cross-sector partnerships, research, policy, advocacy, and assessment.

Nursing has long been recognized as both a science and an art form. The incorporation of social determinants of health, environmental considerations, and health disparities into conscious nursing practice will only further nurses' ability to promote health equity at the individual and population levels. It is the nurse's moral obligation to promote and protect all elements of health in the present and future.

CONCLUSION

The physical, natural, and built environment can improve or impede one's health, quality of life, and overall success. Health cannot be attained independently of the lived environment and the many societal influences, challenges, and barriers. Understanding and appreciating the complexity of the environment in which patients live, work, learn, and play are vital to providing comprehensive patient- and population-centric care. Aspects of the physical, natural, and built environment can create a sense of security, health, and wellness when positive attributes are present. Alternatively, illness, isolation, and food insecurity can result from the environment when unfavorable conditions exist.

A deeper dive is warranted when assessing patients' health behaviors and illness patterns to determine their origins. The root causes of poor health choices and illness can often be found in social determinants of health, such as low income, inadequate housing, food insecurity, inadequate transportation, poor living conditions, less education, and social isolation. The environment in which patients live can ultimately impact morbidity and mortality. As such, the completion of a windshield assessment in the community where one practices can provide the nurse with a unique perspective into the challenges and opportunities patients face daily.

Nurses are perfectly positioned to assess, identify, and act upon complex, social patient needs. At the downstream or midstream levels, this includes helping patients mitigate the risks of living in an unhealthy environment. Investing time in truly understanding an individual's environment outside the healthcare setting can provide significant insight into the many challenges patients must overcome to attain health.

However, the immense work needed to improve the physical, natural, and built environment cannot be accomplished alone and isolated from other social sectors. At an upstream level, this involves partnering with local city leaders, nonprofit agencies, businesses, schools, transportation providers, and congregations to collectively address complex socioeconomic needs. Through cross-sector collaboration, compassion, innovation, and an appreciation of social determinants of health, nurses can significantly impact the overall health and quality of life of individuals, families, and populations.

In summary, the physical, natural, and built environment includes the places where individuals grow, live, work, learn, worship, and play. The physical, natural, and built environment is vital in promoting or hindering health. The physical, natural, and built environment can contribute to morbidity and premature mortality. Health cannot be solely defined as the absence of illness or disease. Social determinants of health significantly impact the way individuals live, learn, work, and access vital resources. Nurses are pivotal in promoting health and advocating for health equity for all.

CASE STUDY

Assume the role of a nursing student completing a clinical rotation with a women's health registered nurse in a low-income community health clinic. The patient assignment for the day includes a patient that has brought her three young children with her to an annual wellness visit with the nurse practitioner. The patient appears disheveled, stressed, and anxious to leave. Her three children, all under the age of 5, appear poorly dressed and have repeatedly verbalized that they are hungry. During the initial intake of demographic data, the patient reports that she is a single mother and has recently moved into a small recreational vehicle park just north of town. She states she is renting a very small camper (recreational

vehicle) from a friend as she is no longer able to afford her previous apartment. She has recently lost her job and is living solely on previous savings and help from her disabled mother.

1. What is the initial assessment of the situation?
2. What socioeconomic factors may be playing into this patient's stress and anxiety?
3. What aspects of the physical, natural, and built environment may pose challenges for this mother and her children to attain health?
4. What resources are available in the community to provide social and emotional support to the patient?

STUDENT REFLECTION ACTIVITIES

1. Collaborative cross-sector community efforts can improve the quality of life and health for vulnerable populations, as shown in the "10 Principles for a Culture of Health."

   Moment of reflection: What are some initial thoughts after reading the "10 Principles for a Culture of Health"? Are these principles practical, attainable, and realistic? Why or why not? What role should the nurse and the entire healthcare community play in this national movement to achieve equity? Discuss the four core action areas and 10 principles in the RWJF Culture of Health framework with your fellow students. Which, if any, of these elements are already present in your community? How can you become involved at the local, state, and national levels outside the traditional nursing role?

2. Environmental justice: Has a question regarding air or water quality been raised in your community? Is there public interest or concern regarding air or water pollution? Where would one find this type of information? To access this information, visit the EPA at https://www.epa.gov/. The EPA website contains invaluable local information about air and water quality, climate change, and lead safety, among others. Spend some time reflecting on local community ratings from the EPA and how they can impact community residents and overall health outcomes.

3. Targeted windshield assessment: Based on the current understanding of the impact of the built environment on health, what potential health issues can be inferred based on this picture? What elements of the SCREEN tool can be identified and documented? Discuss with fellow nursing students the potential health implications for an individual or family living in this home.

4. A Tale of Two Families: The following student reflection activity provides a better understanding of how social determinants can create disparities between individuals, further widening the gap in health equity.

   The Rodriguez family consists of four adults and three young children, ages 10, 7, and 5. The Rodriguez home is multigenerational and includes two elderly grandparents. Mr. and Mrs. Rodriguez are both college educated, work in professional roles, and bring home a combined income of over $150,000 annually. They have a modest home and live in a secure neighborhood with low criminal activity. The children attend a school with excellent academic outcomes and often enjoy playing outside with other neighborhood children. The Rodriguez grandparents walk several times weekly to the local senior citizen center and enjoy socializing with other couples and remaining active. Illness in the Rodriguez home is rare; everyone has health insurance and visits a primary care provider annually for routine checkups. Overall, the quality of life for the Rodriguez family is high, and the family has positive family and social bonds in the community.

   The Jenson family lives just several miles away in the same community. The Jenson family comprises a mother and father and three children, ages 9, 8, and 6. The Jenson family has a limited income, as only the father is currently working. Neither Mr. nor Mrs. Jenson

are college educated, and Mr. Jenson works at a local construction company and has an annual income of $42,000. The Jenson family lives in an older, low-income housing apartment complex, and they do not know any of their neighbors. They live in a two-bedroom apartment, which is crowded but clean and well organized. Mrs. Jenson has concerns about the apartment complex due to recent burglaries in the area and does not allow her children to play outside unless both parents are with them. The children are bussed to a school with poor academic outcomes, as the family lacks transportation to drive them to a different school. Overall, the Jenson family's quality of life is lower, as they feel isolated and insecure in their current environment. No one in the family has health insurance and they infrequently visit a low-income community clinic when someone becomes ill.

   Reflection Questions: Both families comprise two parents and three children. They both live in the same town, only a few miles apart. Yet their quality of life differs greatly.

   1. What are some initial social determinants that stand out and may have an impact on health?
   2. Are there any modifiable living conditions that can be addressed to improve the Jenson family's well-being?
   3. What elements of the physical, natural, and built environment contribute to a lower quality of life for the Jenson family?
   4. What elements of the physical, natural, and built environment contribute to a higher quality of life for the Rodriguez family?
   5. What current and future impacts can the physical, natural, and built environment have on the children in both households?

5. Complete a windshield survey: Consider the overall community health status at the local level. What do local neighborhoods look like when viewed from a health perspective? Is it common to look at the physical, natural, and built environment as it pertains to health? Does it appear that the environment supports or hinders health equity? Is the perception based on where one lives, works, and attends school in the community?

   Take a deeper dive into the overall health and status of the local community by completing a preliminary windshield assessment to help answer these questions and provide a snapshot of the local environment.

Using the previously discussed windshield assessment model (SCREEN) or another windshield survey tool from the literature, complete a preliminary assessment of the immediate or surrounding neighborhood. Assess and evaluate one or more of the following areas of influence: work, home, or school. Or select an area in the community that is unfamiliar and infrequently visited to provide even greater perspective and reflection. Include the following components in your survey for an objective assessment: cleanliness, pollution, safety, grocery store accessibility, public school system, parks, recreational activity opportunities, public transportation infrastructure, healthcare accessibility, religious and political institutions, and overall opportunities for socialization.

Upon completion of the preliminary windshield survey, answer the following questions:

(a) How did the selected area measure up in terms of the selected model?
(b) Were all aspects of the selected model amenable to assessment and evaluation? Or were some unable to be located?
(c) What are some key findings that have an impact at the individual level?
(d) What are some key findings that impact the role of a student nurse or professional nurse in the acute care or community setting?

COMMUNITY-SPECIFIC EXPERIENTIAL LEARNING ACTIVITY

Research local county health rankings data utilizing the RWJF "County Health Rankings & Roadmaps" state report. This report can be accessed using the following link: https://www.countyhealthrankings.org/.

When reviewing local county health rankings, focus specifically on the health outcomes and health behaviors data provided. Make a list of the most pressing data points from a healthcare perspective. Using the local county health rankings, answer the following questions:

1. How does this data impact the role of a nursing student in providing care for patients living in the community?
2. Does this data align with the patient population cared for in current and previous clinical nursing experiences in the hospital and community settings?
3. Is any of the data particularly concerning or alarming? If so, what might specifically impact the health of residents living in the community?
4. Are any of the findings surprising? If so, based on patient health statuses observed in the clinical setting, were the outcomes higher or lower than expected?
5. What type of cross-sector collaborative effort could be derived from a focused/deep-dive approach to population health using the data to guide funding and government decision-making?
6. How might one contribute to this type of collaborative community initiative as a nursing student?

STUDENT REFLECTION QUESTIONS

1. Why should nurses consider the impact of the physical, natural, and built environment on an individual's health status?
2. How can the physical, natural, and built environment contribute to improved health outcomes?
3. What are some examples of how nurses can advocate for improvements in the physical, natural, and built environment?

REFERENCES

10 Essential Public Health Services Futures Initiative Task Force. (2020). *10 Essential Public Health Services EPHS Toolkit.* https://spark.adobe.com/page/Qy1veOhGWyeu5/.

American Nurses Association. (2015). *Code of ethics for nurses with interpretive statements.* https://www.nursingworld.org/coe-view-only.

American Nurses Association. (2022). *ANA acts on climate change and key nursing issues.* Retrieved from https://www.nursingworld.org/news/news-releases/2022-news-releases/ana-acts-on-climate-change-and-other-key-health-care-issues/.

Braveman, P., Arkin, E., Orleans, T., Proctor, D., & Plough, A. (2017), *What is health equity? And what difference does a definition make?* https://www.rwjf.org/en/library/research/2017/05/what-is-health-equity-.html.

Butterfield, P., Leffers, J., & Vasquez, M. D. (2021). Nursing's pivotal role in global climate action. *BMJ, 373,* 1049. doi:10.1136/bmj.n1049.

CDC. (2018). *Social determinants of health: Know what affects health.* https://www.cdc.gov/socialdeterminants/index.htm.

Coleman-Jensen, A., Rabbitt, M., Gregory, C., & Singh, A. (2020). Household food security in the United States in 2019. *ERR-275.* https://www.ers.usda.gov/webdocs/publications/99282/err-275.pdf?v=7049.4.

Cook, C., Demorest, S. L., & Schenk, E. (2019). Nurses and climate action. *The American Journal of Nursing, 119*(4), 54–60. https://doi.org/10.1097/01.NAJ.0000554551.46769.49.

County Health Rankings. (2021). *County health rankings & roadmaps—Texas 2021.* https://www.countyhealthrankings.org/app/texas/2021/rankings/ector/county/outcomes/overall/snapshot.

Crimmins, A., Balbus, J., Gamble, J., Beard, C., Bell, J., Dodgen, D., Eisen, R., Fann, N., Hawkins, M., Herring, S., Jantarasami, L., Mills, D., Saha, S., Sarofim, M., Trtanj, J., & Ziska, L. (2016). The impacts of climate change on human health in the United States: A scientific assessment. http://dx.doi.org/10.7930/J0R49NQX.

Crowley, R. (2016). Climate change and health: A position paper of the American College of Physicians. *Annals of Internal Medicine, 164*(9), 608–610. doi:10.7326/M15-2766.

Health Resources and Services Administration. (2021). *What is shortage designation?* https://data.hrsa.gov/tools/shortage-area/mua-find.

John Hopkins University Center for Applied Public Research. (2020). *Broadband and COVID-19.* https://appliedresearch.jhu.edu/food-insecurity-and-covid-19/broadband-and-covid-19/.

Kava, C. M., Passey, D., Harris, J. R., Chan, K. C., & Hannon, P. A. (2021). The Workplace Support for Health Scale: Reliability and validity of a brief scale to measure employee perceptions of wellness. *American Journal of Health Promotion, 35*(2), 179–185.

Landrine, H., Corral, I., Lee, J. G., Efird, J. T., Hall, M. B., & Bess, J. J. (2017). Residential segregation and racial cancer disparities: A systematic review. *Journal of Racial and Ethnic Health Disparities, 4*(6), 1195–1205.

Leffers, J., & Butterfield, P. (2018). Nurses play essential roles in reducing health problems due to climate change. *Nursing Outlook, 66,* 210–213. doi:10.1016/j.outlook.2018.02.008 pmid:29599047.

Marquet, O., & Hipp, A. J. (2019). Worksite built environment and objectively measured physical activity while at work: An analysis using perceived and objective walkability and greenness. *Journal of Environmental Health, 81*(7), 20–26.

Masten, S. J., Davies, S. H., & Mcelmurry, S. P. (2016). Flint water crisis: What happened and why? *Journal of the American Water Works Association, 108*(12), 22–34. https://doi.org/10.5942/jawwa.2016.108.0195.

Matthews, E., & Lippman, P. C. (2020). The design and evaluation of the physical environment of young children's learning settings. *Early Childhood Education Journal, 48*(2), 171–180. https://doi.org/10.1007/s10643-019-00993-x.

Mehra, R., Boyd, L., & Ickovics, J. R. (2017). Racial residential segregation and adverse birth outcomes: A systematic review and meta-analysis. *Social Science & Medicine, 191,* 237–250.

Minkler, M., Estrada, J., Dyer, S., Hennessey-Lavery, S., Wakimoto, P., & Falbe, J. (2019). Healthy retail as a strategy for improving food security and the built environment in San Francisco. *American Journal of Public Health, 109,* S137–S140. https://doi.org/10.2105/AJPH.2019.305000.

National Academies of Sciences, Engineering, and Medicine. (2021). *The future of nursing 2020–2030: Charting a path to achieve health equity.* https://doi.org/10.17226/25982.

Nurses Climate Challenge. (2021). *Health care without harm.* https://nursesclimatechallenge.org/.

Paine, G., & Thompson, S. (2017). What is a healthy sustainable built environment? Developing evidence-based healthy built environment indicators for policy-makers and practitioners. *Planning Practice & Research, 32*(5), 537–555. https://doi.org/10.1080/02697459.2017.1378972.

Phan, L., Yu, W., Keralis, J. M., Mukhija, K., Dwivedi, P., Brunisholz, K. D., Javanmardi, M., Tasdizen, T., & Nguyen, Q. C. (2020). Google Street View derived built environment indicators and associations with state-level obesity, physical activity, and chronic disease mortality in the United States. *International Journal of Environmental Research and Public Health, 17*(10). https://doi-org.lopes.idm.oclc.org/10.3390/ijerph17103659.

Prüss-Ustün, A., Wolf, J., Corvalán, C., Bos, R., & Neira, M. (2016). *Preventing disease through healthy environments: A global assessment of the burden of disease from environmental risks.* https://apps.who.int/iris/bitstream/handle/10665/204585/9789241565196_eng.pdf;jsessionid=09B-50968F412E8B2DFD3E8FFDA7C200E?sequence=1.

Rider, T. R. (2020). Climate and health in cities: A challenge for the built environment. *North Carolina Medical Journal, 81*(5), 331–337.

Robert Wood Johnson Foundation. (n.d.). *Achieving health equity.* https://www.rwjf.org/en/library/features/achieving-health-equity.html.

Robert Wood Johnson Foundation. (2015). *From vision to action: A framework and measures to mobilize a culture of health.* https://www.rwjf.org/en/cultureofhealth/about.html.

Robert Wood Johnson Foundation. (2021a). *Building a culture of health.* https://www.rwjf.org/en/cultureofhealth.html.

Robert Wood Johnson Foundation. (2021b). *Taking action.* https://www.rwjf.org/en/cultureofhealth/taking-action.html.

Robert Wood Johnson Foundation. (2021c). *How we got here.* https://www.rwjf.org/en/cultureofhealth/about/how-we-got-here.html#ten-underlying-principles.

Ruiz, D. (2020). Population health beyond the classroom: An innovative approach to educating baccalaureate nursing students. *Nursing Education Perspectives, 41*(5), 304–306.

Semega, J., Kollar, M., Shrider, E. A., & Creamer, J. (2020). *Income and poverty in the United States: 2019.* https://www.census.gov/library/publications/2020/demo/p60-270.html#:~:text=The%20official%20poverty%20rate%20in,from%2011.8%20percent%20in%202018.

Smith, M., Hosking, J., Woodward, A., Witten, K., MacMillan, A., Field, A., Baas, P., & Mackie, H. (2017). Systematic literature review of built environment effects on physical activity and active transport: An update and new findings on health equity. *International Journal of Behavioral Nutrition and Physical Activity, 14*, 158. https://doi.org/10.1186/s12966-017-0613-9.

Stoker, P., Chang, H., Wentz, E., Crow-Miller, B., Jehle, G., & Bonnette, M. (2019). Building water-efficient cities: A comparative analysis of how the built environment influences water use in four western US cities. *Journal of the American Planning Association, 85*(4), 511–524. https://doi.org/10.1080/01944363.2019.1638817.

The White House. (2021). Executive Order on Protecting Public Health and the Environment and Restoring Science to Tackle the Climate Crisis.

University of Wisconsin Population Health Institute. (2014). *County health rankings model.* https://www.countyhealthrankings.org/explore-health-rankings/measures-data-sources/county-health-rankings-model.

US Census Bureau. (2019). *American community survey-types of computers and Internet subscriptions.* https://data.census.gov/cedsci/table?q=S2801&tid=ACSST1Y2019.S2801&hidePreview=false.

US Department of Health and Human Services. (2020a). *Healthy people 2030—Environment health.* https://health.gov/healthypeople/objectives-and-data/browse-objectives/environmental-health#cit1.

US Department of Health and Human Services. (2020b). *Neighborhood and built environment.* https://health.gov/healthypeople/objectives-and-data/browse-objectives/neighborhood-and-built-environment.

US Environmental Protection Agency. (2021). *Climate change indicators in the United States.* https://www.epa.gov/climate-indicators.

US Environmental Protection Agency. (2022). *EPA strategic plan.* https://www.epa.gov/system/files/documents/2022-03/fy-2022-2026-epa-strategic-plan.pdf.

US Green Building Council. (2017). *USGBC 2017–2019 strategic plan.* https://www.usgbc.org/about/brand.

Wang, Q., Phillips, N. E., Small, M. L., & Sampson, R. J. (2018). Urban mobility and neighborhood isolation in America's 50 largest cities. *Proceedings of the National Academy of Sciences of the United States of America, 115*(30), 7735–7740. https://doi.org/10.1073/pnas.1802537115.

WHO. (1946). Preamble to the Constitution of WHO as adopted by the International Health Conference, New York, 19 June to 22 July 1946; signed on 22 July 1946 by the representatives of 61 States (official records of WHO, no. 2, p. 100). https://apps.who.int/gb/bd/PDF/bd47/EN/constitution-en.pdf?ua=1.

WHO. (2016a). *Preventing disease through healthy environments: A global assessment of the burden of disease from environmental risks.* https://www.who.int/publications/i/item/9789241565196.

WHO. (2016b). *Deaths attributable to the environment: Data by country.* https://apps.who.int/gho/data/node.main.162.

WHO. (2017). *Human rights and health.* https://www.who.int/news-room/fact-sheets/detail/human-rights-and-health.

Worden, K., Hazer, M., Pyke, C., & Trowbridge, M. (2020). Using LEED green rating systems to promote population health. *Building and Environment, 172*, 106550, 1–8. https://doi.org/10.1016/j.buildenv.2019.106550.

Social and Community Contexts

Teri A. Murray, Pamela Talley, Vanessa Loyd

*The environment and the economy are really both two sides of the same coin.
If we cannot sustain the environment, we cannot sustain ourselves.*
—*Wangari Maathai*

CHAPTER OUTLINE

LEARNING OBJECTIVES

1. Describe the relationship between the social environment and health.
2. Describe the impact of social disorder and community violence on health.
3. Explain how social networks, capital, and cohesion foster community resilience.
4. Describe downstream, midstream, and upstream interventions related to the social environment and health.

THE SOCIAL ENVIRONMENT AND HEALTH

The social environment is a determinant of a population's health. The social factors and physical conditions of the environment impact the community's level of functioning and overall quality of life (US Department of Health and Human Services [USDHHS], Office of Disease Prevention and Health Promotion [ODPHP], 2021). Factors in the social environment that influence health include the availability of adequate resources such as housing, educational and employment opportunities, feelings of safety and security, a sense of belonging and connection to the community via social supports and social networks, sufficient transportation, and public safety. The physical environment, a component of the social environment, comprises elements such as natural and built environments, including aesthetic elements (lighting, green space, parks, and recreational facilities; USDHHS, ODPHP, 2021). While there is no conclusive definition of the term, *social environment*, Barnett and Casper (2011, p. 465) offer a comprehensive definition that merits repeating in its entirety:

Human and social environments encompass the immediate physical surroundings, social relationships, and cultural milieus within which defined groups of people function and interact. Components of the social environment include built infrastructure; industrial and occupational structure; labor markets; social and economic process, wealth; social human and health services; power relations; government; race relations; social inequality; cultural practices; the arts; religious institutions and practices; and beliefs about place and community. The social environment subsumes many aspects of the physical environment given that contemporary landscapes, water resources, and other natural resources have been at least partially configured by human social processes. Embedded within contemporary social environments are historical social and power relations that have become institutionalized over time. Social environments can be experienced at multiple scales, often simultaneously, including households, kin networks, neighborhoods, towns and cities, and regions. Social environments are dynamic and change over time as the result of both internal and external forces. There are relationships of dependency among the social environments of different local areas, because these areas are connected through larger regional, national, and international social and economic processes and power relations.

The WHO defines the social and community context as the complete social and physical conditions in which people live and work, including socioeconomic conditions, demographic characteristics, environmental and cultural conditions, and the healthcare system (WHO, 2012) (Fig. 5.1). Of equal importance in the social and community environment is the nature of the residents' relationships and interactions with family, friends, and community members. These relationships influence health and well-being.

However, not all communities are conducive to health. For example, an unhealthy social environment, such as environments where individuals on the lower rungs of the socioeconomic ladder reside, has been associated with a higher risk of disease. As mentioned, the social environment is comprised of local institutions and social connections between residents, whereas the physical environment includes the built environment, natural green spaces, and food and housing resources. Conditions in the social environment that weigh heavily on the health of the individual and community include the level of violence in the community, the physical or built structure of the community, how the community is designed, and whether the design is health-enhancing.

When assessing the social environment to determine if it is health-enhancing, consider whether the community has access to nutritious and wholesome foods or is a food desert. Does the community have access to sanitized water, adequate sanitation, utilities, adequate schools, school systems, and childcare? What are the ethnicities in the community, the cultural characteristics, and the religious and spiritual beliefs? Are members of the community tight-knit or isolated? Are there strong social networks and supports? Does the community have adequate employment opportunities to generate a sufficient tax base to support the infrastructure? Is it an English-speaking community or do the residents have limited English language proficiency? Is it a primarily heteronormative community or is it an LBGTQ+ community? Is the community safe or does it wreak violence? How do the crime rates compare with other communities? Do community members experience high levels of marginalization, discrimination, or racism? The answers to these questions can determine the level of health in the community and are determinants of health. Health begins in homes, schools, workplaces, neighborhoods, and local communities. The communities where people live can explain why some people lead healthier lives than others and why disparities exist among populations (USDHHS, ODPHP, 2021).

The connections between neighborhood characteristics and health outcomes have long been recognized. Evidence has demonstrated that high crime rates, delinquency, low levels of education, psychological stress, and various health problems are affected by neighborhood characteristics (US Department of Housing and Urban Development, Office of Policy Development and Research, 2011). As discussed in Chapter 2, health and income follow a social gradient. Poorer communities have higher incidences of crime and violence; environmental health threats such as pollutants and toxins; older housing stock, possibly with infestations and walls plastered with lead-based paint; and vendors selling harmful products such as tobacco, alcohol, and high-carbohydrate foods, being located in a food desert (Joint Center for Political & Economic Studies, n.d.) (Figs. 5.2–5.4).

An infant born in the poorest neighborhood of New Orleans is likely to live 25 fewer years than an infant born just 4 miles away in a more affluent neighborhood (Joint Center for Political and Economic Studies, 2012). For example, the subway stops in Chicago corresponded to a 16-year difference in life expectancy (Robert Wood Johnson Foundation [RWJF], 2015). Health varies across and within neighborhoods, based on multiple factors such as educational and employment opportunities, unsafe or unhealthy living conditions, and varying access to quality healthcare facilities—all impacting the quality and length of life (Robert Wood Johnson Foundation

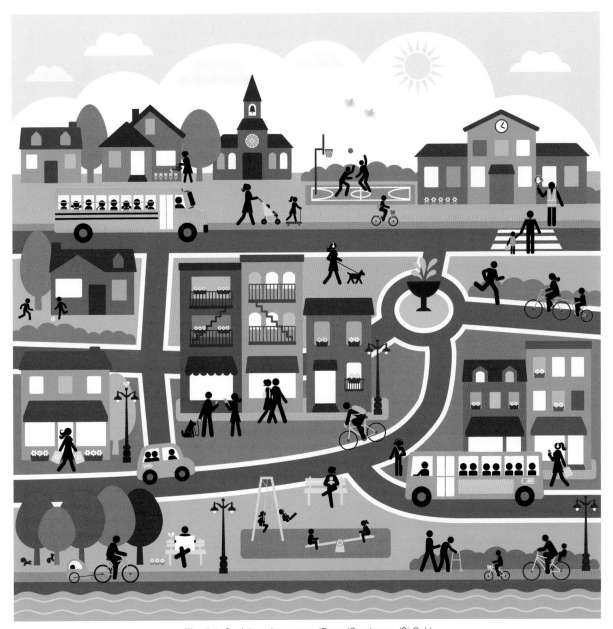

Fig. 5.1 Social environment. (From iStock.com/Si-Gal.)

[RWJF], 2015). Life expectancy differs by nearly 12 years between the Atlanta communities of Buckhead and Northwestern (RWJF, 2015). While these are only three cities, the association between neighborhood characteristics and health outcomes is consistent. Concentrated poverty in neighborhoods affects health, and Blacks and Latinx are more likely than Whites to live in disadvantaged social environments.

Neighborhoods with high concentrations of poverty and segregation are disproportionally burdened with increased morbidity and mortality rates among their members. Box 5.1 highlights the effect of the Delmar Divide in St. Louis, MO.

The social and community context is also determined by whether the area is classified as rural or urban. Urban areas are densely populated cities composed

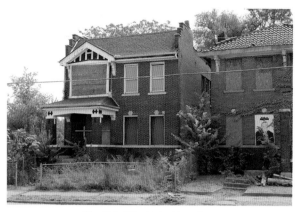

Fig. 5.2 Dilapidated housing.

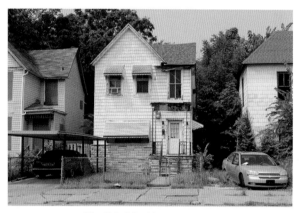

Fig. 5.3 Dilapidated housing.

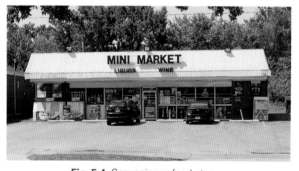

Fig. 5.4 Convenience food stores.

of residential housing that meets minimum density requirements and commercial and other nonresidential types of land uses. Most urban areas are in metropolitan cities with infrastructure and resources to support the city. Rural areas are geographically sparse with few resources, homes, and buildings, and typically have low-density populations.

The "Healthy People 2020" domain, the Social and Community Context, included four specific categories: Civic participation, discrimination, incarceration, and social cohesion (USDHHS, ODPHP, 2018). Each category is explored as it relates to the social determinants of health (SDOH) to better understand how each of these categories has a significant impact on the community's health.

Civic Participation

Civic education supports civic engagement and participation in democratic and participatory governance within communities (Maryland Humanities, 2021). Democratic and participatory governance occurs when community members exercise their right to vote (Fig. 5.5). However, many community members lack an understanding of the significance of voting and how the voting process can influence changes in their community. This absence of understanding can lead to voter apathy and nonengagement in civic participation and democratic processes. Noninvolvement affects the health of the community because to improve the community's health, community members must participate in democratic processes (Maryland Humanities, 2021). Through these processes, voting, and engagement, community members use their voices and vote on matters of concern in the community, whether it is addressing poor lighting and lack of safe walkways, calling for increased protection from rising community crime, or, in rural areas, advocating for increased broadband Internet. Civic engagement empowers community members, and their voices and votes allow them to influence change.

Civic engagement also refers to political activity, membership, and volunteerism in civil society or organizations. Through engagement, individuals can take action to improve the health of their community. Civic engagement is increasingly viewed as a driving force that raises community awareness of issues. Through civic engagement, communities can address unhealthy conditions and take responsibility for changing those conditions. Engagement allows community members to garner increased resources through dialogue with their elected officials. These resources include clean water, improved air quality, better housing stock with increased affordability, and access to healthcare in the community rather than having to travel long distances to seek healthcare (Braveman et al., 2022). The importance of community residents having the ability to vote can never be underestimated. When citizens do not believe their vote counts or believe that voting does not make a difference in their lives, they must be educated on the

BOX 5.1   The Delmar Divide: St. Louis, MO

Delmar Boulevard is a street that runs east to west through St. Louis, MO. It is a dividing line with distinguishing characteristics related to the racial, socioeconomic, and environmental status that impact the entire city of St. Louis.

The neighborhoods immediately south of Delmar are 73% White. The residents live in mansions and affluence, while the residents immediately north of Delmar are 98% Black, with high poverty rates and a high volume of vacant buildings and empty lots. The north side of Delmar is a food desert. The corresponding racial, socioeconomic, and cultural differences became supported by public policy.

Historically, housing has been a contentious issue in St. Louis. In 1911, racial covenants on housing were introduced. These covenants, private agreements among homeowner associations, prevented the sale of houses in specific neighborhoods to Negroes or people that were not Caucasian (National Association of Realtors, 2018).

Racial segregation became legal in 1916 when a citywide segregation ordinance was passed by public vote. According to the National Association of Realtors (2018), restrictive covenants were effective in segregating neighborhoods and stabilizing property values for White families. The federal government supported these discriminatory housing practices through the influential *Underwriting Manual* of the Federal Housing Administration (FHA). From 1934 on, the FHA recommended the inclusion of restrictive covenants in the deeds of homes it insured and instituted a policy known as redlining, refusing to insure homes in Black neighborhoods.

In 1948, the *Shelley v. Kraemer* Supreme Court case overturned these racial covenants and ushered in equal and fair housing (JUSTIA, n.d.). Private agreements that excluded persons based on race or color from the use or occupancy of real estate for residential purposes were not a violation. Still, the state court's enforcement of these agreements violated the equal protection clause of the Fourteenth Amendment. In 1968, the Fair Housing Act prohibited racial discrimination in the sales and rentals of housing. (US Department of Justice, 2021).

Redlining is rejecting a creditworthy applicant's loan for housing in specific neighborhoods even though the applicant may otherwise be eligible for the loan. The courts have upheld redlining as an illegal practice. Although a violation of the law more than 50 years later, housing segregation, discrimination, and redlining continued at the Delmar Divide (US Department of Justice, 2021).

The Delmar Divide, reflective of racially discriminatory practices, has taken a human toll on the Black population on the north side of the divide in every aspect of life. Residents have been significantly impacted by SDOH such as education, income, environmental conditions, the makeup of neighborhoods, and access to community resources like healthy foods and safe public spaces. These determinants have had a significant negative impact on health and health outcomes (JUSTIA, n.d.; National Association of Realtors, 2018; US Department of Justice, 2021).

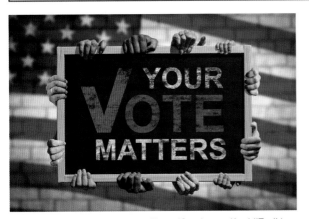

Fig. 5.5 Your vote matters. (From iStock.com/AndriiZorii.)

relationship between voting and health. Nurses should inform patients about the relationship between voting and health and how voting can transform communities. Additionally, if citizens do not vote, elected officials cannot act on their behalf to bring much-needed community resources (Braveman et al., 2022).

Aside from voting, civic engagement encompasses various formal and informal activities that provide direct health-enhancing benefits to communities. Civic engagement is an active process that can take many forms, such as voting, registering people to vote, working as a poll worker on election day, or meeting with an elected official on behalf of the community. Volunteering and participating in community or group activities designed to bring about desired changes to benefit the community and its healthcare also comprise civic engagement activities.

Discrimination

Discrimination is the differential untoward treatment of individuals based on some aspect of their social identities or the intersectionality of those identities, race and ethnicity, sex, sexual orientation and gender identification, socioeconomic status, age, ability, and a host of characteristics or attributes that place individuals into marginalized groups and categories. Structural discrimination within social and community contexts is the creation of conditions that limit opportunities for disadvantaged, racialized, or marginalized groups. These limited opportunities can be imposed in numerous ways through residential occupancy, educational access and quality, healthcare access and quality, and the judicial and justice systems. Insidious forms of structural discrimination can also manifest through financial disinvestments in non-Hispanic White neighborhoods. Noninvestment in communities results in dwindling tax bases and neighborhood socioeconomic disadvantage, biased mortgage lending practices, higher standards to establish creditworthiness, residential redlining, overpolicing, and unfair judicial and legal systems. Discriminatory practices impact health and victims of discriminatory practices often experience psychosocial stressors that lead to increased incidences of hypertension, diabetes, or other health issues (Williams, 2021).

Residential Opportunities

Safe and affordable housing is foundational to good health. Marginalized populations who live in highly segregated and isolated neighborhoods have poorer housing structures that have adverse physical health effects. Housing units may have toxins as a result of mold, dampness, and cold temperatures, thus making occupants susceptible to respiratory diseases. Overcrowding can lead to the spread of infectious diseases and community residents living in overcrowded conditions are at increased risk. This was seen during the coronavirus disease 2019 (COVID-19) pandemic. Some communities could not abide by the social distancing mandate due to limited residential space with many occupants. The stress caused by the risk of being exposed to a potentially deadly virus can lead to mental health concerns among residents. Often, residents of impoverished neighborhoods experience more significant stress and higher incidences of morbidity and mortality (RWJF, 2018; Williams, 2021). Neighborhoods with high concentrations of poverty usually have less access to health-promoting community resources.

Because communities of color often live in close environmental proximity, African Americans and Latinx are more likely to live in neighborhoods with concentrated poverty. The health effects of neighborhood disadvantage are stark. Braveman and colleagues (2022) define environmental injustice as systemic racism that has a direct causal relationship to health. Most disadvantaged and poor communities have higher percentages of power plants that create poor air quality, hazardous waste disposal, and heavy-traffic highways and streets running through the community. A regional study by the United Church of Christ concluded that race was the most important predictor determining the placement of toxic facilities (United Church of Christ, 1987, as cited in Brulle & Pellow, 2006). Evidence points to the differential risk within communities and neighborhoods based on race and socioeconomic status. These risks include noise, residential crowding, exposure to poor air and water quality, and disinvestment in housing and schools (Brulle & Pellow, 2006). The poor, marginalized, disadvantaged, and minoritized bear the brunt of environmental injustices and exposure to unhealthy conditions. For example, heat is the most dangerous weather-related health concern (Crowley et al., 2016). Most urban areas lack tree coverage or canopies to shield residents from the heat. According to *Scientific American,* the lack of trees can raise daytime environmental temperature by 5°F to 7°F and nighttime temperatures by 22°F (Cusick, 2021). Heat-related illnesses include heat rashes, cramps, exhaustion, and stroke. It is estimated that the United States must plant at least 500 million trees to create urban tree canopy equity (Cusick, 2021).

Nursing strategies to address environmental injustices fall into three major foci: research, advocacy, and practice (LeClair et al., 2021). Nurses can engage in partnerships with communities to conduct community-based participatory research that enables community members to elevate the evidence-based concerns of the community to local leaders and politicians who have the power to effect change. Because issues within neighborhoods and committees extend beyond healthcare, the value of partnering with the community and other professionals cannot be understated. Nurses can lead interprofessional teams to address the needs of the community. To be effective, nurses must be immersed in the community in partnership with its residents to understand the lived experience of its members, and how the members can become empowered to translate their concerns to change practices and laws. This collective action to change policies, laws, and actions is an upstream intervention. Partnering with communities to educate legislators on the harmful effects of toxic exposures is a midstream intervention. Downstream interventions include providing direct care to those community members who are experiencing the harmful effects of exposure (e.g., asthma, lead poisoning, hearing deficits, and other health conditions associated with environmental injustices).

Healthcare Access and Quality

The healthcare disparities seen among marginalized populations are caused by a host of factors, discrimination, low levels of educational attainment, low income levels, and a lack of access to healthcare, along with diminished quality of healthcare services.

Most disadvantaged communities are in medically underserved healthcare areas. Medically underserved areas (MUAs) are designated when populations live in areas that have a shortage of primary healthcare providers, high infant mortality rates, high poverty, or a large elderly population (Health Resources and Services Administration [HRSA], n.d.). These shortage areas are geographic and can be an entire county, neighboring counties, urban census tracts, or counties within a municipal division (HRSA, n.d.). Medically underserved populations (MUPs) are groups of people who face economic, cultural, or language barriers to healthcare (Fig. 5.6). Examples include people who are homeless, have low incomes, are eligible for Medicaid, Native Americans and migrant farmworkers, and people who live in rural areas (HRSA, n.d.). Health professional shortage areas (HPSAs) are designated as having shortages of healthcare providers in one of three areas: primary medical care, dental services, and mental health providers. HPSAs can be designated as a specific geographic area, population, or facility (HRSA, n.d.). MUAs/MUPs are provided with federal resources to help establish health maintenance organizations and community health centers in these underserved areas (HRSA, n.d.).

A total of 63% of the counties in the United States have been designated as primary care HPSAs, and these shortages threaten access to services. Rural counties have a disproportionately higher percentage of HPSA designations compared with urban areas (Agency for Healthcare Research and Quality [AHRQ], 2022). Rural residents have limited access to healthcare services, specifically specialty medical services and telehealth, due to the lack of broadband in rural areas. Rural populations have greater health disparities, including higher rates of premature morbidity and mortality, less access to preventive care, and are more likely to engage in unhealthy behaviors than their urban counterparts (Chen et al., 2019) (Fig. 5.7).

There is also the need for increased diversity within the registered nurse (RN) healthcare workforce. This underrepresentation can have serious health consequences for minoritized populations. According to the American Association of Colleges of Nursing (AACN), the RN population is approximately 80% White non-Hispanic, 6.7% African American/Black, 7% Asian, 0.5% American Indian/Alaskan Native, 0.4% Native Hawaiian/Pacific Islander, 2.1% two or more races, and 2.5% other (AACN, 2023). Diverse healthcare providers have experience with diverse populations' cultural and contextual circumstances, which enables them to address the root causes of health disparities more readily (Julion et al., 2019). Diverse providers are more likely to serve diverse populations, increasing access and trust (LaVeist & Pierre, 2014; Neff et al., 2020). Additionally, evidence shows that patients have improved communication and decision-making with providers of the same race, ethnicity, and language (LaVeist & Pierre, 2014; Neff et al., 2020). Diverse providers are also more likely to advocate for vulnerable and diverse populations (LaVeist & Pierre, 2014; Neff et al., 2020). The need for diverse providers is crucial since mounting evidence points to racial discrimination as a risk factor for disease, subsequently contributing to the disparities in health seen

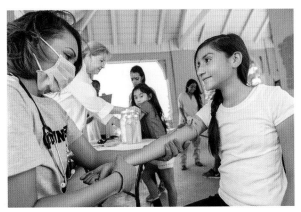

Fig. 5.6 Medically underserved populations. (From iStock.com/SDIProductions.)

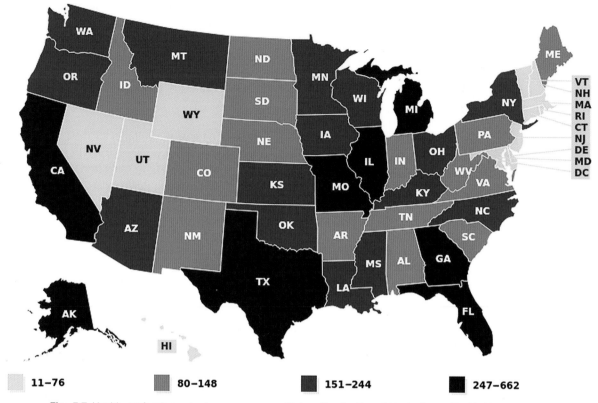

Fig. 5.7 Health professions shortage area map. (Kaiser Family Foundation's State Health Facts, 2023, https://www.kff.org/statedata/ (Accessed on Mar 20, 2024.)

in minoritized populations (Williams et al., 2019). For example, the "2019 National Healthcare Quality and Disparities Report" measured quality in terms of six priorities: patient safety, patient-centered care, care coordination, effective treatment, healthy living, and care affordability (Agency for Healthcare Research and Quality [AHRQ], 2021). The AHRQ Report (2021) documented that Black and American Indian/Alaskan Native patients received poorer care than their White counterparts on 40% of the quality measures. In addition, Latinx and Native Hawaiians/Pacific Islanders received worse care than Whites for more than 33% of quality measures, as did Asians, who also received worse care than Whites for more than 33% of the quality measures (AHRQ, 2021).

Nurse-Led Healthcare

In 2018, according to the National Nurse-Led Care Consortium (NNLC), there were 150 nurse-led clinics nationwide. The NNLC was founded in 1996 as a

nonprofit corporation and is the leading advocacy organization for nurse-managed healthcare. Their mission is to advance nurse-led healthcare through policy, consultation, and programs to reduce health disparities and provide primary and wellness care (NNLC, n.d.). Nurse-led clinics offer primary care and specialty services in underserved communities, improve access to healthcare, and are designed to improve health outcomes and keep people in their communities. In addition, nurse-led clinics and community health workers (CHWs) collaborate to sponsor CHW programs that emphasize health promotion and health education for those populations in the community.

The nurse practitioner (NP) workforce can help improve access to primary care for rural and urban patients. However, NPs cannot always render care because of the different state-by-state scope-of-practice laws, the lack of a diverse NP workforce, and reimbursement policies that favor physicians (Poghosyan & Carthon, 2017). Restrictive practice laws for NPs pose significant barriers and limit the services NPs can provide, further impeding access to quality care for patients. One study showed an association between less restrictive practice guidelines and the growth of retail clinics (Brooks Carthon et al., 2017). NPs are a cost-effective alternative to address the shortages of primary physicians in areas designated HPSAs (Liu et al., 2020).

Community Health Workers

A CHW is a front-line public health worker who frequently works in the community outside health facilities. These CHWs have unique access to the community and the community's local knowledge. Because they work in the community, they can extend health services directly to households and community members. CHWs are seen as trusted members of the community. They understand the community and serve as liaisons or intermediaries between the health and social service sector and the community to facilitate access to services and improve the quality of life and cultural responsiveness of service delivery (American Public Health Association [APHA], 2014).

CHWs engage with communities to improve their health, teach healthcare professionals about their communities, and bridge cultural gaps between health professionals, including nurses, and communities. CHWs are critical in building relationships, mutual respect, and trust between the community and other healthcare team members. Accordingly, CHWs are advocates for the community and can help organize people who share common goals. By doing so, the community gains power and influence over issues impacting their welfare. Strengthening groups at the grassroots level empowers the community to direct their path to some extent, holding government and private organizations accountable for policies and programs that directly impact the health of the community.

Educational Access and Quality

Children who attend lower-resourced schools with limited school nurses and health resources, coupled with low teacher support and increased safety concerns, are likely to have higher incidences of poor physical and mental health than children who attend higher-resourced schools (USDHHS, ODPHP, n.d.). Additionally, the higher the level of education, the more likely a person will live a longer, healthier life. Higher levels of education are tied to higher earnings, and higher wages are linked to the ability to afford the resources needed for good health. Persons with higher incomes usually do not have the social and economic hardship that creates stress and stress-induced illnesses (Center on Society and Health, 2014). Individuals with less education are more apt to live in lower-income communities. Lower-income communities have limited access to grocery stores, less green space, higher crime rates, and less effective political influence to advocate for community needs, leading to community disadvantage (Center on Society and Health, 2014). Thus underperforming schools can impact educational outcomes, economic success, social environments, and access to quality healthcare (Center on Society and Health, 2014). The effects of education on health are discussed in more detail in Chapter 3.

Judicial and Criminal Justice Systems

Discriminatory practices in the judicial and criminal justice systems against minoritized populations are long-standing and structural. Structural reasons underlying these practices include the legacy of subordination from the country's historical enslavement practices of Blacks and Native Americans, overpolicing in minoritized communities, and drug policies that unfairly disadvantage poor and urban communities (The Sentencing Project, 2018). The pervasive, unfair challenges associated with the criminal justice system begin with policing, arrests, and pretrial bail policies and persist through pleas, conviction, incarceration, and beyond (Inman, n.d.) There are also post-prison collateral damages, such as barriers to securing steady employment resulting from having a criminal conviction (The Sentencing Project, 2018). The inability to obtain decent work leads to cycles of repeat offending and repetitive incarcerations. The absence of a parent in the home thus contributes to an intergenerational cycle of poverty (Acker et al., 2019). To begin to solve this cycle, Brink (2021) suggested that the Biden presidential administration focuses on four primary areas: "1) reduce incarceration, 2) root out racial, gender, and income-based disparities, 3) refocus the system on redemption and rehabilitation, and 4) eliminate profiteering off of the criminal justice system" (paragraph 1).

Incarceration

Incarceration has been deemed a structural determinant of individual health that worsens a community's health (Peterson & Brinkley-Rubinstein, 2021). The historical legacy of racism has led to an overrepresentation of minoritized populations in jails and prisons. Reasons for the higher incarceration rates of Black men can be attributed to them having been portrayed as predators, the negative racial imagery often depicted in media, segregated residential living, and the government's hypocrisy, which celebrates freedom and equality yet denies them both, often based on the color of their skin (Alexander, 2020).

Racial and ethnic minorities are arrested, convicted, and incarcerated for criminal offenses at much higher rates than Whites. Black men are 6 times more likely to be incarcerated than Whites, and Latinx are 2.5 times more likely to be incarcerated than Whites (Fig. 5.8) (The Sentencing Project, 2021). Disparities in surveillance, arrests, and sentencing contribute to the disproportionate rate of and risk for incarceration in marginalized communities. The mass incarceration of racial and ethnic minorities has been called the *new Jim Crow*, the declaration that the racial caste system has not ended in the United States but has merely been redesigned through the overpolicing of Black and Brown communities (Alexander, 2020). Mass

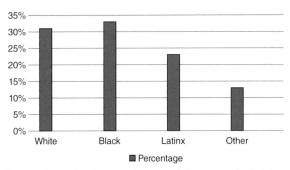

Fig. 5.8 Federal and state prison trends by race and ethnicity. (Adapted from: The Sentencing Project, 2021.)

incarceration resulted from the "war on drugs," which targeted Black and Brown men leading to their arrest and conviction based on stringent mandatory sentencing requirements. Most offenders arrested under these harsh sentencing regimes will spend most of their lives under the control of the criminal justice system—whether in jail or prison, or on probation or parole (Alexander, 2020). This period of control can last a lifetime. Once released, incarcerated individuals are usually discriminated against for the remainder of their lives in employment, housing, education, and public benefits (Alexander, 2020). Most never overcome these circumstances, hence the high rates of recidivism. Key findings related to mass incarceration can be found in Box 5.2.

Residents who live in communities with high incarceration rates likely experience poor mental health (Peterson & Brinkley-Rubinstein, 2021). In addition, the families of those incarcerated experience fragmented families and disruption of their social ties, which further compromises individual and family mental health. As mentioned, among those incarcerated, prospects for employment, economic stability, and affordable housing are greatly diminished (Acker et al., 2019). When imprisoned individuals return to their communities, their health can be further compromised by stigmatization, denial of employment opportunities, unaffordable housing, and minimal education. Furthermore, high incarceration rates within communities disrupt social and family networks, decrease the potential for economic development, and generate distrust toward law enforcement officials (Acker et al., 2019). The fragmentation of families and disruption of social ties further compromise individual, family, and community mental health (Peterson & Brinkley-Rubinstein, 2021).

BOX 5.2   Key Findings Related to Mass Incarceration

- The effects of mass incarceration on health have far-reaching consequences and extend beyond the period of incarceration.
- Mass incarceration causes lifelong stigmatization and the damage of restricting future employment opportunities.
- Parental incarceration increases children's chances of disease; decreases their economic, educational, and social opportunities; and has a lifelong consequence of untoward effects on their health.
- Marginalized groups are disproportionately incarcerated compared with Whites.
- Political processes and practices are behind the disparities in incarceration rates.
- Mass incarceration harms communities.
- A just criminal justice system should be grounded in evidence-based policies.

Adapted from Acker, J., Braveman, P., Arkin, E., Leviton, L., Parsons, J., & Hobor, G. (2019). *Mass incarceration threatens health equity in America*. Executive Summary. Robert Wood Johnson Foundation.

Policing Practices

Marginalized and minoritized communities have viewed policing practices as a threat rather than a service to the community. The current systems of policing are an outgrowth of slave patrols in the South, and these practices have resulted in structural violence that continues to oppress and harm communities of color.

When communities are overpoliced, residents are subject to increased "stops and frisks," these frequent stops and frisks have been associated with depression, anxiety, posttraumatic stress disorder (PTSD), suicidal ideation, hypertension, asthma, and obesity (Theall et al., 2022). These practices have devastating consequences for individual and community physical and mental health. Community residents exposed to hostile policing practices have been found to have shorter telomere lengths, biological markers of aging (Fleming et al., 2022). Decreased telomere length has been associated with increased susceptibility to and faster progression of aging-related diseases such as cardiovascular and coronary artery disease (Chae et al., 2020). Additionally, residents living in frequently policed neighborhoods do not have to have direct contact with officers to be affected by the stress of policing; just knowing of the experience of others places them at risk for increased cardiovascular disease and other adverse health outcomes (Theall et al., 2022).

Between 2015 and 2021, the rate of police shootings of Black Americans was 37 per million people and 28 per million people for Hispanics; this compares to 15 per million people for Whites (Statista Research Department, 2021). This is alarming considering that Black/African Americans comprise 13.4% of the population, Hispanics/Latinx comprise 18.5%, and Whites comprise 76.3% (US Census Bureau, 2021). Policing practices have resulted in the untimely deaths of numerous African Americans. From January 1, 2020, through March 6, 2023, there were 83 unarmed Black men killed by police (Wikipedia, 2023).

Police officers have also acted as immigration enforcement agents to increase the surveillance, arrests, removal, detention, and deportation of undocumented community residents. Such policing practices have been found to result in adverse birth outcomes for infants born to Latina mothers (Novak et al., 2017), cardiovascular problems (Torres et al., 2018), poor healthcare utilization (Doshi et al., 2020), and increased stress with consequent adverse health effects (Valentín-Cortés et al., 2020).

Discriminatory policing practices occurring over the life course have an intergenerational impact on health and socioeconomic and political consequences. Hypervigilance (heightened alertness and self-protection against trauma, often based on race, transgender status, or sexual orientation) is a key feature of PTSD. PTSD has been found to cause poor cardiovascular and metabolic health and sleep disturbances (Davis, 2020).

COMMUNITY VIOLENCE AND SOCIAL DISORDER

Community disorder is when a neighborhood environment has observable signs of a lack of social control, and the appearance of little concern for maintaining a safe and orderly physical environment. In disordered communities neighborhoods are plagued by dilapidated buildings, graffiti, litter, public drinking, drug use, and vandalism. There are visual cues that crime occurs at frequent intervals, including the frequent arrest of occupants and regularly seeing crime scene tape (Turner et al., 2013) (Fig. 5.9). Residential instability and frequent evictions also increase the likelihood of crime.

Residents of socially disordered communities often experience adverse health due to the stress of living in an unhealthy environment. These repetitive, stress-inducing events undermine physical health. Chronic stress causes elevations in allostatic load causing biological aging and wear and tear on the body, which explains why individuals exposed to community disorder and violence exhibit greater mental and physical health problems (Jackson et al., 2019).

The extent of disadvantage within a community can be determined by the level of education of community

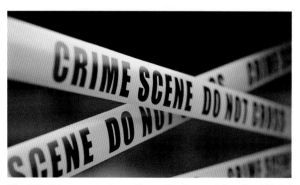

Fig. 5.9 Crime scene tape. (From iStock.com/MicroStockHub.)

residents, the number of individuals actively participating in the labor market, the quality of the housing, and the degree of poverty. These community characteristics play an essential role in health outcomes, above and beyond individual characteristics (Chamberlain et al., 2020). Living in a disadvantaged community increases morbidity and can greatly diminish life expectancy.

The social impact of living in disadvantaged and disordered communities is substantial. Community disadvantage undermines the ability to build social relationships between and among residents, which results in decreased social capital (Laurence, 2019). Younger people who live in disadvantaged communities reported fewer positive social interactions but an increase in the number of negative relations in the community, which ultimately diminished their sense of well-being. Feelings of powerlessness, alienation, and mistrust are common in disordered neighborhoods. Community disorder reduces available social support; residents are less likely to form social ties with neighbors because of the transient nature of the community, which results from the high turnover of tenants. Communities with a high degree of social disorder have increased susceptibility to a host of adverse health outcomes (Jackson et al., 2019). Signs of disordered communities include a high number of vacant and abandoned buildings, numerous liquor stores, and easy access to illicit drugs. Historically troubled relationships with police officers, officers' expressed bias toward marginalized communities, and community mistrust of officers hinder law enforcement's ability to curtail violence and crime. When there is a perceived or actual lack of safety in the community, residents avoid outdoor activities, thus reducing their physical activity. Residents may also engage in maladaptive coping patterns, such as substance use (cigarettes, alcohol, and drugs), becoming at risk for substance use disorder (Kondo et al., 2018).

Community violence and disorder can considerably impact residents' physical and psychological health. When there is concentrated poverty, high neighborhood turnover, overcrowded housing, and the absence of a sense of community, there is a high probability of crime (Kondo et al., 2018). In addition, the lack of a sense of community leads to diminished collective efficacy, a primary risk factor for violence. "Collective efficacy is defined as social cohesion among neighbors and their willingness to intervene for the common good" (Office of Policy Development & Research, 2016, paragraph 16).

SOCIAL COHESION, SOCIAL NETWORKS, AND SOCIAL CAPITAL

According to "Healthy People 2030," social cohesion describes the relationships and solidarity expressed among community members (USDHHS, ODPHP, n.d. a). Definitions of social cohesion have evolved. The following definitions highlight the essence of community social cohesion as cited in Fonseca and colleagues (2019, p. 235):

"Social cohesion involves building shared values and communities of interpretation, reducing disparities in wealth and income, and generally enabling people to have a sense that they are engaged in a common enterprise, facing shared challenges, and that they are members of the same community (Maxwell, 1996, p. 235)." And this definition was further expanded by (Jeannotte, 2003, p. 235) to, "the ongoing process of developing a community of shared values, shared challenges and equal opportunity within Canada, based on a sense of trust, hope and reciprocity among all Canadians." The OECD presents its concise definition that relies on three independent pillars: social inclusion, social capital, and social mobility: "A cohesive society works towards the wellbeing of all its members, fights exclusion and marginalization, creates a sense of belonging, promotes trust, and offers its members the opportunity of upward mobility" (Organisation for Economic Co-operation and Development [OECD], 2012, p. 235). Lastly, Peterson defines social cohesion as a construct linked to community participation with notions of trust, shared emotional commitment, and reciprocity (Peterson & Hughey, 2004).

These definitions provide an overall view of what social cohesion means concerning the community. Social cohesion comprises social trust and active participation in community activities and events. Social cohesion is a set of attitudes and norms that include trust, a sense of belonging, and the willingness to participate and help (Pérez et al., 2020). A cohesive community is necessary to attain common goals and solidarity among community members, and this collective efficacy enables the community to achieve their desired outcomes (Fonseca et al., 2019). An example of social cohesion within a community is illustrated by the establishment

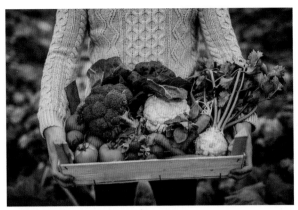

Fig. 5.10 Community garden. (From iStock.com/hobo_018.)

of a community garden. In one urban community in St. Louis, MO, community members came together to plan and build a community garden of vegetables with the goal of distributing the harvest to community members since the community was in a food desert (Fig. 5.10). Another example of what cohesive communities do is projects such as "Neighbor Helping Neighbors." The Neighbor Helping Neighbors Project is a mutual aid program in which neighbors provide services for each other. Neighbors in one local community who needed landscaping and grass-cutting services worked with another neighbor who needed work. The project was mutually beneficial.

Consider the following questions when determining the level and sense of cohesion in a specific community. First, what is the extent of neighborhood problems? What is the frequency of interactions among neighbors? What is the predominant race and ethnicity of the community? Do neighbors interact? What is the level of perceived safety in the community? Is there a sense of community or trustworthiness among community members? Is there civic engagement among community members? Are there planned community events? Finally, what is the sense of "self" in relation to the community?

Residents are more likely to have a sense of belonging and share feelings, aspirations, and goals in communities that establish trust, hold frequent meetings, invite community members to participate in community events and activities, welcome newcomers to the community, and create opportunities for community members to become engaged in activities and events. Social interaction and integration in communities have been associated with positive health outcomes (National

Research Council [US], Institute of Medicine, 2013). Social cohesion is known to build resilient communities. The success of communities depends on the relationships between and among members and their willingness to work toward mutual goals (Fonseca et al., 2019). Essential components of social cohesion include social capital, social networks, and forms of social support.

Social Capital and Social Networks

Social capital can be perceived as an individual, group, or community attribute. When viewed as an individual attribute, there are three types of social capital: bonding, bridging, and linking. Bonding occurs in homogenous groups where demographic characteristics, attitudes, and beliefs are similar. There are strong ties within the network. This type of social capital is usually seen among emotionally close individuals such as relatives and friends and most often provides needed social support. Social support is when people believe they are cared for, esteemed, and valued (Moore & Carpiano, 2020). A social network of family and friends promotes social and psychological health and is priceless when responding to stressful events (Rector, 2018). Bridging occurs through loosely connected social networks. Bridging is tied to professional networks, organizations, and associations and is helpful for sources of information and accessing resources. For example, bridging social capital can be seen in participation in community organizations where individuals access information about prospective employment, how to write a resume, or get the resources needed to help with a specific project. Linking is related to formal authoritative positions. Linking is when a community resident is connected to someone in power, such as a town hall council member, an alderman, or a mayor, to leverage their power and influence. The bonding, bridging, and linking framework can help map the types of networks available when conceptualizing social capital as a community.

In viewing social capital as a community attribute or collective, social capital refers to characteristics such as trust, norms, and networks that can influence the community's self-efficacy. Social capital depends on the ability of those living in the community to form and maintain positive relationships and networks with their neighbors. It involves resources and benefits accrued by memberships, connections, and interactions among community members (Westpbaln et al., 2020). According to Moore and Carpiano (2020), social capital is considered a group's network-based resources. Moore and Carpiano (2020) also suggest that social capital is a feature of a social organization that involves civic participation, norms of reciprocity, and trust in others. These characteristics are the property of the geographic locales and not individuals. Finally, social capital can be described as the relationships among people who live within a defined geographical territory or community, and those relationships enable the community to function effectively.

The National Social Capital Benchmark Community Survey is used to measure social capital. Elements of the survey capture a person's sense of belonging in relation to the community, frequency of connections to community members, community participation and involvement in activities and events related to community projects, spiritual events, social and recreational activities, and volunteerism. Social capital fosters norms of trust in the community, is based on reciprocity, and facilitates the attainment of collective or mutual goals. It is based on networks, norms, trust, and action-driven cooperation to accomplish community goals. Therefore, another essential step when attempting to engage communities is to harness social networks, such as faith communities, neighborhood associations, or block units, whose social capital can steer the collective approaches needed to improve community health (Clinical and Translational Science Awards Consortium, 2011).

Community churches are gathering places for residents, specifically Black communities, and are a source of information for those who reside there (McIntosh & Curry, 2020). Powell and colleagues (2021) found that 50% of Black Americans attend church weekly and 79% reported the significance of religion in their lives. Churches are well-established institutional structures in the community, well-respected, and viewed as advocates for the community.

Larger congregations, even those amid impoverished communities, offer programs that help strengthen the community (Fig. 5.11). For example, a large suburban church in North St. Louis County, a predominantly Black community, offered health education programs at their women's monthly fellowship meetings. A congregation member was a doctorally prepared nurse educator who presented educational information on various health-related topics, including high blood pressure, breast health and self-examinations, weight, obesity, diet, cholesterol, and the benefits of daily exercise. These classes, a midstream intervention, provided

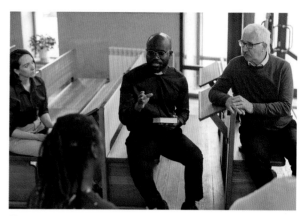

Fig. 5.11 Church congregants discussing community issues. (From iStock.com/shironosov.)

basic knowledge on health issues that plague Black communities and wellness strategies, including risk reduction.

In addition to health-related programs, many churches offer daycare services, tutoring programs for school-aged children, and GED classes for adults. Some churches focus on financial management to help communities pursue debt-relief strategies and more effectively manage their finances. Wong and colleagues (2018) found that many pastors provided counseling on substance use disorders. As a midstream intervention, nurses working in these communities could connect the pastor and the congregant with treatment referral centers. McIntosh and Curry (2020) illustrate how a partnership between a church and a high school positively influenced the educational attainment of students through relationship and community bridging.

Churches can play a crucial role in building community cohesion and resilience. Pastors can readily mobilize their members against social injustices in the community. Many significant civil rights leaders emerged from the church: Reverend Martin Luther King Jr., Congressman John Lewis (an ordained Baptist minister), Reverend Al Sharpton, and Reverend William Barber, the cofounder of the Poor People's Campaign—all activists—out of the church. This advocacy and activism led by church leaders could build greater resilience in communities with high levels of social disadvantage. This should involve pastors working collaboratively with local officials and cross-sector stakeholders to develop agendas, strategies, and tactics to improve the conditions of the community and advance health.

Interestingly, when disasters occur, such as floods, tsunamis, and hurricanes, federal responses are mostly related to shoring up physical infrastructure. This shoring up entails building flood walls, raising buildings on stilts, and requiring more stringent building codes; but seldom, if at all, does it focus on building community resilience, which is enhanced through social capital (Aldrich & Meyer, 2015). Community resilience is the ability to prepare, plan, absorb, and recover from an adverse event and the collective capacity of the community to address stressors and ultimately resume normal functioning (Aldrich & Meyer, 2015; National Academies of Sciences, Engineering, and Medicine [NASEM], 2021).

CONCLUSION

In conclusion, the social environment is a synthesized concept that incorporates the immediate physical infrastructure including the built environment, surrounding landscape, social relationships, and the people and their culture. It consists of individuals, families, and businesses in the community, including social networks, social capital, and cohesion (NASEM, 2017). Nurses must look beyond the downstream clinical care of an individual into the broader social and community contexts in which a person is born, grows, lives, works, and ages, and connect this context to their health and well-being. For marginalized communities, community stressors such as the lack of resources, the presence of environmental toxins and hazards, unemployment, and exposure to violence can have negative effects on health. This also includes children growing up in stressful environments with high levels of violence and crime who are at risk for a host of adverse health effects created by adverse childhood experiences. While social networks, capital, and cohesion can buffer some of the effects of stressed communities, they are not a panacea for restoring communities to a healthy state.

Nurses can engage in downstream, midstream, and upstream activities to help strengthen communities. An example of a downstream activity is when the nurse renders healthcare to a homeless individual who falls on broken glass when walking through a dilapidated vacant building and suffers a laceration. This care could be given in a homeless shelter or a hospital emergency room. Regardless of the setting, caring for the injury is a downstream intervention. A midstream intervention would be if the client were unhoused and perhaps sleeping on the streets and the nurse makes a referral or works with a caseworker to find a homeless shelter for the individual. The nurse refers him for services to meet his social needs. An upstream intervention is when the nurse works with local officials to ask why the dilapidated buildings have not been torn down. Going further, the nurse attends town hall meetings to increase the community's awareness of issues regarding derelict buildings and advocates for municipal solutions. At the grassroots level, the nurse, in concert with communities that have strong collective efficacy, could put pressure on city officials to address the issue. Upstream interventions focus on the fundamental issues that affect communities and look toward policies to resolve those issues. Examples of other advocacy opportunities for nurses to become involved in upstream interventions that address social and community contexts include helping community members learn how to set up voter registration booths so that community members can become more civically engaged or working with community networks to support summer programs for young children in disadvantaged communities. These interventions require multisector engagement with community residents, local businesses, and community officials, and working with interprofessional partners.

While nurses have been taught to practice holistic care, few learn about the social and community contexts of their patients. As mentioned, health is more than clinical services; it is linked to social and environmental contexts. Nurses have a role and duty to work with other professionals to address social and environmental contexts to achieve health equity (NASEM, 2021a). Nonprofit hospitals should assess and respond to the needs of the community where the hospital is located. However, there is currently no accountability for nonprofit hospitals to address the SDOH within communities (Swider et al., 2017). Nurses can raise awareness among leaders in the community, advocates, and activists for health about the potential for community benefit investments to address the SDOH in the community and improve the overall health of the community (Swider et al., 2017). Nurses should engage with their interprofessional partners and other sectors to advance health (NASEM, 2021a). This includes addressing congressional leaders about community investments that would improve the health of the community. Nursing education must learn to create opportunities for students to become more involved in interprofessional collaborative partnerships and advocacy if nurses are ever to move beyond caring for the individual before them without considering the patient's social environment.

BOX 5.3   Community Immersion Exemplar

Exemplar: Learning the Social and Community Context through a Community Immersion Experience

Experiential learning opportunities where people are born, grow, live, work, and age can facilitate the student's under-standing of the conditions that impact health. Optimal sites for this type of learning include, but are not limited to, hair salons, homeless shelters, housing projects, schools, churches, community recreation centers, public libraries, and parks. When time is spent in spaces where people live, insight into the social and structural factors that impact the individual's health and community's health is gained.

In one private university, students were enrolled in a social determinants of health course that used the flipped classroom concept. Students prepared beforehand through assignments and readings and then spent the scheduled class time discussing the content. This active learning approach sparks deeper learning than learning through passively listening to lectures.

The course consisted of two in-class sessions, the initial and the last. Between these two sessions, students were expected to spend the regularly scheduled class time in the community, which enabled them to avoid scheduling con-flicts since that class time was already committed. In the first-in-class session, students received the course orientation, an overview of the SDOH, and information on a final course project. In the final in-class session, students presented the course project. Between class sessions, students engaged in weekly online discussions to facilitate their understanding of the SDOH and allow them to consider upstream approaches for improving health.

Through established networks, course faculty connected students with a community mentor in an under-resourced community. The community mentor knew the community and the community's needs and resources and agreed to serve as a mentor for the student. Over the semester, the community mentor facilitated the student's connection with additional community members, professionals within the community, business leaders, and civic leaders. By the third week of the course, students worked collaboratively with the community mentor, assigned faculty, and other community members to develop a community project based on a community-identified need. The final in-class session was held in the evening, dinner was provided, and the mentor was invited to attend the session. The focus was the course deliverable, the student's presentation of the community project. The evaluation component consisted of faculty feedback, mentor input, and the student's assessment of their level of knowledge recognizing the SDOH and the relationship of the SDOH on health and health outcomes, in addition to their overall satisfaction with the course.

From Schroeder, K., Garcia, B., Phillips, R. S., & Lipman, T. H. (2019). Addressing social determinants of health through community engagement: An undergraduate nursing course. *Journal of Nursing Education, 58*(7), 423–426. Reprinted with permission from SLACK Incorporated.

STUDENT REFLECTION QUESTIONS AND LEARNING ACTIVITIES

1. How could nurse-led clinics and CHWs improve social and community environments?
2. How does civic participation impact health?
3. What is the impact of the social environment on health?
4. Box 5.3 highlights a student's experiential learning experience.

REFERENCES

Acker, J., Braveman, P., Arkin, E., Leviton, L., Parsons, J., & Hobor, G. (2019). *Mass incarceration threatens health equity in Amer-ica. Executive summary.* Robert Wood Johnson Foundation.

Agency for Healthcare Research and Quality. (2021). *2019 National healthcare quality and disparities report.* Agency for Healthcare Research and Quality. https://www.ahrq.gov/research/findings/nhqrdr/nhqdr19/index.html.

Agency for Healthcare Research and Quality. (2022). *2022 National healthcare quality and disparities report.* Agency for Healthcare Research and Quality. https://www.ahrq.gov/sites/default/files/wysiwyg/research/findings/nhqrdr/2022qdr-final-es.pdf.

Aldrich, D. P., & Meyer, M. A. (2015). Social capi-tal and community resilience. *American Behavioral Scientist, 59*(2), 254–269. https://doi.org/10.1177/0002764214550299.

Alexander, M. (2020). *The new Jim Crow: Mass incarceration in the age of colorblindness* (Tenth Anniversary Edition). The New Press.

American Association of Colleges of Nursing (AACN). (2023). Enhancing diversity in the nursing workforce. https://www.aacnnursing.org/news-data/fact-sheets/enhancing-diversity-in-the-nursing-workforce#:~:text=Considering%20racial%20backgrounds%2C%20the%20RN,report%20their%20ethnicity%20as%20Hispanic.

American Public Health Association [APHP]. (2014). *Support for community health workers to increase health access and to reduce health inequities.* American Public Health Association. https://www.apha.org/policies-and-advocacy/public-health-policy-statements/policy-database/2014/07/09/14/19/support-for-community-health-workers-to-increase-health-access-and-to-reduce-health-inequities.

Barnett, E., & Casper, M. (2011). Research: A definition of "social environment. *American Journal of Public Health, 91*(3), 465.

Braveman, P. A., Arkin, E., Proctor, D., Kauh, T., & Holm, N. (2022). Systemic and structural racism: Definitions, examples, health damages, and approaches to dismantling. *Health Affairs, 41*(2), 171–178. https://doi.org/10.1377/hlthaff.2021.0139.

Brink, M. (2021). *The next four years: What Biden should prioritize on policing and criminal justice reform.* American Bar Association. https://www.americanbar.org/groups/crsj/publications/human_rights_magazine_home/the-next-four-years/policing-and-criminal-justice-reform/.

Brooks Carthon, J. M., Sammarco, T., Pancir, D., Chittams, J., & Wiltse Nicely, K. (2017). Growth in retail-based clinics after nurse practitioner scope of practice reform. *Nursing Outlook, 65*(2), 195–201. https://doi.org/10.1016/j.outlook.2016.11.001.

Brulle, R. J., & Pellow, D. N. (2006). Environmental justice: Human health and environmental inequalities. *Annual Review of Public Health, 27*, 103–124. https://doi.org/10.1146/annurev.publhealth.27.021405.102124.

Center on Society and Health. (2014). *Why education matters to health: Exploring the causes. Issue Brief 2.* VCU. Retrieved from https://societyhealth.vcu.edu/work/the-projects/why-education-matters-to-health-exploring-the-causes.html.

Chae, D. H., Wang, Y., Martz, C. D., Slopen, N., Yip, T., Adler, N. E., Fuller-Rowell, T. E., Lin, J., Matthews, K. A., Brody, G. H., Spears, E. C., Puterman, E., & Epel, E. S. (2020). Racial discrimination and telomere shortening among African Americans: The Coronary Artery Risk Development in Young Adults (CARDIA) study. *Health Psychology, 39*(3), 209–219. https://doi.org/10.1037/hea0000832.

Chamberlain, A. M., Rutten, Finney, L., J., Wilson, P. M., Fan, C., Boyd, C. M., Jacobson, D. J., Rocca, W. A., & St. Sauver, J. L. (2020). Neighborhood socioeconomic disadvantage is associated with multimorbidity in a geographically-defined community. *BMC Public Health, 20*(1), 13. https://doi.org/10.1186/s12889-019-8123-0.

Chen, X., Orom, H., Hay, J. L., Waters, E. A., Schofield, E., Li, Y., & Kiviniemi, M. T. (2019). Differences in rural and urban health information access and use. *The Journal of Rural Health, 35*(3), 405–417. https://doi.org/10.1111/jrh.12335.

Clinical and Translational Science Awards Consortium. (2011). *Principles of community engagement.* National Institute of Health, Publication No. 11-7782.

Crowley, R. A. Health and Public Policy Committee of the American College of Physicians. (2016). Climate change and health: A position paper of the American College of Physicians. *Annals of Internal Medicine, 164*(9), 608–610. https://doi.org/10.7326/M15-2766.

Cusick, D. (2021). Trees are missing in low income neighborhoods. *Scientific American.* https://www.scientificamerican.com/article/trees-are-missing-in-low-income-neighborhoods/.

Davis, B. A. (2020). Discrimination: A social determinant of health inequities. (Health Affairs Blog). *Primary Care Collaborative.* Retrieved from https://thepcc.org/2020/02/26/discrimination-social-determinant-health-inequities.

Doshi, M., Lopez, W. D., Mesa, H., Bryce, R., Rabinowitz, E., Rion, R., & Fleming, P. J. (2020). Barriers & facilitators to healthcare and social services among undocumented Latino(a)/Latinx immigrant clients: Perspectives from frontline service providers in Southeast Michigan. *PloS One, 15*(6), e0233839. https://doi.org/10.1371/journal.pone.0233839.

Fleming, P. J., Lopez, W. D., Spolum, M., Anderson, R. E., Reyes, A. G., & Schulz, A. J. (2022). Policing is a public health issue: The important role of health educators. *Health Education and Behavior, 48*(5), 553–558. https://doi.org/10.1177/10901981211001010.

Fonseca, X., Lukosch, S., & Brazier, F. (2019). Social cohesion revisited: A new definition and how to characterize it. *Innovation: The European Journal of Social Science Research, 32*(2), 231–253. https://doi.org/10.1080/13511610.2018.1497480.

Health Resources and Services Administration (HRSA). (n.d.). *MUA Find.* https://data.hrsa.gov/tools/shortage-area/mua-find.

Inman, S. N. (n.d.). Racial disparities in criminal justice: How lawyers can help. American Bar Association. https://www.americanbar.org/groups/young_lawyers/publications/after-the-bar/public-service/racial-disparities-criminal-justice-how-lawyers-can-help/.

Jackson, D. B., Posick, C., & Vaughn, M. G. (2019). New evidence of the nexus between neighborhood violence, perceptions of danger, and child health. *Health Affairs (Project Hope), 38*(5), 746–754. https://doi.org/10.1377/hlthaff.2018.05127.

Jeannotte, M. S. (2003). Singing alone? The contribution of cultural capital to social cohesion and sustainable communities. *The International Journal of Cultural Policy, 9*(1), 35–49.

Joint Center for Political and Economic Studies. (2012). *Place matters for health in New Orleans parish: Ensuring opportunities for good health for all*. Joint Center for Political and Economic Studies.

Joint Center for Political and Economic Studies. (n.d.). *Place matters: Advancing health equity*. Joint Center for Political and Economic Studies.

Julion, W., Reed, M., Bounds, D. T., Cothran, F., Gamboa, C., & Sumo, J. (2019). A group think tank as a discourse coalition to promote minority nursing faculty retention. *Nursing Outlook, 67*, 586–595.

JUSTIA. (n.d.). *Shelley v. Kraemer*, 334 U.S. 1 (1948). https://supreme.justia.com/cases/federal/us/334/1/.

Kaiser Family Foundation (KFF). (2023). Primary healthy care HPSA designations as of September 2022. https://www.kff.org/other/state-indicator/primary-care-health-professional-shortage-areas-hpsas/?activeTab=map&currentTimeframe=0&selectedDistributions=total-primary-care-hpsa-designations&sortModel=%7B%22colId%22:%22Location%22,%22sort%22:%22asc%22%7D.

Kondo, M. C., Andreyeva, E., South, E. C., MacDonald, J. M., & Branas, C. C. (2018). Neighborhood interventions to reduce violence. *Annual Review of Public Health, 39*, 253–271. https://doi.org/10.1146/annurev-publhealth-040617-014600.

Laurence, J. (2019). Community disadvantage, inequalities in adolescent subjective wellbeing, and local social relations: The role of positive and negative social interactions. *Social Science & Medicine (1982), 237*, 112442. https://doi.org/10.1016/j.socscimed.2019.112442.

LeClair, J., Watts, T., & Zahner, S. (2021). Nursing strategies for environmental justice: A scoping review. *Public Health Nursing, 38*(2), 296–308. https://doi.org/10.1111/phn.12840.

LaVeist, T. A., & Pierre, G. (2014). Integrating the 3Ds–social determinants, health disparities, and health-care workforce diversity. *Public Health Reports, 129*(Suppl. 2), 9–14. https://doi.org/10.1177/00333549141291S204.

Liu, C. F., Hebert, P. L., Douglas, J. H., Neely, E. L., Sulc, C. A., Reddy, A., Sales, A. E., & Wong, E. S. (2020). Outcomes of primary care delivery by nurse practitioners: Utilization, cost, and quality of care. *Health Services Research, 55*(2), 178–189. https://doi.org/10.1111/1475-6773.13246.

Maryland Humanities. (2021). *Civic participation and the social determinants of health*. https://www.mdhumanities.org/2021/03/civic-participation-and-the-social-determinants-of-health/.

Maxwell, J. (1996). *Social dimensions of economic growth*. University of Alberta.

Mcintosh, R., & Curry, K. (2020). The role of a Black church-school partnership in supporting the educational achievement of African American students. *School Community Journal, 30*(1), 161–189.

Moore, S., & Carpiano, R. M. (2020). Introduction to the special issue on social capital and health: What have we learned in the last 20 years and where do we go from here? *Social Science and Medicine, (1982), 257*, 113014.

National Academies of Sciences, Engineering, and Medicine (NASEM). (2021a). *Enhancing community resilience through social capital and connectedness: Stronger together!*. The National Academies Press. https://doi.org/10.17226/26123.

National Academies of Sciences, Engineering, and Medicine (NASEM). (2021). *The future of nursing 2020–2030: Charting a path to achieve health equity*. The National Academies Press. https://doi.10.17226/25982.

National Academies of Sciences, Engineering, and Medicine (NASEM); Health and Medicine Division, Board on Population Health and Public Health Practice; Committee on Community-Based Solutions to Promote Health Equity in the United States. In Baciu, A., Negussie, Y., Geller, A., & Weinstein, J. N. (Eds.) (2017). *Communities in action: Pathways to health equity*. National Academies Press (US).

National Association of Realtors. (2018). You can't live here: Enduring impacts of restrictive covenants. https://www.nar.realtor/sites/default/files/documents/2018-February-Fair-Housing-Story.pdf

National Nurse-Led Care Consortium (NNLC). (n.d.). About us. https://nurseledcare.phmc.org/about/about-us.html

National Research Council (US), Institute of Medicine (2013). In Woolf, S. H., & Aron, L. (Eds.), *US health in international perspective: Shorter lives, poorer health*. National Academies Press.

Neff, J., Holmes, S. M., Knight, K. R., Strong, S., Thompson-Lastad, A., McGuinness, C., Duncan, L., Saxena, N., Harvey, M. J., Langford, A., Carey-Simms, K. L., Minahan, S. N., Satterwhite, S., Ruppel, C., Lee, S., Walkover, L., De Avila, J., Lewis, B., Matthews, J., & Nelson, N. (2020). Structural competency: Curriculum for medical students, residents, and interprofessional teams on the structural factors that produce health disparities. *MedEdPORTAL: The Journal of Teaching and Learning Resources, 16*, 10888. https://doi-org.ezp.slu.edu/10.15766/mep_2374-8265.10888.

Novak, N. L, Geronimus, A. T., & Martinez-Cardoso, A. M. (2017). Change in birth outcomes among infants born to Latina mothers after a major immigration raid. *International Journal of Epidemiology, 46*(3), 839–849. https://doi.org/10.1093/ije/dyw346.

Office of Policy Development & Research. (2016). *Evidence matters: Neighborhoods and violent crime*. https://www.huduser.gov/portal/periodicals/em/summer16/highlight2.html

Organisation for Economic Co-operation and Development (OECD). (2012). *Social cohesion in a shifting world. Perspectives on global development 2012*. https://www.oecd-ilibrary.org/development/

perspectives-on-global-development-2012_persp_glob_dev-2012-en

Pérez, E., Braën, C., Boyer, G., Mercille, G., Rehany, É., Deslauriers, V., Bilodeau, A., & Potvin, L. (2020). Neighbourhood community life and health: A systematic review of reviews. *Health & Place, 61*, 102238. https://doi.org/10.1016/j.healthplace.2019.102238.

Peterson, M., & Brinkley-Rubinstein, L. (2021). Incarceration is a health threat. Why isn't it monitored like one. *Health Affairs Blog.* https://doi:10.1377/hblog20211014.242754.

Peterson, N. A., & Hughey, J. (2004). Social cohesion and intrapersonal empowerment: Gender as moderator. *Health Education Research, 19*, 533–542. https://doi:10.1093/her/cyg057.

Poghosyan, L., & Carthon, J. M. B. (2017). The untapped potential of the nurse practitioner workforce in reducing health disparities. *Policy, Politics & Nursing Practice, 18*(2), 84–94. https://doi.org/10.1177/1527154417721189.

Powell, T. W., West, K. R., & Turner, C. E. (2021). Size matters: Addressing social determinants of health through black churches. *Journal of Racial and Ethnic Health Disparities, 8*(1), 237–244. https://doi.org/10.1007/s40615-020-00777-9.

Rector, C. (2018). *Community and public health nursing: Promoting the public health* (9th ed.). Wolter Kluwer. https://pubhtml5.com/dhqc/dldj/basic.

Robert Wood Johnson Foundation (RWJF). (2015). *Babies born just miles apart face large gaps in life expectancy.* https://www.rwjf.org/en/library/articles-and-news/2015/04/babies-born-just-miles-apart-in-cities-across-the-u-s-face-larg.html

Robert Wood Johnson Foundation (RWJF). (2018). What's the connection between residential segregation and health? *Culture of Health Blog.* https://www.rwjf.org/en/blog/2016/03/whats-the-connection-between-residential-segregation-and-health.html.

Schroeder, K., Garcia, B., Phillips, R. S., & Lipman, T. H. (2019). Addressing social determinants of health through community engagement: An undergraduate nursing course. *Journal of Nursing Education, 58*(7), 423–426.

Statista Research Department. (2021). *Rate of fatal police shootings in the United States from 2015 to November 2021, by ethnicity.* https://www.statista.com/statistics/1123070/police-shootings-rate-ethnicity-us/

Swider, S. M., Berkowitz, B., Valentine-Maher, S., Zenk, S. N., & Bekemeier, B. (2017). Engaging communities in creating health: Leveraging community benefit. *Nursing Outlook, 65*(5), 657–660. https://doi.org/10.1016/j.outlook.2017.08.002.

The Sentencing Project. (2018). *Report of the Sentencing Project to the United Nations special rapporteur on contemporary forms of racism, racial discrimination, xenophobia, and related intolerance: Regarding racial disparities in the United States criminal justice system.* The Sentencing Project.

The Sentencing Project. (2021). *Fact sheet: Trends in U.S. Corrections.* The Sentencing Project.

Theall, K. P., Francois, S., Bell, C. N., Anderson, A., Chae, D., & LaVeist, T. A. (2022). Neighborhood police encounters, health, and violence in a Southern city. *Health Affairs, 41*(2), 228–236. https://doi.org/10.1377/hlthaff.2021.01428.

Torres, J. M., Deardorff, J., Gunier, R. B., Harley, K. G., Alkon, A., Kogut, K., & Eskenazi, B. (2018). Worry about deportation and cardiovascular disease risk factors among adult women: The Center for the Health Assessment of Mothers and Children of Salinas study. *Annals of Behavioral Medicine, 52*(2), 186–193. https://doi.org/10.1093/abm/kax007.

Turner, H. A., Shattuck, A., Hamby, S., & Finkelhor, D. (2013). Community disorder, victimization exposure, and mental health in a national sample of youth. *Journal of Health and Social Behavior, 54*(2), 258–275. https://doi.org/10.1177/0022146513479384.

US Census Bureau. (2021). Quick facts. https://www.census.gov/quickfacts/fact/table/US/RHI225219

US Department of Health and Human Services (USDHHS), Office of Disease Prevention and Health Promotion (ODPHP). (n.d.). *Discrimination.* https://health.gov/healthypeople/objectives-and-data/social-determinants-health/literature-summaries/discrimination

US Department of Health and Human Services (USDHHS), Office of Disease Prevention and Health Promotion (ODPHP). (n.d. a). *Social cohesion.* https://health.gov/healthypeople/objectives-and-data/social-determinants-health/literature-summaries/social-cohesion

US Department of Health and Human Services (USDHHS), Office of Disease Prevention and Health Promotion (ODPHP). (2018). *Social and community context.* https://www.healthypeople.gov/subtopics-of-sdoh/social-and-community-context.

US Department of Health and Human Services (USDHHS), Office of Disease Prevention and Health Promotion (ODPHP). (2021). *Determinants of health.* https://www.healthypeople.gov/2020/about/foundation-health-measures/Determinants-of-Health

US Department of Housing and Urban Development. (2011). Office of Policy Development and Research. In *Evidence matters: Transforming knowledge into housing and community development policy.* https://www.huduser.gov/portal/periodicals/em/winter11/highlight2.html.

US Department of Justice. (2021). *The Fair Housing Act.* https://www.justice.gov/crt/fair-housing-act-1.

Valentín-Cortés, M., Benavides, Q., Bryce, R., Rabinowitz, E., Rion, R., Lopez, W. D., & Fleming, P. J. (2020). Application of the minority stress theory: Understanding the mental health of undocumented Latinx immigrants. *American Journal of Community Psychology, 66*(3–4), 325–336. https://doi.org/10.1002/ajcp.12455.

Westpbaln, K. D., Fry-Bowers, E. K., & Gorges, J. M. (2020). Social capital: A concept analysis. *Advances in Nursing Science, 43*(2), E80–E111. https://doi:10.1097/ANS.0000000000000296.

WHO. (2012). *Social and environmental determinants of health and health inequalities in Europe: Fact sheet.* https://www.euro.who.int/data/assets/pdf_file/0006/185217/Social-and-environmental-determinants-Fact-Sheet.pdf

Wikipedia. (2023). List of unarmed African Americans killed by law enforcement officers in the United States. https://en.wikipedia.org/wiki/List_of_unarmed_African_Americans_killed_by_law_enforcement_officers_in_the_United_States

Williams, D. R. (2021). Why discrimination is a health issue. *Culture of Health Blog.* Robert Wood Johnson Foundation. https://www.rwjf.org/en/blog/2017/10/discrimination-is-a-health-issue.html.

Williams, D. R., Lawrence, J. A., & Davis, B. A. (2019). Understanding how discrimination can affect health. *Health Services Research, 54,* 1374–1388.

Wong, E. C., Derose, K. P., Litt, P., & Miles, J. N. V. (2018). Sources of care for alcohol and other drug problems: The role of the African American church. *Journal of Religion and Health, 57*(4), 1200–1210. https://doi.org/10.1007/s10943-017-0412-2.

Race, Racism, Bias, Discrimination, and Privilege

Roberta Waite, Deena A. Nardi

We are haunted in America by our history of racial inequality.
—Equal Justice Initiative (2021, paragraph 1)

CHAPTER OUTLINE

LEARNING OBJECTIVES

1. Explore the relationships between racism, race, racialization, and the consequences of White settler colonization.
2. Describe the direct and indirect influences of racism on mental and physical health and healthcare.
3. Identify actions that nurses in education and clinical practice can take to advance health equity.
4. Explain the groundwater approach and its use as a template to understand and challenge structural racism.
5. Examine an antiracism action that can be useful to you in healthcare practice or education. Explain why and how you would use it and for what outcomes.

RACISM AND HEALTH

Dr. Susan Moore, University of Michigan Medical School graduate, member of Delta Sigma Theta sorority, internist, mother, caregiver, Black woman, activist, and 52 years old, was hospitalized after testing positive for coronavirus disease 2019 (COVID-19). She had a long history of sarcoidosis, a chronic, inflammatory disease of the lungs and lymph nodes, documented in her medical records. Yet she maintains in a videotape from her first hospital bed, "he did not even listen to my lungs, he didn't touch me in any way" and suggested she just go home (Maybank et al., 2020, paragraph 3). She videotaped her unanswered requests for pain medications for comfort and to help her breathe, and to receive treatment with Remdesevir, the antiviral treatment used in

COVID treatment. Responses she received included: "You are not even short of breath." "Yes, I am!" she responded (CNN, 2020, paras 3–4). She says, "[The doctor] made me feel like I was a drug addict … and he knew I was a physician" (Lewis, 2020, paragraph 5). She was discharged but then rushed to a different hospital 12 hours later in distress with a high fever and drop in blood pressure, bacterial pneumonia, COVID pneumonia, and new lymphadenopathy. She was transferred to the ICU the next day, where she died 2 weeks later. In an interview in the *Times*, her son said, "Nearly every time she went to the hospital, she had to advocate for herself, fight for something in some way, shape or form, just to get baseline, proper care" (Eligon, 2020, para. 19). *Note: Dr. Moore's name is used in this case study to honor her activism for equality in healthcare; her story is a matter of public record, so we say her name. See "Say her name"* (Maybank et al., 2020).

Dr. Moore's struggle to be heard did not occur centuries ago as part of the US history of enslavement, the Civil War to end it, or the extended Jim Crow era of segregation and discrimination that followed it. It happened during the development of Healthy People 2030's overarching goal, which was to eliminate health disparities and achieve health equity (Health.Gov, 2021).

Coordinated actions between all areas of healthcare—education, prevention, access, treatment, and follow-up—are needed to prevent the inequities and disparities prevalent among historically marginalized and racialized groups. Health disparities, or critically uneven health outcomes, are often linked synergistically (e.g., depression can worsen anxiety and anxiety can worsen depression; poverty and abuse potentiate both). Disparities can be caused and potentiated by inequities in health resources and access to healthcare across society. Health equity is the fair and just opportunity to live the healthiest life possible (Pastor et al., 2018). The use of a health equity framework, which targets racism, poverty, discrimination, and other social and structural determinants of health (SDOH), can guide coordinated actions to directly target these influencers to mitigate or eliminate them and their effects (Table 6.1). An example of coordination of action and purpose to pursue health equity in patient care is as follows: (1) At the personal, individual level, nurses can improve their understanding of the healthcare needs and values of the populations they work with, so they can support their patients' voices and choices. They must identify and access resources needed to add to their patients' health capital and thus reduce illness burden as much as possible. (2) At the institutional level, these resources used by direct care nurses include policies and practices that should be regularly critiqued, audited, developed, and applied to identify known SDOH and guide healthcare practice. (3) At the structural, systemic level, nursing leaders in education, research, administration, and direct healthcare practice and policy positions are uniquely situated to direct the needed coordination between direct healthcare, primary and specialty care, and planned follow-up to mitigate the risks associated with SDOH in patients' lives.

Health equity requires valuing all individuals and populations equally and an equal distribution of resources, which are the structural and SDOH. As illustrated in Fig. 6.1, SDOH are the conditions—structural, environmental, and cultural—in the various settings or places in which everyone functions, including schools, housing, places of employment and worship, and where we live, work, eat, learn, pray, and play, that influence our health, quality of life, and overall physical, mental, emotional, and social functioning. These SDOH are shaped by influences outside healthcare, such as policies and political structures, internal biases, sex (globally, females are more likely than males to be poor, unemployed, and work in places with no healthcare benefits), economics, education and its absence, wars, and the displacement of peoples. The WHO formed a Commission on the Social Determinants of Health in 2005 that recommended that the unequal distribution of power, money, and resources, the structural drivers of health inequities, be tackled locally, nationally, and globally. Noting that "health systems will not naturally gravitate towards equity," they called for health and health equity to be a marker for the performance of government policies and programs (WHO, 2021, paragraph 4).

The latest pandemic of the severe acute respiratory syndrome COVID-19 uncovered persistent inequities in access to quality healthcare, health and wellness resources, providers, and treatments for historically marginalized minorities in the United States. In July 2020, Black and Latina women comprised 70% of pregnant women infected with COVID-19 in the United States (Bowen, 2020). By December 2020, Black and Latina women with COVID-19 were hospitalized 4.7 times more often than White patients, with Black patients twice as likely to die from the infection (Klugman & Patel, 2021). These statistics should not be surprising to providers familiar with what is already known about the impact of significant disparities in the United States among racialized people of color.

Disparities in prevalence, treatment, and outcomes for Black, Latinx, Indigenous, and other historically marginalized populations with hypertension, diabetes, asthma, stroke, major depressive disorder, and breast and other cancers (Mobula et al., 2020) confound the body's response to pandemics, stressors, and COVID-19; this is why they are termed *chronic, complex diseases*. A summary of health outcomes from a 2020 report on disparities by race and ethnicity by the Center for American Progress is presented next, providing a snapshot of the egregious lack of progress in eliminating disparities for African Americans (AA), Hispanics or Latin (H/L), Asian Americans (AS) Native Hawaiian or Pacific

TABLE 6.1   Social and Structural Determinants of Health: Considerations to Guide Assessment

Determinants	Considerations
Discrimination	The realities of discrimination can traumatize and shape physical and mental health, and affect a person's trust in a system and its providers and one's willingness to use primary care resources, such as vaccinations, to support health. *How are individuals engaged to ascertain if they have been treated disrespectfully or judged unfairly?*
Early child development	Learning opportunities for very young children are crucial to their social development and lifelong health. *What form of early child development activities are children engaged in?*
Education and higher education	*Enrollment in higher education decreases risks to health since it provides access to more resources.* Are children regularly in school? If not, what prevents their regular attendance? Do they perceive school as a positive resource or negative obligation?
Employment	Being employed and earning a living wage mitigate risks to health since sources of access are increased. Is there accessibility of working full or part time? Are healthcare benefits provided by the employer? Is there a threat of unemployment? Are wages at the povorty level? *All these determinants affect the amount and quality of resources used to support health.*
Environmental	Landscape architecture informs conservation, construction, and preservation of spaces, which has implications for one's health. *Are individuals exposed to toxic waste, garbage dumps, disposals, or waste or chemical processing plants? Is lead exposure probable? Are there green spaces (parks) or playgrounds to exercise?*
Access to healthy food	Food deserts are areas and communities that do not have a full-service food/grocery store, limiting access to or making it difficult to find healthy food choices on a regular basis. *Are there local farmers markets? How many grocery stores?*
Health systems	*Access to quality healthcare across the lifespan is important to support overall health.* Is there a primary care provider accessible? Does the family have and use insurance? What is the type and can they afford to pay premiums? Does it provide adequate coverage for health visits and events? What is their health literacy?
Housing	*Residing in a comfortable and safe place has health implications.* Is housing adequate? Is it temporary or otherwise unstable? Is it close to public transportation and school(s)? Are conditions sanitary?
Social exclusion	*One's relational stance to resources impacts health.* Are they involved and engaged in the social life of the community or their family? Are they part of a spiritual, social, or education group in comfortable and welcoming contexts?
Racism	*A system of beliefs and practices that anchors power and well-being of dominant races at the expense of historically excluded races; this impacts health disproportionately.* Is there segregation of schools, neighborhoods, and workplaces? Are redlining practices by lending institutions operational? Are voting restrictions and immigration policies racially inequitable?
Crime, violence, and incarceration	*Living in an unsafe environment and exposure to crime and violence comprise a critical public health issue.* It can lead to a host of physical and mental health conditions, including posttraumatic stress disorder, anxiety, depression, behavioral problems in children, and increased risk of death and disability. Is policing of crime disproportional based on location? Are effective strategies for community policing enforced? Are adequate resources provided for nonviolent offenses?

Islanders (NH-PIA), and American Indians and Alaska Natives (AI/AN) compared with non-Hispanic Whites (NHW) (Carratala & Maxwell, 2021).

- Maternal mortality for AA both during and after birth is three times higher than for NHW.
- Infant deaths for AA are twice as high, at 11.0. There are 11 infant deaths per 1,000 live births among Black Americans. This is almost twice the national average of 5.8 infant deaths per 1000 live births.

- 42% of AA over 20 have hypertension compared with 28.7% of NHW over 20.
- 12.6% of AA children under 20 have asthma compared with 7.7% of NHW under 20.
- 21.5% of H/L over 20 have diabetes compared with 13% of NHW over 20.
- AS are 40% more likely to be diagnosed with diabetes than NHW.

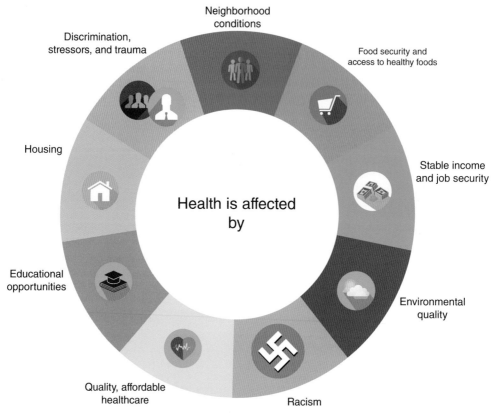

Fig. 6.1 Social and structural determinants of health.

- AS are 80% more likely to be diagnosed with end-stage renal disease than NHW.
- NH-PIA are 3 times more likely to have diabetes than NHW and 2.5 times more likely to die from diabetes.
- The rate of infection with HIV for NH-PIA is twice as high as in NHW.

If these chronic conditions are not seen as confounding each other and intersecting with other diseases and environmental contexts, then the severity of manifestations of illness intensifies, because assessment, treatment, and needed follow-up become inadequate to care or cure. Health providers at all levels of practice must take these disparities and the structural conditions that cause and aggravate them into account to provide, as Dr. Moore's son said, "basic, proper care" (Associated Press, 2020, p. 11). The role of racism in the creation and persistence of these health disparities has been long acknowledged and well documented. Racism has been called a web of "actions, beliefs, and economic, political, social and cultural structures" that

allocate power and privilege to benefit the dominant (majority) racial group (Thurman et al., 2019). Racism is a SDOH named one of several types of discrimination in Healthy People 2030 (Health.Gov, 2021); but without addressing racism forthrightly as a root cause of these disparities, substantive movement toward health equity will not occur.

Racism has been most recently recognized as such by the American Association of Colleges of Nursing (AACN) in its "Essentials: Competencies for Professional Nursing Education" (AACN, 2021), calling for nurse educators to promote social justice by removing systemic racism, inequities, and discrimination in how students are prepared for practice. Yet it does not clearly and directly advocate the use of an antiracism approach to reach this goal, which is *essential* for undoing racism, the powerful and persistent SDOH that it has already identified. There remains much work for the profession to directly acknowledge, uncover, and target these inequities and do so forthrightly.

An antiracist framework can be used to understand how SDOH can be assessed and mitigated equally across all patient population groups, including Indigenous peoples, migrants, immigrants, and refugee groups. Antiracism operationally employs a process of recognizing and exterminating racism by decisively appraising and reforming systems, institutional structures, policies, and language to reallocate power equitably. This requires nursing programs to not focus merely on cultural competency but to apply this learning explicitly to address racism and mobilize antiracism efforts. Furthermore, a structural competency skill set is needed to perceive how profoundly rooted social dynamics of power, opportunity, and wellness are drawn along racial lines. Germane to structural competency is recognizing social and environmental structures that affect clinical encounters, cultivating insights into structures from other branches, learning beyond nursing courses, fostering critical consciousness of structural humility, and recognizing structural violence—social provisions that are detrimental to individuals and populations. Nursing must adopt an antiracist framework applying structural competency skills if we truly aspire to dismantle, reimagine, and redesign healthcare and the promotion of health justice in our society. Indisputably, health is a right, and applying an antiracist approach is its right bearer (Crear-Perry et al., 2020).

To advance these efforts it is important to empower yourself, ask the right questions, reach out, and use resources at hand to mitigate risk, promote trust, and improve health outcomes. The National League for Nursing's (NLN) vision series directs faculty to integrate SDOH into the nursing curriculum (NLN, 2019). This also requires updating of teaching tools and resources used in teaching therapeutic communication with diverse patients; assessment of not only the identified patient but the neighborhood, family, and cultural context; how to partner in direct care provision; and follow-up care after direct care. These SDOH would then be better integrated into the teaching of holistic assessment and understood as an essential part of clinical education experiences.

Types of Racism

When black people are killed by the police, "racism" isn't the right word.

—*Kihana Miraya Ross (2020, p. 1)*

Racism has been used as a catch-all or umbrella term for discrimination, bias, and unfair and inequitable treatment, but it is much more than that. Racism is a complex system of actions—personal, in institutions, and across systems and society—the purpose of which is to dehumanize, exploit, and/or eliminate the "other." These actions are based on a learned refusal to acknowledge the humanity and equal rights of another group of people or person. There are many forms of racism often simultaneously intersecting with one another and environmental and social contexts. They function by driving disparities, potentiating trauma, decreasing resources, and adding to the schism between those who have and use privilege (advantage) and those who do not and cannot. *White privilege* describes this unearned and invisible but real advantage of being considered a White person in the United States; this built-in advantage is race based and separate from anyone's effort, education, or social status. It can be accompanied by *White fragility* (D'Angelo & Dyson, 2018), which is the denial and awkwardness often accompanied by defensiveness expressed by a White person during race-based conversations.

Anti-Black racism is the most virulent form of racism, evidenced as an often violent hostility toward and hatred of people identified as Black or African American. Ultimately, inherent to Whiteness and its construction as superior is not just the racism that logically follows that construction but specifically *anti-Blackness*. By silently framing Whiteness as a prize (intentionally or not, though truthfully its intent is irrelevant), we contribute to what more of us are finally seeing as a worldwide adherence to the ideology of anti-Blackness, with Black people seen as property and not fully human (see *Dred Scott* decision of 1857; USHistory.org, 2021), which was embedded in the US Constitution. Without the creation of race and Whiteness and the values aligned with it, we would not have anti-Blackness.

Anti-Black racism was sown in the soil of chattel slavery because the very practice of enslavement, chaining, beating, and bonding of other human beings requires a denial of their humanity. This disavowal of humanity in another person silences or compartmentalizes one's moral compass to profit from another's exploitation, trauma, pain, and even death. These foundational sentiments have been cemented into the American narrative and are perpetuated today.

One example of this is the killing of George Floyd, an unarmed 46-year-old Black man in Minneapolis, MN who bought cigarettes one night in May 2020 with a $20 bill at his neighborhood convenience store. The bill was counterfeit, and the cashier called the police. Mr. Floyd was sitting in his SUV in the parking lot, the passenger door open, smoking his cigarette and talking to two other passengers in the back seats. Two officers arrived and one approached with his gun drawn. Court transcripts describe Mr. Floyd as cooperative and apologizing to the officers, but this soon changed as he was pulled out of the car and handcuffed. He objected and said he was claustrophobic and fell to the ground as they scuffled and tried to pull him over to the squad car. Another squad car arrived. This time the officers restrained Mr. Floyd, still facedown on the asphalt. The third officer put his knee on Mr. Floyd's neck, and knelt there, with his hands in his pockets, telling Mr. Floyd to "stop talking, stop yelling, it takes a heck of a lot of oxygen to talk." The officer knelt on his neck for 9 minutes and 29 seconds, with Mr. Floyd crying out more than 20 times that he could not breathe, saying "You're going to kill me, man," and finally, "Mom, I love you. Love you. Tell my kids I love them. I'm dead." Several bystanders pleaded with the officers to let him up. Seventeen minutes from the beginning of this event, he was still facedown but now unconscious on the asphalt in cardiac arrest. The officer with his knee on Mr. Floyd's neck and another officer at the scene had histories of excessive force and other past involvements with the Minneapolis Police Internal Affairs Department (BBC News, 2020, paras. 9–11).

Emmett Till, a 14-year-old Black teenager, was visiting his uncle in Mississippi during his summer vacation in 1955, helping him harvest his crop. Till was accused of flirting with a White woman in a general store, then a week later was kidnapped by the woman's husband and another adult, brutally beaten, and killed at point-blank range with a shotgun, tied up, and dumped in the Tallahatchie River. His body was discovered a week later, so badly beaten that the only means of identification was his father's ring on his finger. His mother chose an open casket for Emmett's funeral to "show mourners and the world" the violence he had endured (Byrne, 2021, p. 4). The two men who killed him were tried and acquitted by an all-White jury. One year later they were paid for their story of abduction and murder by *Look* magazine (Ray, 2021).

Personal racism is sometimes called individual racism: the negative actions and attitudes, biases and beliefs, and stereotypes and prejudices individuals have absorbed about another group or themselves. It can be

outwardly focused as *interpersonal racism,* comprising the individual's prejudicial, racist, or discriminatory beliefs or actions toward others whether alone or as a member of a group, or *internalized racism,* including the negative actions and attitudes, biases and beliefs, stereotypes and prejudices individuals have absorbed about themselves regarding their abilities or personal value. These adverse attributes are internalized over time through experiences such as role modeling of beliefs and behaviors by parents, authority figures, or people at school; family culture; neighborhood play and bullying; social media and other telecommunication platforms; and other means of learning about social behaviors, respect for or categorization of people, and "how to be" with people who remind you of yourself and those who do not. These abhorrent internalized attributes all begin with this learning of "disdain, disregard and disgust" (Ross, 2020, p. 1) that drives the horrific violence of anti-Black racism, the prejudice and "thingification" of interpersonal racism, and the appropriated racial oppression of internalized racism, also called "internalized White racism," "intracultural racism," and "internalized oppression" (Pyke, 2010, pp. 552–555).

Internalized racism is a "very real and insidious" consequence of racism (Pyke, 2010, p. 558) and is a phenomenon becoming more frequently understood as appropriated racial oppression (Versey et al., 2019). It is a social-psychological phenomenon of identification with one's oppressor, in this case with a White-run society's privileges (advantages), discriminations, prejudices, race-based restrictions, and stereotypes (White supremacy), which allows for internal negotiations between one's personal values and the values of the society in which one must live, work, and thrive (Versey et al., 2019). This negotiation occurs through a "taking in" of society's messages that are centered on Whiteness and allows one to "navigate and cope with racism" (Versey et al., 2019, p. 296) using a range of actions, some healthy and ego-supportive, some including a world view that one's race is inferior, and some using a "defensive othering" response. These responses involve distancing oneself from another who, because of personal behaviors or circumstances, seems farther from the Whiteness ideal than oneself. It is a symptom of the disease of racism, but "not the disease itself" (Pyke, 2010, p. 558). One example of defensive othering is a group of Asian American students who shun the newly arrived student, calling her "FOB" or "fresh off the boat" and ridiculing her accent; another example is the Latinx who casually exclaims, "We don't need any more wetbacks—they just take away our jobs" (Padilla, 2001, paragraph 3). Padilla likens defensive othering to a ladder, with Whiteness at the top of the ladder, along with success, prestige, privilege, and opportunities. The bottom of the ladder represents the racialized self and racial group one is in and, with it, self-criticism, self-doubt, loss of opportunities, and powerlessness. Is it any wonder, then, that the racialized person can want to distance themselves from someone or a group that seems to be farther from the idealized White power standard?

Thus internalizing these attributes of the White-run society (see "White privilege" earlier in this chapter) as one's own by someone who does not self-identify as White (Paradies, 2018) is an instinctive response to a racist society by racially marginalized populations such as Black, Brown, and Indigenous people of color (BIPOC), and other racialized groups, such as the Jewish people, tribes of Native Americans, or First Nations and Indigenous people. These two racialized groups have endured oppression, forced relocations, and genocide over centuries (see "Network Advocates" for links to the Indian peoples/tribes lost to enslavement in the Americas, plus the *Encyclopaedia Judaica* for historical information about the persecution of Jewish peoples since before the common era) (Skolnik & Berenbaum, 2007; Network Advocates, n.d.). It has both subconscious and deliberately strategic components and is an adaptive response to the cultural osmosis of constant exposure to "normative Whiteness" or racial oppression in a historically White-dominated society (Versey et al., 2019). This cultural osmosis is examined more fully in the section describing the groundwater approach later in this chapter.

Internalized racism can also take the form of altering one's physical characteristics through actions such as skin bleaching, eyelid slashing to create a double lid, or hair straightening to resemble privileged Whiteness more closely. This is done to better identify with and seemingly succeed in a perceived White-dominant society.

Kurt Lewin, the father of social psychology, studied this internalized racism, or appropriated racial oppression, and described a self-hatred, which he said can result when a people are persecuted, traumatized, and stereotyped historically or over time by a more privileged cultural group. He observed that self-hatred occurred among "entirely normal" people and said the following about one of these historically oppressed groups, the Jewish people: "Self-hatred will die out only when actual equality of status with the non-Jew is achieved … there is nothing so important as a clear and fully accepted belonging to a group whose fate has a positive meaning." He explained that oppressed and traumatized people need a "past of courage" and a "future of hope" to regain the self-respect and self-love historically stripped from them through stereotyping, oppression, and religion and race-based brutalities (Jewish Virtual Library, 2021, paragraph 6).

This understanding of internalized racism can be applied to all racialized people and becomes a template for antiracist actions. This subconscious acceptance of the values and beliefs of a group that has power over you (this power could be social, financial, legal, educational, etc.) to the extent that you self-identify with the oppressor and in turn discriminate against your own cultural group is described by Kurt Lewin:

> *In a minority group, individual members who are economically successful … usually gain a higher degree of acceptance by the majority group. This places them culturally on the periphery of the underprivileged group and makes them more likely to be 'marginal' persons. They frequently have a negative balance and are particularly eager not to have their 'good connections' endangered by too close contact with those sections of the underprivileged group which are not acceptable to the majority. Nevertheless they are frequently called on for leadership by the underprivileged group because of their status and power. They themselves are usually eager to accept the leading role in the minority, partly as a substitute for gaining status in the majority, and partly because such leadership enables them to have and maintain additional contact with the majority. (Jewish Virtual Library, 2021, paragraph 4)*

Brief examples of the two types of personal racism, *interpersonal* and *internalized*, are presented in Table 6.2. *Institutional racism* refers to racism embedded in the policies and practices of institutions, such as schools, businesses, healthcare institutions and hospitals, prisons, and places of worship, that exclude a racialized group or put them at a disadvantage. These behaviors are routinely practiced by the people living

TABLE 6.2   Examples of Interpersonal and Internalized Racism

Action	Type of Racism
A White man rammed his car into a crowd of racial justice demonstrators in Iowa, striking several. When asked why he did it, he said because the protestors needed "an attitude adjustment" (Press, 2021).	Interpersonal
A Black man bird-watching in Central Park tells a White woman to leash her unleashed dog. She calls 911 and tells them that "There's a man, an African American man, threatening my life … he is recording me and threatening me and my dog. Please send the cops immediately." The videotape of the encounter shows no threatening moves or speech on his part, and that he had spoken to her calmly and kept his distance (Massingale, 2020).	Interpersonal
"When I grew up my parents would hate me hanging out with anyone Asian … I guess they have a preconception of them being gang members … Maybe it is the way my parents influenced me because the whole time I was with anyone Asian I just felt uneasy. I can't stand Vietnamese people or just Asians in general" (group interview with Vietnamese American males) (Pyke, 2010).	Internalized
Results of a 2011 survey of Indigenous students at a university in Australia showed that 60% had experienced lateral violence in the workplace from fellow indigenous colleagues. *Lateral violence* describes the phenomenon of a person or persons from a racially discriminated against group discriminating against or stereotyping another racialized person. This reaction often takes the form of insults, social excluding, sabotage, undermining, and scapegoating or backstabbing from members of one's own cultural/ethnic group, also seen as the *defensive othering* of internalized racism (Paradies, 2018).	Internalized

and working in these institutions. Racial profiling, by the criminal justice system or, in this next case, the news media, is just one example, as described in this recent news item: In its blunt self-assessment, the [*Kansas City*] *Star* found that for many decades of its 140 year history, "Black residents were rarely mentioned in anything but crime stories" (Alder, 2020, para 1). Just a few of the many examples of this form of racism are: the shrinking numbers of full-service hospitals serving Black communities in cities across America, making it more difficult for people dependent on public transportation to find and get to and from healthcare; hiring and retention practices that minimize or ignore the work of racialized people; and the profound lack of academic mentors that historically marginalized young adults who are the first members of their families to attend college can identify with to improve their chances of academic success. The trial for Emmett Till's murder is yet another example of this form of racism; Blacks and women were not legally permitted by Jim Crow laws to serve as jurors at that time, so the two men on trial who later published an account of their act were acquitted by an all-White, all-male jury.

Structural racism is sometimes called *systemic racism*. It is an intersectionality of racist policies and practices across all components of society, including institutions such as schools, the criminal justice system, hospitals, religious institutions, political systems at all levels, and social groups of people, families, and even neighborhood block clubs. This intersectionality magnifies the harm done to the historically marginalized and potentiates the racial burden for an already racialized group of people. Because it persists in part due to its history of longevity and the covert nature of much of it, it is difficult to detect, requiring a deep-dive examination of the outcomes of racist or inequitable policies, practices, or socially held behaviors over time. Emmett Till's story is an example of how various forms of racism intersected to support the brutal beating and murder of a child: (1) interpersonal racism (the perpetrators who tortured and murdered him), (2) institutional racism (Jim Crow policies that restricted jury selection to White males only for the trial of the perpetrators), and (3) structural racism (societal beliefs that BIPOC should "know their place" and that anybody with White epidermal skin color can strip Black and Brown racialized persons of their rights to life). Lastly, the evidence the jury saw and heard yet ignored to reach their verdict speaks of the level of inhumanity that remains today and is often state sanctioned. The following narrative presents another example of structural racism:

A social worker of over 20 years comes home from work and is in the middle of changing clothes when she hears a knock on her door. A group of 12 police burst in, breaking her front door, and handcuff her with guns drawn, with a warrant "improperly done" on the wrong house. She was now frantic, crying out over 40 times that they had the wrong house, all the time being videotaped by a police bodycam with her hands cuffed behind her, not allowed to dress until a female officer arrives 13 minutes later. She was told by the police to stop shouting and to relax. The target of that raid was a young man on house arrest, wearing an electronic ankle bracelet, living next door to her. In this incident, the callousness of the police intersected with the department's now-uncovered institutional lack of oversight of search warrant procedures to produce a bungled raid with risk to a woman's safety, her mental health, and her right to privacy (Chicagotribune.com, 2021).

Groundwater Approach

Particularly in my community, the saying is, you only go to the physician when you are about to die.
—*Lawrence (2020, paragraph 11)*

Understanding the roots of racism can be challenging due to the systemic and inconspicuous nature by which it operates in society (Fig. 6.2). To enhance awareness of how systemic racism works, a metaphor is applied to describe the structural biases in society that predictably affect downstream factors. The approach promotes structural clarity to distinguish how a multitude of concerns described clinically as symptoms, points of view,

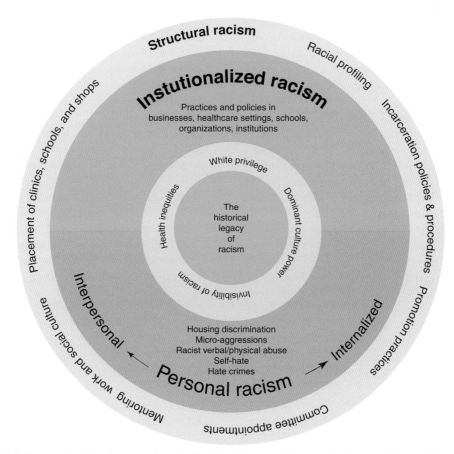

Fig. 6.2 Intersectionality of personal, institutional, and structural racism. (Adapted with permission from Nardi, D. et.al., (2020). *Achieving HealthEquity Through Eradicating Structural Racism in the United States: A Call to Action for Nursing Leadership.* John Wiley and Sons.)

or ailments also characterize the downstream effects of numerous inequitably allocated upstream obstacles and structural violence (Love & Hayes-Green, 2018). Racial bias and the inequities it upholds epitomize a metaphorical *groundwater,* adept at tainting numerous policy areas. Thus racial bias affects every part of daily life. Efforts to tackle this bias in individual policy areas while not attending to the root sources will not generate effective solutions.

It may be less challenging to examine some of the most difficult matters related to advancing health equity when the groundwater metaphor is applied. These concerns are not isolated events but are instead interconnected by systemic racism. For example, the groundwater of environmental racism produces poorer respiratory outcomes such as asthma for Black populations in the United States. Treating asthma without addressing the cause is not only ineffective; it is also an ethical concern. Residences for many Blacks are located where more harm from environmental factors occurs, and this is not accidental. Research has illuminated that industries involving waste disposal, toxic dumping, power plants, and factories are located disproportionately in areas where Blacks are concentrated (Berkovitz, 2020; Love & Hayes-Green, 2018). Importantly, environmental racism is indivisible from racial segregation leading to residential segregation. These segregated areas are inextricably linked to personal and systemic racism as well as public policy decisions made at the governmental level and exclusionary preferences by the financial arena. For example, in the 1940s and 1950s, the American government rejected access to money and would not underwrite loans for aspirant homeowners who were Black. However, these loans were secured by White individuals and were substantially more economical compared with the uninsured loans accessible to Black homeowners. This led to the government building housing developments where most Black Americans who sought employment in urban areas resided. These governmental policies were intentionally constructed to produce generational wealth and protection for homeowners who were White while relegating many Black families to live in segregated locales (Pratt-Chapman, 2020). Unsurprisingly, racially Black and Brown populations tend to be clustered in communities that have often been disempowered politically and financially (Berkovitz, 2020). In contrast, policy adoptions have functioned together with financial factors to push these adverse environmental conditions away from more affluent, racially White communities, due to inequities in political power. The interconnectedness of discriminatory practices reveals the systemic nature of racism. The groundwater metaphor proposed by Love and Hayes-Greene (2018) states:

> If you have a lake in front of your house and one fish is floating belly-up dead, it makes sense to analyze the fish. What is wrong with it? Imagine the fish is one student failing in the education system. We'd ask: Did it study hard enough? Is it getting the support it needs at home? But you come out to that same lake and half the fish are floating belly-up dead, what should you do? This time you've got to analyze the lake. Imagine the lake is the education system and half the students are failing. This time we'd ask: Might the system itself be causing such consistent, unacceptable outcomes for students? If so, how? Now … picture five lakes around your house, and in each and every lake half the fish are floating belly-up dead! What is it time to do? We say it's time to analyze the groundwater. How did the water in all these lakes end up with the same contamination? On the surface the lakes don't appear to be connected, but it's possible—even likely—that they are. In fact, over 95% of the fresh water on the planet is not above ground where we can see it; it is below the surface in the groundwater (p. 4).

This metaphor is established based on three observations. The first is that racial disparity appears to be consistent across systems. The second is that socioeconomic differences do not account for racial disparity. The third observation is that inequalities are produced by systems irrespective of a population's culture or behavior (Love & Hayes-Greene, 2018).

Racism impinges on every level and part of American society (Van Cleve, 2020). Racism (i.e., the groundwater) is sustained in every system and institution (i.e., the lakes), causing harm to individuals (i.e., the fish) (Van Cleve, 2020). Among the lakes, unequal outcomes predominate based on race (Bailey et al., 2017; Dave et al., 2021). In the United States this is consistent and universal; however, we narrate these differences using terminology such as health disparities in society, since this is more palatable for many to reckon with as it relates to racism (Egede & Walker, 2020). Patterns of fish (individual) well-being show

Black Americans having the worst outcomes, followed by Native Americans, Latinx, and Asian Americans fluctuating in the middle (Van Cleve, 2020). Racially White individuals show the best outcomes across systems (lakes), including health, wealth, educational attainment, criminal justice, and so on. (Van Cleve, 2020). With this reality, disparities cannot be ascribed merely to individuals' behavior, which is often done in the US context. For example, the norm of simply focusing on a fish's (individual's) nutrition, fitness routine, or level of resilience will not address the root causes of these inequities. Disparities are fed by a history of failing to reckon with the original sin of the United States—racism. Racism was a premise upon which the United States was founded. Consequently, this premise has enabled individuals in power (predominately White men) to maintain power. As a result of the ideology and practices stemming from White settler colonizers, structuring opportunities for persons with White epidermal skin, especially those that were men and wealthy, while other groups were not valued (e.g., genocide of Native Americans and chattel slavery in the case of racially Black individuals) and basic human rights were denied. Over time, these ideals have been rooted in society, supported through policy, and penetrated our groundwater so deeply that the toxicity has become normalized. Thus problems in society must be analyzed systemically and historically. We must also recognize and emphasize that the harmful consequences of a system are not problems. They are symptoms of a flawed, corrupt, failing system.

Literature tends to present research and other information using a Eurocentric universalism lens when describing disparities and race. *Eurocentric universalism* presents descriptions of the social world positioning European experiences as universal models (Williams, 2020). However, as discussed in the next section, using this approach to race in literature, repressing colonial history, has significant effects on how readers cognize what race denotes and how outcomes and conclusions are deduced. Suppressing this aspect of colonial history obscures the historical inequities that make race possible (Williams, 2020). Inequity is precisely the justification for race from a historical stance. Notably, race did not produce inequity; inequity produced race (Williams, 2020). Ignoring this reality undercuts the social construction of race, which obfuscates fundamental social features

of racialized groups. These truths permit us to confront the realism that systems, institutions, and outcomes originate from the racial hierarchy rooted in the founding of the United States. That said, a groundwater problem exists, requiring groundwater solutions (Love & Hayes-Green, 2018).

Individual approaches (or taking a myopic focus) lack sustainable effective outcomes, therefore if we are committed to addressing deep-rooted health-related issues, a comprehensive approach is necessary. For instance, healthcare leaders often try to solve health inequities from individual and health system perspectives. Equity requires leaders to peer beyond the health facility doors to societal divides (e.g., racism and poverty) as the basis of inequities in health outcomes. Healthcare leaders must reflect on how they use their position(s) in one system to affect a structural racial composition that may be deeper than any single system. Leaders in health systems are well positioned to make meaningful contributions and lead a groundwater approach beyond repairing the fish but rather targeting the fundamental system influencing the health of communities they should partner with to create wellness (Dave et al., 2021). Health systems can leverage their financial power, policy influence, and prominent leadership to deal with not only the disproportionate distribution of adverse SDOH but also practices, policies, and behaviors that uphold racism at all levels. An approach that incorporates the core mission and community stewardship role often stated by health systems can expedite momentous action to deal with the groundwater conditions that have the greatest effect on people's health and community well-being. To repair the fish or fix one lake at a time will not be effective, since the result would be returning the mended fish to toxic water or a cleaned-up lake that is rapidly polluted again by the toxic groundwater. In the lake-versus-fish analogy, using the groundwater approach, placing blame on the fish (individual) is not only wrong but goes against ethical and social justice principles that are pivotal to the nursing profession. If pervasive harm is impacting half the fish (individuals), look at the source—the groundwater, or system (systemic racism) (Dave et al., 2021). The pervasive inequities in American society continue to be reproduced, and race is a colonial doctrine formed to validate and normalize those exploitative relations (McLean, 2020).

RACE

The greatest difficulty we face is first of all to excavate our actual history.

—*James Baldwin (McLean, 2020, p. 1)*

Colonialism and Race

For professional nurses to understand race relations and the pervasive inequities in our country, they must begin with an understanding of chattel slavery and its effects on our society, including that systems operating in the United States, from academics to healthcare, were originally constructed by and for White Americans (Thurman et al., 2019). W.E.B. Du Bois, an American sociologist, understood the color line as a colonial invention rooted in the European operation of chattel slavery (i.e., trans-Atlantic slave trade). Chattel slavery was supported by extracting Black individuals from Africa with the purpose of colonizing them in what would be the United States (Williams, 2020). The colonial exploit that became the United States occurred because of the European (most pointedly British) empire-building process (Wilson, 2018). English aristocrats or want-to-be aristocrats indentured servants and enslaved individuals from Africa and other groups of settlers who migrated by choice or by force. They all discovered themselves in unusual conditions with an unfamiliar ecology to contend with and existing on land already occupied by native populations. During the 17th century, about one-half to two-thirds of immigrants in North America were indentured servants, since indentured servitude subsisted before chattel slavery. Of note, Africans and Europeans in indentured roles possessed similar rights (Wilson, 2018). For instance, these groups were permitted to own property and get married and, after the terms of their servitude, were released and had the status of free men. Subsequently, demands for labor deepened, Europeans in servitude procured more legal rights, and the status of Africans was degraded with the associated reliance on African laborers.

Chattel slavery (i.e., complete ownership of one human being by another; a human caught, sold, or born into permanent servitude as the master's property) of Africans was far more atrocious than the intertribal slavery that subsisted in Africa before European influence. W.E.B. Du Bois described the reality quite vividly:

They could own nothing; they could make no contracts; they could hold no property, nor traffic in property; they could not hire out; they could not legally marry nor constitute families; they could not control their children; they could not appeal from their master; they could be punished at will. They could not testify in court; they could be imprisoned by their owners, and the criminal offense of assault and battery could not be committed on the person of a slave . . . The slave owed to his master and all his family a respect "without bounds, and an absolute obedience." This authority could be transmitted to others. A slave could not sue his master; had no right of redemption; no right to education or religion; a promise made to a slave by his master had no force nor validity. Children followed the condition of the slave mother. The slave could have no access to the judiciary. A slave might be condemned to death for striking any white person. (Taifa, 2020, pp. 25–26)

Chattel slavery in the Americas not only launched the vexing feature of race into the master/slave relationship, but dark skin also became the engrained mark of chattel slavery. Moreover, as a means of rationalizing this twist to an ancient tradition, enslavers and their benefactors crafted a race-specific system of condemnation. This fabricated pomposity not only eliminated the ability of slave and master to interchange roles from the realm of cultural and political possibility, but it endures to this very day (Brooks, 2003). For example, interchangeability of power and prestige between master and slave existed in Africa wherein a slaveholder could lose his fortune in gambling and then become enslaved to one of his prior slaves. The traditional system of slavery in Africa then vastly shifted. Chattel slavery of Africans in the United States was more self-sustaining compared with ancient systems (traditional slavery or indentured servitude). The latter usually functioned as an adjunct or afterthought to another event/issue such as the rewards of continuous civil wars. Chattel slavery, however, was different. It was an independent operation that comprised the vicious and cruel transoceanic haulage of human beings with millions of Black individuals dying during the Middle Passage (Brooks, 2003).

While early on the distinction between slave and servant was to a certain degree imprecise, with the fear of slave rebellion, White aristocrats established a shared sense of Whiteness with White servants, especially after Bacon's Rebellion in 1676 (Williams, 2020). Brooks (2003) related how White settlers perceived persons identified as Black as beings of an inferior order, unsuited to be with the White race socially or politically and so inferior that they should not have any rights that the White man was compelled to acknowledge. Being enslaved was for life, whereas generational while servants were indentured for a set period (Parisot, 2019).

Chattel status operated via the juridical law of *partus sequitur ventrum*; this denotes that the child follows the status of the mother, therefore persons enslaved became locked in for life, cementing their fate (McLean, 2020). Human beings were trafficked from one region to the next lacking regard for family ties and cultural traditions including language. The enslaved were not permitted to marry and were subjected to physical and mental torture. For example, enslaved Africans were brutally raped, beaten with all forms of equipment including leather whips, murdered, disfigured by chopping off limbs, branded, commercially bred like livestock, and prohibited from learning to read, practice cultural rituals, or

maintain their cultural name (McLean, 2020). These are only some of the ways in which race relegated Blacks to the plantation. Such brutality was structured in a system of race with great intention. Moreover, the foundation and starkest example of oppression in the United States stems from chattel slavery.

Conceiving the idea of race in the 17th century permitted justification for colonialism. The following section includes a critical understanding of why race was constructed in the manner that it was in the United States (Fig. 6.3).

Why Race Was Constructed

In the United States specifically, White settlers committed genocide and confiscated land from Native Americans and enslaved individuals from Africa, which was justified through their lens by racial or biological differences between groups of people (Mize, 2009). Not only is there no gene prescribed to indicate if a person is Black

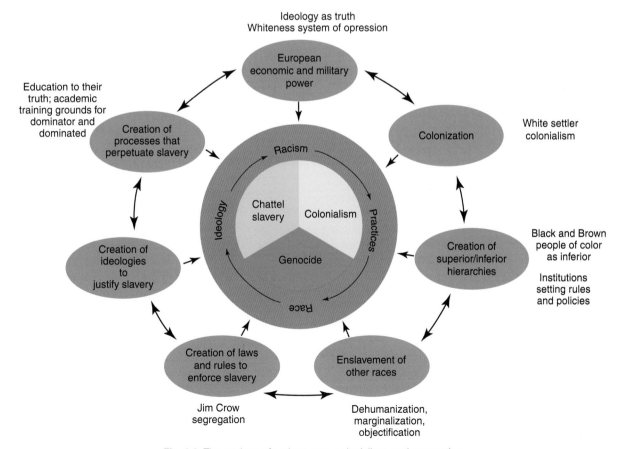

Fig. 6.3 The ecology of racism, race, colonialism, and oppression.

or White, but research also establishes that intraracial genetic differences are greater than interracial genetic differences (Wilson, 2018). That said, no gene or group of genes relate to the classification of culturally significant racial groups (e.g., Black or White). Thus nothing is biologically inherent about being racially designated as Black that would limit a person's capabilities and lead them to a position where they would have less wealth or political representation compared with a person who is racially White. In fact race is completely socially constructed, lacking any consequential basis in biological verity; both race and the characteristics linked to it are the results of social customs rooted in the practices of White settler colonization (Wilson, 2018). Consequently, the narrative constructed through a biological lens was that White was considered the ideal, perfect, or superior race, and Black was perceived and treated as the most inferior of all other skin hues (Parisot, 2019). Consequently, *colorism* is inextricably linked to racism, yet distinct. Colorism includes bias against individuals based on their characteristics irrespective of their perceived racial identity. The hierarchy used in colorism is comparable to the one that governs racism—light skin with less melanin is valued over heavily melanated dark skin, European facial structures and body shapes are cherished over African characteristics and body shapes, and colorism bears ranks of advantage and disadvantage even within racialized groups. Of note, the origin of colorism in the United States is directly linked to Atlantic chattel slavery. Race is ocular and corporeal and, as a social phenomenon, epitomizes the rootedness of social conflict around human bodies. Of note, race is described in terms of negation, specifically, as what it is not instead of what it is. That said, the social construction of race centers on the making of the racial hierarchy and racial disparity. Settler colonialism is therefore an ongoing structure, not an event that has ceased to exist. Settler colonialism captures material conditions such as land and labor that are vital in the creation of racialized groups; the stealing of land by White settler colonialists through Indigenous genocide and the enslavement of Africans not only leads to the inequitable allocation of resources, but it establishes a socially constructed racial hierarchy between racialized groups (Williams, 2020).

White settlers in the United States needed to address the ideals of freedom, democracy, and individual liberties while at the same time constructing the hierarchical inequities characteristic of capitalism (e.g., stealing of land and labor). As a result, the conception of race was historically invented to suit an ideological need of the dominant groups (White heteronormative men) to justify disparate access and position. Early settlers and slaveowners like Thomas Jefferson were the creators of the Declaration of Independence and these officials had to reconcile the statements: "We hold these truths to be self-evident, that all men are created equal, that they are endowed by their Creator with certain unalienable rights, that among these are Life, Liberty, and the pursuit of Happiness" (Seabrook & Wyatt-Nichol, 2016, p. 23). They led with a justification using a perceived practical outlook for the dominant power structure, that slavery was essential because Africans were inferior and the financial and political effects of its elimination made slavery an obligatory evil. In Jefferson's "Notes on the State of Slavery of Virginia," he further asserted that (1) Black inferiority exists since Blacks were less attractive than Whites and (2) the emotional life of Blacks was less complex. Enslavement was pervasive among the elite—55 delegates at the Constitutional Convention were slave owners and slavery was apparent in numerous passages of the Constitution (three-fifths clause that counted those enslaved toward the Southern population increasing the South's political strength; the slave trade clause that permitted and taxed the sale of slaves until 1808; and the fugitive slave clause that codified the return of runaway slaves to their masters) (Seabrook & Wyatt-Nichol, 2016). The Constitution surely has economics infused into its framework, which was clearly intended to protect the economic interests and property rights of the White colonial aristocracy (Seabrook & Wyatt-Nichol, 2016). Slaveholders held positions of power across the three branches of government at the genesis of our nation. Most US Presidents owned slaves, as did Supreme Court justices and Southern speakers of the House. Therefore courts were impediments to the eradication of slavery, evident in the *Scott v. Sanford* decision in 1857, which alleged that Dredd Scott could not take legal action because slaves were not citizens, they were subhuman (Seabrook & Wyatt-Nichol, 2016).

Race and economic domination were inextricably fused to chattel slavery and the treatment of racially identified Black individuals as property (or subhuman) (Mize, 2009). Racialization is the social reproduction of racialized characteristics or, more applicably put, race in action. Racialized groups are created for individuals to authorize political control of others, for example, through forms of economic exploitation, dispossession, displacement, genocide, and chattel slavery. Thus people come to their racial identity by way of the interactions between them racializing themselves (self- or internalized racialization) and being racialized by others (externalized racialization) (Williams, 2020). While the systems of domination of Black and Native Americans varied in appearance, reinforcing both was a radicalized conception of property executed by a powerful force that was sanctioned by the rule of law (Mize, 2009). For example, Virginia lawmakers introduced English law and adapted it to suit the pressures of capital growth in the colony. This consisted of producing a legal structure that would impose the collection of debts, chasten indentured servants' deviance, and defend the development and expansion of chattel slavery (Parisot, 2019). This led to the making of Blackness and the entrenchment of White supremacy. As Williams (2020) notes,

> Scholars who frame race in the context of settler colonialism points out how the racialization process—given meaning to otherwise meaningless categories (e.g., phenotypical features)—was contingent upon the colonial relationship with Europeans.…we cannot simply say that settler colonialism or genocide have been targeted at particular races, since a race cannot be taken as given. It is made in the targeting. Black people were racialized as slaves; slavery constituted their blackness. Correspondingly, Indigenous North Americans were not killed, driven away, romanticized, assimilated, fenced in, bred White, and otherwise eliminated as the original owners of the land but as Indians. (p. 152)

McLean (2020) describes that without White settlers from Europe there are no Indians or Natives. The Native American race was produced in contrast to European settlers. Relatedly, Blackness materialized over intergenerational dimensions of time where different groupings became a homogenous mass via the shared history of displacement and chattel slavery (McLean, 2020). Race, as a social problem, has its explanatory power in racism. The function of race is its maintenance of colonial and imperial power accumulated because of historical and continuing displacement and denial in an intensifying global fashion. Notably, the first step of separating humans into groups is a political practice. Liberal tactfulness, niceties, and intentions lack competitiveness compared with

state-sanctioned racialization of biology. Furthermore, these tactics lack power against the continued use of biological concepts of race in the natural, social, and applied sciences. Race persists with revered utility since it provides social, political, and economic benefits to dominant groups with power, both historical and present-day actors (individuals and institutions). We must always remember that race is a product of racism and subjugation of persons with melanin, especially Black individuals (McLean, 2020).

The ideology of slaves as property extended to health-related matters. Enslaved Black persons were used for medical experimentation across all age groups; however, the bodies of Black women were exploited on numerous levels (e.g., reproduction and rape). A timeline from 1619 to 2018 (https://www.liebertpub.com/doi/10.1089/heq.2017.0045) highlights the exploitation and healthcare experiences of Black women that contribute to health disparities. For slave owners, enslaved women on southern plantations with vaginal fistulas were a problem that endangered profits since the forced brutal labor could not be carried out. Enslaved women with fistulas no longer had reproductive capacity, which meant no slave capital (for producing more children that would be enslaved) and that these women could not be raped for sexual exploitation by their White male slaveholders. Difficult and prolonged labor contributed to the high frequency of fistulas and since women were forced to breed, this was a frequent occurrence. Thus the political economy of slavery produced marked experiences of nonexistent bodily integrity for enslaved women who were required to procreate and be sexually accessible as a stipulation of their oppression. A distinct example of medical experimentation was conducted by Dr. Sims, an Alabama surgeon who performed investigational operations on Black women (1845–1849) who endured injuries during childbirth causing vesicovaginal fistula. Dr. Sims received permission from slave owners who had women with this condition and was permitted to try tools and procedures to repair these fistulas without anesthesia. In fact, one enslaved woman, Anarcha, endured 30 operations before Sims honed a method to repair the injury (Lederer, 2005). The scientific progress of the present is constructed upon a foundation of medical exploitation and experimentation on Blacks. Colonized individuals served as research subjects from the beginning of colonialism. There is likely no domain of American medicine that was not affected by the use of Blacks in research (Lederer, 2005).

Afterlife of Chattel Slavery: Reconstruction, Civil Rights, Redlining, and Mass Incarceration

The United States is built on narratives of captivity via the colonization of native lands, massacre and forced relocation of Native populations, and chattel slavery. Following the Civil War and the emancipation of enslaved Blacks, there was a tsunami of new challenges Blacks encountered. Freedom is a relative term given the context. Postemancipation most Blacks had nothing except the garment on their backs. They lacked livestock, seeds for food, land to farm, shelter, money, and were not able to read or write. Pertinent areas are highlighted in the subsequent sections making manifest the ongoing structure of settler colonialism. The era of reconstruction and Jim Crow, the Civil Rights Movement, redlining, and mass incarceration are discussed, illuminating a range of inequities that were structurally enforced via legal policies and embedded as normalized operational processes in day-to-day living in the United States, all of which disproportionately and adversely target and work to destroy historically subjugated individuals.

Reconstruction

Moving from the era of chattel slavery to reconstruction (1865–1877) produced a challenge for the potency of racial subornation and oppression. Reconstruction arose with the Confederate admission of defeat that halted the Civil War. While America needed to come together, heal, and change course from White settler colonial oppression, these practices continued, especially for Black individuals and anyone who agreed with their termination. This led to the assassination of President Lincoln by a Southern supporter who did not want this change to be realized. The burning question faced the nation during Reconstruction, with the emancipation of those enslaved, would Black individuals now be accepted as equals and given the same rights, liberties, and advantages that White persons enjoyed? The answer was a resounding "no." Emancipation and new rights for Blacks only initiated a different relationship with the state; that is instead of evading the coercive control of the state, domination was enacted employing new institutional clothes. The end of chattel slavery did not end the trauma and shame experienced by Black individuals. Black codes, legal acts, and state constitutional revisions ratified by ex-Confederates

to control the freedoms of emancipated slaves took root (Nisa, 2019). Thus in the land of the free and the home of the brave, Black individuals and communities remain plagued by the permanency of racial oppression made manifest in numerous ways after the Civil War (1861–1865). These codes restricted where Blacks could live, controlled their work lifestyles even apprehending and incarcerating them if they vacated their jobs, banned Blacks from opposing anything White individuals wanted to enforce, and regulated Black mobility and all-inclusive freedoms to the point of forbidding interracial marriages. White supremacy and patriarchy upheld power over and control of Black bodies (Williams, 2020).

Power and finances deepened the brutality against Black persons since Whites in the South faced major loss of land, life, and financial resolve due to wartime liabilities, the fall of confederate money, and poor effects from cropping (Nisa, 2019). Compared with the aristocracy, less advantaged White Americans were now in competition with recently released Black individuals for scarce opportunities. For Whites to maintain their social dominance in the South, unfettered violence and Jim Crow laws were enforced—these were laws that legally supported segregation of public facilities between Blacks and Whites. Blacks who defied these laws were beaten, killed, and often lynched and burned with spectators looking on (Nisa, 2019). Violence and horror were employed as extralegal deterrents to uphold Black subjugation and protect racial control. Lynching became a widespread practice terrorizing Blacks to conform with Jim Crow laws. Between the end of Reconstruction and the contemporary civil rights period, in one state alone (Mississippi) 539 Blacks were murdered by lynching. During the late 19th and early 20th centuries, on average, two or three Black individuals in the South were hung, burned, or murdered weekly; these actions were fueled by the ideology that Black individuals were not only inferior but subhuman—the same perspective lauded to justify chattel slavery (Graff, 2015). Murders by lynching occurred in public spaces, largely allowed by state and federal representatives, and frequently in the presence of large groups of people in the context of a carnival-like atmosphere. This included having vendors selling food, printers generating postcards showing pictures of the lynching and dead body, and body parts kept as mementos. These acts of torture and terrorism traumatized Blacks nationwide (Graff, 2015). Furthermore, the current authors contend that White individuals posed for photos underneath the bodies of Black-raced humans beings hanging from a tree or adjacent to the burnt remains of their body. Practices of terror also mutated with gendered and sexual oppression, such as White men's customary practice of levying White supremacy and male-controlled domination by raping Black women (Fleming & Morris, 2015).

Jim Crow (an era where Blacks were not enslaved yet were not free) is a tripartite system of domination. Jim Crow practices manifested in the control of Blacks politically and socially and economic exploitation of them. Specifically, in the southern part of the United States, political exclusion deprived Blacks of constitutional rights. Similarly, economic corruption limited control over any financial advancement, pushing Black individuals to work in farming as sharecroppers entrenched in a debt bondage system, functioning as a new structure of slavery (Fleming & Morris, 2015). Likewise when Black persons traveled to cities, they were typically consigned to segregated labor markets taking on manual labor and service work lacking the safeguards of unions and the rule of law.

The advantages of Whites and disadvantages of Blacks were viewed as mutually constitutive; thus the well-being of White persons is the manifestation of a hierarchal system resulting in their overall advancement; the structural relations of race advantage, reward, and empower them. As Williams (2020) argued, "Whiteness has been constructed and defended as a rigidly exclusive category precisely because it is not a descriptor of national origin but a marker of entitlement to colonial power, privilege and property" (p. 156). Because the White settler colonial structure has persisted overtime, White-presenting individuals have lived experiences that contrast with individuals racialized as Black because of the variance in material and psychological experiences between these populations (Nisa, 2019). While this part of American history can be challenging to read, this is indeed our history. Images that may surface and thoughts that may emerge can test "our sense of who we are and who we have been" (Graff, 2015, p. 121). It is not surprising that these egregious actions occupy negligible parts of history books or awareness among many Americans; however, intentional exclusion allows us not to wrestle with how we have treated fellow humans, resulting in continuing this egregious behavior in different formations

and enabling a process of double lynching since exclusion also murders any memory of the original crime (Graff, 2015).

Policies that produce inequities in daily life also promote health inequities. The systematized oppression inflicted upon Black Americans lays the groundwork for multiple interacting determinants that drive inequities in health and are reinforced by the US political system and professional organizations. During the years of segregation, explicit racism endured and existed in America's healthcare system. Segregation was upheld (*Plessy v. Ferguson*, 1896) and the healthcare enterprise supported the *Plessy* ruling and the Jim Crow law that trailed; thus Blacks were banned from medical schools necessitating the development of historically black colleges and universities. What's more, Black physicians already carrying out their professional roles were precluded from practicing medicine in hospitals run by White Americans. Southern hospitals completely prohibited Blacks from entering their buildings. Hospitals in the North often operated by separating Blacks and Whites on different wards. Consequently, Blacks had to establish their own hospitals, medical schools, and healthcare facilities. Black physicians were chased out of communities, received death threats, and were denied membership to the American Medical Association (AMA; founded in 1847) without which Black physicians had no admitting privileges to local hospitals or access to continuing education, income, and status in their communities. This led to the creation of the National Medical Association (founded in 1895), which became the voice of Black physicians. When the AMA eventually allowed Black physicians into the organization, they lacked the power to vote; they could only serve as scientific members. This meant they had to leave before the business meeting and dinner with White colleagues (Washington et al., 2009). Similarly, professional nursing in the United States appeared in the late 19th century and deeply rooted racism only permitted a limited number of Black women to enter nursing schools in the northern United States using quotas, and they were denied admission in southern states. Mary Eliza Mahoney was the first Black person in the United States to earn a professional nursing license in 1879 and, because of discrimination encountered in the Nurses Associated Alumnae of the United States and Canada, later known as the American Nurses Association, she formed the National

Association of Colored Graduate Nurses, later becoming the National Black Nurses Association. Individual attitudes created exclusion practices and structural policies. These all promoted health inequities in American society.

Also during the Jim Crow era, Blacks continued to be subjected to medical experiments without their knowledge. The most well-known experimentation on Blacks during this period is the Tuskegee Syphilis Study, which began in 1932. This study, devised to assess the effect of untreated syphilis on the male body and sponsored by the US Public Health Services, included about 400 Black men affected by syphilis and 200 Black men not affected by syphilis (Akpan, 2013). Most were from low socioeconomic background, illiterate sharecroppers and farmers, and they were not informed that they had contracted syphilis; they were told they were engaged in the experiment because they had bad blood. Their sustained engagement was supported by bribery—promised free healthcare and therapy, transportation to and from the hospital, hot meals, and burial insurance (Akpan, 2013). Even after penicillin, an effective treatment for syphilis, was discovered, medical authorities withheld this information from these Black men for 40 years. Physicians had no intention of offering any treatment to the infected men during this study. It was not until 1972 that these men were informed they had syphilis; this was the longest medical experiment to deny treatment to humans in documented US history (Akpan, 2013). As James Baldwin stated,

> It is dangerous to be an American Negro male. America has never wanted its Negroes to be men, and does not, generally, treat them as men. It treats them as mascots, pets, or things. (Akpan, 2013, p. 1123)

History has elucidated the distinct relationships the Black community has had with the American legal system. It has historically maintained institutionalized, racist limitations that have mired Black populations' ability to be recognized equally with White populations. From the foremost interactions with the White population, Blacks were deemed intrinsically inferior subhumans whose presence was taken only to serve and be subjected to atrocious inhuman brutality. American law and its officials have buttressed Blacks to endure this position and associated experiences (Akpan, 2013).

Civil Rights Movement

By the 1950s Blacks, especially in the South, were subjected to stern segregation and oppression contributing to a collective identity rooted in subordination. This led Blacks to develop necessary skills and resilience—for example, to manage brutal pain—stemming from a communal history of resistance, extending from slave rebellions, to the Underground Railroad, boycotts, and social movements (Fleming & Morris, 2015). This Civil Rights Movement was a colossal challenge to norms of racial inequality in the United States. As a major undertaking, the Civil Rights Movement depended on the use of diverse tactical methods such as litigation, community organizing, and mobilization to engage in political empowerment. Additionally, the Civil Rights Movement emphasized the need to expand economic opportunities, integrate major institutions, change social relations, and transform the cultural landscape (Fleming & Morris, 2015).

The Civil Rights Movement reflects the many manifestations of uprising against racial oppression displayed by many Black Americans and other supporters, a continuation of the legacy of racism and inequality. This movement predictably conveyed both inequity and freedom in rights-based conditions, such as the right to contract, possess property, racially integrate schools, have privacy, vote, and join in matrimony with an individual of a different race, ethnicity, or sexual orientation. With the ratification of civil rights laws, the expectation was that White supremacy would fritter away. Antidiscrimination laws passed; however, they did not dismantle racial subordination. The Supreme Court described discrimination as interpersonal with an emphasis on explicit interpersonal discrimination. The equal protection section of the 14th Amendment of the US Constitution, which is exceedingly influential with regard to American antidiscrimination law, only prohibits actions that are carried out by state actors with the deliberate "intent" to harm another on account of race. This does not include implicit bias, institutional racism, or structural racism. This intent clause was part of the Constitution and applied to a range of nonconstitutional antidiscrimination doctrines, including key provisions of the Civil Rights Act of 1964. Ultimately these laws sustained White supremacy since explicit directives to dismantle racism were nonexistent, therefore default whiteness and colorblindness (i.e., no recognition of racial distinctions) were endorsed.

This strips the historical meaning of beliefs about and actions taken on account of race, which is a problem since race in the United States is not a benign concept (Wilson, 2018).

The Civil Rights Movement fueled protests, sits-in, and boycotts that were nonviolent but challenged racial boundaries and inequalities, which endangered the social position and unearned advantages of White individuals. A predictable fact in US history is that any instance of genuine progress toward advancement for the Black population results in a stern backlash and White rage. Civil rights activity incited countermovement dynamics by Whites including the creation of segregationist schools and the formation of hate groups such as the Ku Klux Klan, which inflicted horror (e.g., Emmitt Till). Moreover, social-psychological forces of FBI informants, schemes, collusions, and assassination reports were frequent and carried out (e.g., Dr. Martin Luther King and Medgar Evers). If real progress is desired, one certain approach to undo structural inequity (e.g., racism) and promote civil rights is to focus on revamping all state action that preserves *caste*—a man-made structure using a rigid and entrenched ranking of human value that positions the alleged supremacy of one group (Whites) against the supposed inferiority of other groups (Black and Brown) based on ancestry and often fixed features. The features are neutral conceptually but nonetheless assigned life-and-death significance in a hierarchy preferring the dominant caste (racially White individuals) whose ancestors conceived of it.

The Civil Rights Movement has implications that also affect the health of individuals. Explicit segregation in the space of healthcare stayed completely intact until Congress passed the Civil Rights Act (1964), which outlawed discrimination based on race by federally funded systems and establishments. The subsequent year Medicare was created making nearly all hospitals the beneficiaries of federal funding; thus they were forced to accept the conditions of the Civil Rights Act of 1964. Though Blacks could not be denied entrance to hospitals, they were often denied care by White health professionals. Dr. Martin Luther King called out organizations, for example, lambasting the AMA for a conspiracy of inaction in the preservation of a medical apartheid that continued even into the late 1960s. King stated, "Of all the inequalities that exist, the injustice in health care is the most shocking and inhuman" (Dhar & Gebreyes, 2020, p. 1). King was a staunch leader in human rights and fought for those who were historically excluded; a core pillar in his campaign as part of the Civil Rights Movement was that healthcare is a right (Dhar & Gebreyes, 2020).

Even today, civil rights in health can support a health justice framework; that is, developing a structural awareness of the SDOH along with civil rights activism. The civil rights effort, focused on antidiscrimination law, is distinctively vital (Harris & Pamukcu, 2020). Legal tools and justice movements to promote empowerment are necessary; this prioritizes one's right to contribute to decision-making and policymaking and considers legal engagement an addition to political action. This is relevant since there are limits to laws. Specifically, law ascribed in books does not necessarily transform into law on the street, in our communities, and in professional groups. In fact, organizations and structures of the law can at times extend or intensify subjugation. Positive aspects of laws are that they can serve as a channel to foster power, provided it is recognized as ancillary, to the end goal of supporting personal agency and collective efficacy, and this is essential for health and well-being. (Harris & Pamukcu, 2020).

Redlining

Homeownership is one of the greatest contributors to wealth for Americans (Wilson, 2018). Unequal opportunities to gain homeownership between Blacks and Whites is accredited chiefly to the racialized wealth gap that has been fueled over centuries by policy. For example, after the Great Depression (1929–1939) the federal government established programs to support home ownership broadly via initiatives such as the Home Owners' Loan Corporation (Wilson, 2018). Structural barriers were entrenched and the ability to gain access to funding was not race neutral. The suitability of properties and communities was assessed using a four-color Residential Security Map comprising green (most desirable/likely to obtain loan assistance), blue, yellow, and red (least desirable/likely to receive loan assistance); this practice was also assumed by private institutions providing loans. Communities were reduced in rank if residents were racially Black or Brown, immigrant, or both, and of course these were rated red (i.e., redlining) (Wilson, 2018).

Furthermore the federal government funded the Federal Housing Administration (FHA) lending program. This entity tendered insurance to private lenders to assist them in financing residential mortgages (Wilson, 2018); therefore if the mortgagee failed to pay, FHA insurance would cover the amount of money loaned. By the early 1970s the FHA helped 11 million families to purchase homes and 22 million families to render home improvements (Wilson, 2018). Again, structural racism penetrated the process. The FHA applied race-conscious policies in determining who to lend to, refusing Black borrowers' access to loans, equating to blocking opportunities for the homeownership that was made widely available to White individuals and families. Of note, they adopted the redlining process, which lead the FHA to not cover loans in areas indicated by red on the map, which is where Black residents lived, and more desirable blue and green areas had preventive racial pledges that precluded Blacks from buying homes in those areas (Wilson, 2018). In addition to the Residential Security Map, the Home Owners' Loan Corporation also agreed to an underwriting policy. This policy also comprised race-conscious language signaling they should indemnify loans that would support maintaining communities, preserving alike racial makeup and imposing segregation (Wilson, 2018). Consequently, Blacks were refused access to conventional resources to finance their homes, and this was endorsed by institutionalized procedures (i.e., institutional racism). These practices deliberately excluded Blacks and favored Whites in terms of where they were able to build equity and subsequently employ that equity to establish businesses, finance education, or purchase an additional home (Wilson, 2018). Race-conscious housing policies engrained White supremacy (Wilson, 2018).

Segregating low-income, low-resourced individuals concentrates poverty, which was an expected result of redlining and subsequent residential segregation. Low land value and low political power attract industrial and polluting dangers including landfills, incinerators, and power plants, locating them near residential areas of Black and Brown racialized populations. The landscape of social, economic, environmental, and cultural determinants of health of segregated communities includes elevated rates of poverty, lower home ownership, soaring unemployment, more violent crime, higher levels of industrial pollution, and are more likely to be classified as medically underserved compared with nonsegregated communities. Moreover, persons living in communities

designated red suffer from higher levels of asthma, cancer, obesity, neurotoxicity/neurodegenerative disorders, and cardiac disease (Patterson & Harley, 2019). These adverse health effects are not accidental; creating an ecosystem with toxicity produces a breeding ground for ill health. As stated by Schneider and colleagues (2020), "Every system is perfectly designed to get the results it gets" (p. 486).

Mass Incarceration

Mass incarceration has roots in how Black bodies are policed. Modern-day US policing has origins in slave patrols, originally formed in 18th-century colonial Virginia, enforcing imprisonment on enslaved Black individuals and suppressing rebellions by those enslaved. Postemancipation, police and prisons functioned as important institutions for reaffirming White dominance, particularly in the South. Law enforcement also authorized, allowed, and partook in the lynching of Black individuals, which White crowds habitually supported, deceptively stating it was reprimand for a crime. Southerners also employed police and prisons to implement homelessness laws and the convict-leasing and sharecropping systems to force previously enslaved Blacks to work in the fields (another guise for slavery) (Bailey et al., 2017).

Policing has long been entwined with other structures that breed racism, including residential segregation, racial restrictions in "sundown" towns where Black individuals were prohibited except during working hours, and harassing Black individuals who had a presence in communities where White individuals resided (Bailey et al., 2017). Over the years, incarceration has been linked to rhetoric such as "law and order," "tough on crime," "superpredator," and "war on drugs." The drug epidemic gave rise to incarceration not like any that history had formerly seen, and of course all these structurally devised mechanisms flagrantly racialized Black individuals as offenders, instead of victims of the drug pandemic. The previously mentioned terms were imported as politically correct language, yet they all had an investment in the removing of Black populations from American society as a way of upholding White supremacy. Even with equivalent use of drugs, Blacks are arrested more often. Laws also have a disproportionate penalty for Blacks, for example, when punishing crack (primarily used by Blacks) versus cocaine (primarily used by Whites) use. The first federal criminal law, the

Anti-Drug Abuse Act of 1986, distinguished crack from other forms of cocaine, creating a 100:1 weight ratio as the level for drawing the mandatory 5-year minimum punishment upon conviction of possession; the penalty for holding 500 g of powder cocaine was analogous to holding only 5 g of crack (Palamar et al., 2015). This was indeed a race-conscious law. Similarly, the recent narrative on opioid use has altered with increased representation of Whites who have been harmed. Instead of imprisonment, a focus on rehabilitation and support has become a common lexicon, with associated resources.

Michelle Alexander has appropriately called the trend of mass incarceration of Blacks, "the New Jim Crow." There are more Black men incarcerated or on probation than there were Blacks enslaved in 1850 (Powell, 2019). Thus to comprehend how mass incarceration could attain its present-day peak, there must be an understanding of the factors that contributed to its development. The prison industrial complex produces an underclass (like subhuman status), stripped of civil rights, analogous to both chattel slavery and Jim Crow laws. The chains are just invisible now. Intriguingly, the actual amendment that eliminated caste-based oppression in America has been converted to a license to privatize the prison system and commodify mass incarceration. As stated in Powell (2019):

> If neither slavery nor involuntary servitude shall exist within the United States, then punishment for crime should not be a new form of slavery. The Thirteenth Amendment should be employed to eradicate all badges and incidents of slavery with present-day effects. A stark vestige of slavery's indelible impact is the criminal justice system and mass incarceration (p. 35).

A total of 40% of the incarcerated population in the United States is of African American descent, while African Americans only account for 13% of the total population. The United States has made the prison industrial complex a business that profits on crime (Powell, 2019). Moreover, America's incarcerated populace comprises approximately 25% of the incarcerated population worldwide, although the American population only represents roughly 5% of the world's population (Mays, 2017). This creates a society in decline because incarceration and criminalization are fundamental to the removal of citizenship in the United States. This is revealed by

Black women being twice as likely to be imprisoned as White women and Black men being almost six times more likely to being imprisoned than White men. There is no doubt that America has made a distinct investment in Whiteness, employing mass incarceration as its latest method of colonization, moving Black individuals back into the wretched "other" position that enslaved Africans were subjected to (Mays, 2017).

Policing and incarceration also have profound adverse health effects. The consequences are direct and indirect. Obvious direct implications include the deadly force that disproportionately kills hundreds of Black individuals annually (e.g., Breonna Taylor, Michael Brown, Tamir Rice, Walter Scott, Alton Sterling, Philando Castile, Stephon Clark, Ronell Foster, Jordan Edwards, and Nathaniel Pickett II) and nonfatally injures thousands more (e.g., Jacob Blake). Prisons and jails are key locations for disease transmission and this was especially true during the COVID-19 pandemic. Indirect effects include police violence causing harm to the mental health of entire communities and unceasing surveillance and threat of violence contributing to a vast range of psychological traumas (Bailey et al., 2017).

Understanding how structural racism operates permits us to perceive how policing and prisons have accomplished their projected purpose of social control of the Black population, which has historically been imposed by violence. For any effective transformation, appropriate mental health and social services and other supports must be engaged equitably in directing public safety without needing a police response (Bailey et al., 2017). Moreover, the struggle against settler colonialism structure is not simply one of structural or policy change, but true transformation of mental consciousness to eradicate the toxic anti-Black sentiments that are engrained in American life.

CONCLUSION

Using an antiracism framework to achieve health equity is essential to eliminating the persistent racism that remains unacknowledged yet virulent in medical and nursing education, its professional organizations, and its policies and practices. Antiracism work in the nursing profession is a long-term process that requires commitment, humility, and a willingness to be uncomfortable while learning who you are in the context of racism, what you can do and when, and what you do and do not control. It involves coordinated actions between all domains of healthcare to identify, deconstruct, and eliminate it. This is requisite to prevent the critical disparities in healthcare and outcomes that continue to plague racialized people of color. Antiracism work requires:

1. An understanding of the historical roots and characteristics of racism;
2. A commitment to promote learning about the history and legacy of race, racism, and the location of privilege (i.e., advantage);
3. An examination of the direct and indirect effects of personal or individual, institutional, and structural racism; its manifestations within organizations; and its cumulative effect on individuals, public health, and society; and
4. Intentional actions to integrate antiracism into one's personal life and professional work.

As the groundwater metaphor illustrates, antiracism work consists of organization-linked actions that target the upstream, midstream, and downstream political, economic, and environmental determinants of health. Upstream determinants include the lack or presence of toxic and stressful influencers of health to an entire community, family, or group, such as poverty; lack of jobs; scarce affordable housing; food deserts in BIPOC communities; limited childcare; scarce, inconsistent healthcare; inadequate public transportation; chronic, stressful exposure to discriminatory practices, racism, and biases in job recruitment and placement; and so on. They can be mitigated and targeted for change through community, political, educational, and healthcare advocacy (see the Case Study that follows). Midstream determinants are the learned and reinforced human behaviors, such as nutrition and exercise practices, tobacco use, and drug and alcohol abuse, that increase risk for chronic diseases such as cardiovascular disease, obesity, diabetes, stroke, and so on. Keep in mind that midstream determinants are open to change through individual counseling and education, and many types of public–private partnerships to, say, improve the high school graduation rate for ethnic minority students or to prevent/defuse violence and improve safe public transportation in a community. Downstream determinants are how these cumulative, evidenced incidences of chronic illnesses are identified and effectively treated by the medical and nursing professions using best practices for all people. These best practices include comprehensive, evidence-based holistic treatment of those people with no insurance or who are underinsured, including follow-up programs to prevent recurrence or worsening of conditions.

Antiracism work can be put into practice through individual, group, and organizational efforts that begin with the following self-work necessary to understand the holistic needs of the increasingly diverse patient and provider populations nurses teach, treat, and collaborate and work with:

1. Strengthen personal understanding of the social construction of race and the role of racism in healthcare administration, policies and practice, delivery, access, and outcomes of care for racialized people. Educate yourself. Do not wait for someone else to do it for you. Start with your own professional and personal organizations; the questions in the Learning Activity and Case Study at the end of this chapter can be used to guide your path.
2. Do a self-assessment and critical self-inquiry into nursing education and/or practice (depending on your background and field of interest) and conduct a structured critique of the profession. There are many tools available to guide such self-assessments and organizational critiques, for instance, the many writings about race and racism by Kenneth V. Hardy, such as his chapter on antiracial approaches to shaping theories (Hardy, 2016), and the antiracism toolkit by Jackson and colleagues (2020).
3. Contribute to honest, respectful dialogue, called "difficult conversations," about discrimination, racial biases, stereotyping, microaggressions, and untested, unchallenged assumptions about who people are and what they value and want. *Microaggressions* are a more subtle and hidden part of the spectrum of racism, bias, and discrimination. They are demonstrated in a woman smilingly commenting about her daughter's new friend from school, who is a member of a racialized group, "oh, I didn't know her kind was accepted to your_____ (school, sorority, study group, housing subdivision, country club)," fill in the blank, and they continue growing in lethality and venom to the macroaggressions (e.g., anti-Black racism) of the lynching and shooting of racialized people to this day.
4. Use new knowledge to build empathy and the ability to truly "see" people, patients, and neighbors in the context of their histories, family roles, and supports; environmental contexts; and the doors to health and wellness that are open or closed to them by

discrimination, racist beliefs and practices, and the exclusive barriers of White privilege.

Antiracism work in all areas of healthcare and education is very late in coming and, to date, has not found its place as a significant focus of attention by nursing, nor is it a central guide to nursing assessment, treatment, and follow-up actions in nursing education programs, or in practice. Applying an antiracism framework, however, is critical to the development of a new pipeline for the updated preparation of nurses to provide full-service health care for the 21st century, fully recognizing and valuing the vast diversity and humanity of all populations we work with and the diversity and humanity within the profession.

CASE STUDY

The Chicago Southside Shredder Project

If (the shredder) wasn't good enough for Lincoln Park, why is it good enough for the Southeast Side?
—**Michael Hawthorne, 2021b, p. 3**

General Iron closed its scrap shredder plant in the wealthy, predominantly White, Lincoln Park neighborhood after the company was cited on multiple occasions and taken to court for "emitting pungent odors of sweet metals that burn [my] nostrils." The Chicago Department of Public Health also noted that pollution-control equipment required by the USEPA was not working properly to control "noxious emissions" from the shredder. General Iron then merged with Reserve Marine Terminals, applied for key state permits from the Illinois EPA, and were cleared by the state of Illinois to build a new shredder at a southeast site in Chicago on former Republic Steel property on the Calumet River.

The proposed site is in a "low-income, predominantly Latino neighborhood on Chicago's Southeast Side." It is within sight of a high school and elementary school, the Calumet River, less than 2 miles from Indiana, and where state monitoring equipment routinely detects the city's "dirtiest air." The proposed site is also surrounded by three Southside neighborhoods, with dozens of backyards, baseball fields, and playgrounds contaminated with "lead pollution and other metals" from past and present industries such as US and Republic Steel, which were operating in the area for decades. The neighbors formed a group, hired lawyers, and petitioned for federal intervention to prevent construction of that business in the area. The petition stated that the Illinois EPA had "colluded with developers to concentrate industries in a corner of the city where residential yards already are contaminated by heavy metals and toxic chemicals." The Illinois EPA, however, said that the state law "gave them no choice" but to approve the permit. Meanwhile, legislation to combat "environmental racism" was stalled and had died in state government committee a year earlier. At the time of this writing, the USEPA had announced an investigation into the "granting of approval in a polluted area," and community members had started a hunger strike to bring attention to their cause. Notably, this shredder comes with the promise of employment for many who have faced unemployment for years since the manufacturing plants left the area. It might also help decrease the overwhelming deficit the state faces. It is also right next door to Indiana, and close to Lake Michigan, a major recreation site and supplier of drinking water to multiple counties in Illinois and other states (Hawthorne, 2021a, 2021b, p. 3).

1. What do you think "environmental racism" means in these two news reports?
2. What are the upstream determinants of environmental health for this Southside community and what are their downstream effects?
3. What are the types of racism at work in this case study and how do they intersect?
4. How does this problem relate to the role of nursing in the community?
5. If you were a community nurse working in this neighborhood and the residents, your patient population, came to you for help with blocking this shredder, what would your response be?
6. In what ways does this situation relate to the social and structural determinants of health?
7. As a representative of the profession of nursing, you have an opportunity to speak to all the listed players in this situation. What would you want to say to each?

STUDENT REFLECTION AND LEARNING ACTIVITIES

Reflective practice is at the core of all professional practice and is the creative engine that informs the application of evidence and science-based actions. Nursing shares this practice attribute with physicians, social workers, educators, therapists, clergy, artists, and other professionals to remain relevant and authentic to the populations they serve. Reflective practice can be used to develop a trauma-informed lens, which provides a deeper understanding of how one's own racial identity, whether it is "being White" or "being Black" or "being Latinx" or "being Indigenous," or being a member of another historically marginalized group, categorizes people into social groups that are more likely to be privileged or oppressed, entitled or dominated and abused, and the consequences of such categorization. Building this understanding is done by asking oneself critical-thinking questions such as "How does this help my client or benefit this population, this person, or this neighborhood?" "If what I am doing is not helping, then why am I doing it?" "If not this, then what needs to change, what should be done, and what is my role in strategic change for the better?" The overarching question used to focus on upstream determinants of health inequities is "What needs to happen to prevent this (illness/condition/situation/inequity) from ever happening again?" The next section includes reflective practice questions that can be used in private or in small group settings with an experienced mentor or coach in developing an antiracist perspective and a better understanding of the values and expressed needs of patients and populations in your care.

STUDENT REFLECTION QUESTIONS

Take some time to think about each of these questions, their purposes, and the meaning of your written, verbal, or emotional responses to them. Think about how this self-examination can be used to grow your understanding of yourself and the patient populations you serve.

1. When were you first aware of race and yourself as a *racial being*? Describe the context of that experience and your thoughts and feelings about that racial identity.
2. What do the terms "health inequities," "health disparities," "racism," and "race" mean to you? How do you negotiate your experiences with them in your practice?
3. An exchange student is spending a semester at the college of nursing near you. He says he has heard the terms "White privilege," "White supremacy," and "White fragility" in class and asks you to interpret or explain them to him. What do you say?
4. What can be done locally or politically to advance *health equity* in your location?
5. What antiracist actions have you taken to respond to *racism* in healthcare or nursing?
6. How is the saying, "you can't be neutral on a moving train" related to the *racial justice* approach to healthcare in the United States?
7. Select one health disparity discussed in this chapter that is particularly troubling to you and use the *groundwater metaphor* to explain its upstream causes and propose solutions. Using this metaphor as a practicing nurse, how can you contribute to health equity outside your day-to-day care?
8. What is meant by "difficult conversations"? Describe a time you were involved in one, the context and your role, how you responded, and what you were thinking and feeling.
9. What is your understanding of, or experience with, *White privilege*? What strategies can the nursing profession adopt to mitigate the influence of White privilege on the nursing profession and healthcare delivery and access?
10. What is your takeaway from this chapter on *race, racism, discrimination,* and *privilege* in nursing?

REFERENCES

Akpan, A. M.-A (2013). Dark medicine: How the National Research Act has failed to address racist practices in biomedical experiments targeting the African-American community. *Seattle Journal for Social Justice, 11*(3). https://digitalcommons.law.seattleu.edu/sjsj/vol11/iss3/11.

Alder, E. (2020). 'Brute' and murderers: Black people overlooked in KC coverage – except for crime. The Kansas City Star. Retrieved from https://www.kansascity.com/news/local/article247235584.html.

American Association of Colleges of Nursing. (2021). *The essentials: Core competencies for professional nursing education.* https://www.aacnnursing.org/Education-Resources/AACN-Essentials.

Bailey, Z. D., Krieger, N., Agénor, M., Graves, J., Linos, N., & Bassett, M. T. (2017). Structural racism and health inequities in the USA: Evidence and interventions. *The Lancet, 389*(10077), 1453–1463. https://doi.org/10.1016/S0140-6736(17)30569-X.

Bauderap, D. (2020). Kansas City newspaper reckons with its racial mistreatment. Breitbart. https://www.breitbart.com/news/kansas-city-newspaper-reckons-with-its-racial-mistreatment/.

BBC News. (2020). *George Floyd: What happened in the final moments of his life.* BBC News. https://www.bbc.com/news/world-us-canada-52861726.

Berkovitz, C. (2020). *Environmental racism has left black communities especially vulnerable to COVID-19.* The Century Foundation. https://tcf.org/content/commentary/environmental-racism-left-black-communities-especially-vulnerable-covid-19/.

Bowen, A. (2020). Of the COVID-19 pregnancy cases reported in Illinois, Black and Latina women make up over 70%. *Chicago Tribune.* https://www.chicagotribune.com/coronavirus/ct-life-coronavirus-hispanic-black-moms-pregnant-women-covid-20200702-opoekt3avvbqvfkf3caxtvrnkm-story.html.

Brooks, R. L. (2003). Ancient slavery versus American slavery: Distinction with difference. *University of Memphis Law Review, 33*(2), 265–276.

Byrne, J. (2021). *Emmett Till's Chicago home granted city landmark status.* Chicago Tribune.

Carratala, S., & Maxwell, C. (2021). *Health disparities by race and ethnicity.* Center for American Progress. https://www.americanprogress.org/issues/race/reports/2020/05/07/484742/health-disparities-race-ethnicity/.

CNN. (2020). *Black Indiana doctor died of coronavirus weeks after accusing hospital of racist treatment.* ABC7 Chicago. https://abc7chicago.com/9094278/.

Crear-Perry, J., Maybank, A., Keys, M., Mitchell, N., & Godbolt, D. (2020). Moving towards anti-racist praxis in medicine. *The Lancet, 396*(10249), 451–453. https://doi.org/10.1016/S0140-6736(20)31543-9.

D'Angelo, R., & Dyson, M (2018). *White Fragility: Why it is so hard for white people to talk about race.* Beacon Press.

Dave, G., Wolfe, M. K., & Corbie-Smith, G (2021). Role of hospitals in addressing social determinants of health: A groundwater approach. *Preventive Medicine Reports, 21,* 101315. https://doi.org/10.1016/j.pmedr.2021.101315.

Dhar, A., & Gebreyes, K. (2020). *Racism is a public health crisis.* Modernhealthcare.com. https://www.modernhealthcare.com/patient-care/racism-public-health-crisis.

Egede, L. E., & Walker, R. J. (2020) That Structural racism, social risk factors, and COVID-19—A dangerous convergence for Black Americans. *New England Journal of Medicine, 383*(12), e77. https://doi.org/10.1056/NEJMp2023616.

Eligon, J. (2020). *Doctor who complains of racist care dies of COVID 19* (para. 19). New York Times, https://www.nytimes.com/2020/12/23/us/susan-moore-black-doctor-indiana.html.

Encyclopaedia Judaica. Michael Berenbaum and Fred Skolnik, editors. 2nd edition. Detroit: Macmillan Reference USA, 2007. 22 vols. (18,015 pp.). ISBN 978-0-02-865928-2.

Equal Justice Initiative. (2021). *Public Education.* https://eji.org/public-education/.

Fleming, C. M., & Morris, A. (2015). Theorizing ethnic and racial movements in the global age: Lessons from the Civil Rights Movement. *Sociology of Race and Ethnicity, 1*(1), 105–126. https://doi.org/10.1177/2332649214562473.

Graff, G. (2015). Redesigning racial caste in America via mass incarceration. *The Journal of Psychohistory, 43*(2), 120–133.

Hardy, K. V. (2016). Antiracist approaches for shaping theoretical and practice paradigms. In Carten, A., Siskind, A., & Green, M. P. (Eds.), *Strategies for deconstructing racism in the health and human services* (1st ed., pp. 392). Oxford University Press, 125–139. https://irp-cdn.multiscreensite.com/226e693c/files/uploaded/Ken%20Hardy%20PAST%20Model%20article%20-%20Anti-Racist%20Approaches%20(1)%20(1).pdf.

Harris, A. P., & Pamukcu, A. (2020). The civil rights of health: A new approach to challenging structural inequality. *UCLA Law Review, 67*(5), 758–832.

Hawthorne, M. (2021a). *Pritzker's EPA probed for OK of S. Side shredder.* Chicago Tribune.

Hawthorne, M. (2021b). Southeast side activists go on hunger strike to stop scrap shredder. *Chicago Tribune.*

Jackson, A., O'Brien, M., & Fields, R. (2020). Anti-racism: A toolkit for medical educators. Retrieved from https://hivtrainingcdu.remote-learner.net/pluginfile.php/934/mod_page/content/43/AntiRacism_A%20toolkit%20for%20Medical%20Educators%20UCSF.pdf.

Klugman, C., & Patel, A. (2021). *Commentary: Who gets the COVID-19 vaccine first? Social justice must be a factor.* Chicago Tribune. https://www.chicagotribune.com/opinion/commentary/ct-opinion-coronavirus-vaccine-order-black-hispanic-20201202-oivauayforghlhwpeuhtyw7zim-story.html.

Lawrence, E. (2020). Activists prescribing change for curriculums. Chicago Tribune.

Lederer, S. (2005). Experimentation on human beings. *OAH Magazine of History, 19*(5), 20–22. https://doi.org/10.1093/maghis/19.5.20.

Lewis, S. (2020). *Black doctor in Indiana dies of COVID-19 after publicly complaining of racist treatment at hospital.* CBS News. https://www.cbsnews.com/news/black-doctor-susan-moore-indiana-dies-covid-19-facebook-video-racist-treatment-iu-hospital/.

Love, B., & Hayes-Green, D. (2018). *The groundwater approach: Building a practical understanding of structural racism.* The Racial Equity Institute. https://static1.squarespace.com/static/578fa7e3d482e9af82f8f507/t/5c1b08a50eb-be8eec9f38d21/1545275564106/REI+Groundwater+Approach.pdf.

Massingale, B. N. (2020). The assumptions of white privilege and what we can do about it. *National Catholic Reporter.* https://www.ncronline.org/news/opinion/assumptions-white-privilege-and-what-we-can-do-about-it.

Maybank, A., Jones, C. P., Blackstock, U., & Perry, J. C. (2020). Opinion. Say her name: Dr. Susan Moore. *Washington Post.* https://www.washingtonpost.com/opinions/2020/12/26/say-her-name-dr-susan-moore/.

Mays, E. (2017). *Repositioning criminal justice in the American settler colony.* Stanislaus State. https://www.csustan.edu/sites/default/files/groups/University%20Honors%20Program/Journals/mays.pdf.

McLean, S.-A. (2020). Isolation by distance and the problem of the 21st century. *Human Biology Open Access Pre-Prints, 91*(2). https://digitalcommons.wayne.edu/humbiol_preprints/159.

Mize, K. (2009). What teachers should know about racism, prejudice, and privilege: A literature review. *Northwest Journal of Teacher Education, 7*(1), 38–48. https://doi.org/10.15760/nwjte.2009.7.1.5.

Mobula, L. M., Heller, D. J., Commodore-Mensah, Y., Walker Harris, V., & Cooper, L. A. (2020). Protecting the vulnerable during COVID-19: Treating and preventing chronic disease disparities. *Gates Open Research, 4,* 125. https://doi.org/10.12688/gatesopenres.13181.1.

National League for Nursing. (2019). *A vision for integration of the social determinants of health into nursing education curricula.* http://www.nln.org/docs/default-source/default-document-library/social-determinants-of-health.pdf?sfvrsn=2.

Network Advocates. (n.d.). Recommit to racial justice: The legacy of injustices against Native Americans, Retrieved from https://networkadvocates.org/recommittoracialjustice/legacy/.

Nisa, K. (2019). *Historical events in Jim Crow laws era as reflected in Kathryn Stockett's novel The Help.* UIN Sunan Ampel Surabaya. https://core.ac.uk/download/pdf/227286228.pdf.

Padilla, L. M. (2001). Internalized oppression and Latinos. *Race, Racism and the Law.* https://racism.org/index.php?option=com_content&view=article&id=314:latinos01a&catid=65&Itemid=236.

Palamar, J., Davies, S., Ompad, D., Cleland, C., & Weitzman, M. (2015). Powder cocaine and crack use in the United States: An examination of risk for arrest and socioeconomic disparities in use. *Drug Alcohol Depend, 149,* 108–116. 10.1016/j.drugalcdep.2015.01.029.

Paradies, Y. (2018). *Racism and Indigenous health.* Oxford Research Encyclopedia of Global Public Health. https://doi.org/10.1093/acrefore/9780190632366.013.86.

Parisot, J. (2019). *How America became capitalist: Imperial expansion and the conquest of the West.* Pluto Press. https://library.oapen.org/bitstream/handle/20.500.12657/25934/1004147.pdf?sequence=1&isAllowed=y.

Pastor, M., Terriquez, V., & Lin, M. (2018). How community organizing promotes health equity, and how health equity affects organizing. *Health Affairs, 37*(3), 358–363. https://doi.org/10.1377/hlthaff.2017.1285.

Patterson, R. F., & Harley, R. A. (2019). Effects of freeway rerouting and boulevard replacement on air pollution exposure and neighborhood attributes. *International Journal of Environmental Research and Public Health, 16*(21). https://doi.org/10.3390/ijerph16214072.

Powell, C. M. (2019). *The structural dimensions of race: Lock ups, systemic chokeholds, and binary disruptions.* University of Louisville Law Review. https://racism.org/articles/law-and-justice/criminal-justice-and-racism/137-prison-industrial-complex/2571-the-structural-dimensions-of.

Pratt-Chapman, M. (2020). *Race and America: How did we get here, and what can we do about it?* https://aonnonline.org/expert-commentary/aonn-blog/3066-race-and-america-how-did-we-get-here-and-what-can-we-do-about-it.

Press, T. A. (2021). *White man who drove into Iowa protesters avoids prison.* KCCI Des Moines. https://www.kcci.com/article/white-man-who-drove-into-iowa-protesters-avoids-prison/35165584.

Pyke, K. D. (2010). What is internalized racial oppression and why don't we study it? Acknowledging Racism's hidden injuries. *Sociological Perspectives, 53*(4), 551–572. https://doi.org/10.1525/sop.2010.53.4.551.

Ray, M. (2021). Emmett Till. Death, mother, grave, & facts. *Encyclopedia Britannica.* https://www.britannica.com/biography/Emmett-Till.

Ross, K. M. (2020). Opinion. Call it what it is: Anti-Blackness. *The New York Times.* https://www.nytimes.com/2020/06/04/opinion/george-floyd-anti-blackness.html.

Schneider, E., Malina, D., & Morrissey, S. (2020). Fundamentals of the US health policy; A basic training perspective series. *The New England Journal of Medicine, 383,* 486–487. doi:10.1056/NEJMe2023287.

Seabrook, R., & Wyatt-Nichol, H. (2016). The ugly side of America: Institutional oppression and race. *Journal of Public Management & Social Policy, 23*(1), 20–46.

Taifa, N. (2020). Let's talk about reparations. *Columbia Journal of Race and Law, 10*(1). https://doi.org/10.7916/cjrl.v10i1.5182.

Thurman, W. A., Johnson, K. E., & Sumpter, D. F. (2019). Words matter: An integrative review of institutionalized racism in nursing literature. *Advances in Nursing Science, 42*(2), 89–108.

US Department of Health and Human Services Office for Disease Prevention and Health Promotion. (2021). *Healthy People 2030 Framework—Healthy People 2030,* health.gov. https://health.gov/healthypeople/about/healthy-people-2030-framework

UShistory.org, The Dred Scott decision (2021). *US history pre-Columbian to the new millennium.* https://www.ushistory.org/us/32a.asp.

Van Cleve, S. (2020). *Groundwater problems, groundwater solutions.* Blue Garnet. https://bluegarnet.net/blog/2020/07/17/groundwater-problems-groundwater-solutions/.

Versey, H. S., Cogburn, C. C., Wilkins, C. L., & Joseph, N. (2019). Appropriated racial oppression: Implications for mental health in Whites and Blacks. *Social Science & Medicine, 230,* 295–302. https://doi.org/10.1016/j.socscimed.2019.03.014.

Washington, H. A., Baker, R. B., Olakanmi, O., Savitt, T. L., Jacobs, E. A., Hoover, E., & Wynia, M. K. (2009). Segregation, civil rights, and health disparities: The legacy of African American physicians and organized medicine, 1910–1968. *Journal of the National Medical Association, 101*(6), 513–527. https://doi.org/10.1016/S0027-9684(15)30936-6.

WHO. (2021). *Inequities are killing people on grand scale, reports WHO's commission.* WHO. https://www.who.int/news/item/28-08-2009-inequities-are-killing-people-on-grand-scale-reports-who-s-commission.

Williams, D. (2020). Rethinking Black families in poverty: Postcolonial critiques and critical race possibilities. In Martin, L. L. (Ed.), *Introduction to Africana demography* (pp. 143–164). Brill. https://doi.org/10.1163/9789004433168_008.

Wilson, E. (2018). The legal foundations of White supremacy. *DePaul Journal for Social Justice, 11*(2). https://via.library.depaul.edu/cgi/viewcontent.cgi?article=1168&context=jsj.

Strategies to Promote Health Equity

Policy, Politics, and the Political Determinants of Health

Teri A. Murray

The moral test of government is how that government treats those who are in the dawn of life, the children; those who are in the twilight of life, the elderly; and those who are in the shadows of life, the sick, the needy and the handicapped.
—*Hubert H. Humphrey*

CHAPTER OUTLINE

LEARNING OBJECTIVES

1. Explain the interrelatedness of politics and health.
2. Synthesize how the political determinants of health shape the social determinants of health (SDOH).
3. Describe the dynamics among power, influence, advocacy, and politics.
4. Employ communication and empowerment strategies to influence policy.
5. Design upstream measures to influence policy.

INTRODUCTION

The first law to address the SDOH can be traced back to the Bureau for the Relief of Freedmen and Refugees (Dawes, 2018). The Bureau for the Relief of Freedmen and Refugees provided food, education, employment, housing, and healthcare to marginalized populations displaced by the Civil War (Dawes, 2018). The law was short-lived, and it would take another 100 years before it was recognized that the health of minoritized and marginalized populations lagged the general population's health. This recognition of health disparities led to the passage of the Disadvantaged Minority Health

Improvement Act and the Minority Health and Health Disparities Research and Education Act under the George H.W. Bush and Clinton administrations, respectively (Dawes, 2020). The Disadvantaged Minority Health Improvement and Minority Health and Health Disparities Research and Education Acts raised awareness of health disparities and garnered national attention for the study of minority health and minority health disparities (Dawes, 2018). The next most significant piece of legislation that addressed health disparities and health equity was signed into law under the Obama administration, the Patient Protection and Affordable Care Act (ACA). Although highly controversial, the

151

ACA transformed the healthcare landscape in the United States. The ACA was designed to address the significant shortcomings in the healthcare system: access to care, poor health outcomes, inconsistent quality of care, and the high cost of healthcare.

Laws and policies are essential in shaping the health and health status of the US population. Health policy can have a major bearing on the health and well-being of a population. Accordingly, "Healthy People 2030" focuses on keeping the population safe and healthy through laws and policies at the local, state, territorial, and federal levels (US Department of Health and Human Services [USDHHS], Office of Disease Prevention and Health Promotion [ODPHP], n.d.). "Healthy People 2030" established a goal of using health policy to prevent disease and improve health.

Laws and policies are influenced by and through political processes, termed the *political determinants of health.* The political determinants of health are the systematic processes of structuring relationships, distributing resources, and administering power, all of which operate simultaneously in ways that mutually reinforce or influence one another to shape the opportunities that advance health equity or exacerbate health inequities (Dawes, 2020). Laws and policies provide evidence of the extent to which a country can and will promote health equity or support a system of inequities that ultimately results in health disparities.

The impact of politics, political views, and political players on health was seen in the presidential changes from the Obama to the Trump administration. Trump's views on the ACA sparked national debates concerning whether to repeal or replace the ACA despite the benefits seen from the law's passage (Dawes, 2020). When the ACA was enacted, more than 46 million individuals were uninsured. The ACA extended health insurance to more than 20 million Americans, effectively decreasing the number of uninsured (Center for American Progress, 2020; The Commonwealth Fund, 2020). The ACA further codified protections for people with preexisting conditions by prohibiting health insurance plans from denying coverage or raising rates for people with preexisting illnesses, in addition to placing limits on the out-of-pocket costs that individuals need to pay for yearly deductibles, coinsurance, and copayments (Silberman, 2020). The ACA further eliminated cost sharing for high-impact preventive healthcare services (Center for American Progress, 2020; The Commonwealth Fund, 2020). Other provisions

of the ACA included addressing the needs of breastfeeding mothers who work by implementing a federal law that mandated employers provide reasonable break times and a private place shielded from the view of others to express breast milk (US Department of Labor, n.d.). There were many provisions under the ACA, all aimed at improving health. The provisions included nutritional labeling and calorie information for standard menu items in restaurants and retail establishments so people can be more conscious of their food choices (US Food and Drug Administration, 2018). The full extent of the benefits provided by the ACA lies beyond the scope of this chapter. However, the ACA was not without criticism. The two major criticisms of the ACA centered on the individual health insurance mandate and Medicaid expansion.

The individual insurance mandate was designed to expand coverage by requiring that most people have health coverage and, if they did not, they would have to pay a tax penalty. However, this mandate was repealed under the Trump administration when Congress reduced the penalty to $0 and expanded short-term, limited-duration, and associated health plans. Short-term limited-duration plans were designed for people who experience a temporary gap in health insurance (Pollitz et al., 2018). The plans provide major medical coverage for a fixed term of less than 1 year and offer limited types of service with a maximum dollar amount (Pollitz et al., 2018).

The Medicaid expansion program under the ACA allowed states to expand their Medicaid program to nonelderly adults with incomes up to 138% of the federal poverty line. The poverty level was $16,243 for a single person and $33,465 for a family of four in 2016. The Medicaid expansion program increased access to care for low-income individuals, which is associated with greater use of healthcare services (The Commonwealth Fund, 2020). A lack of health insurance coverage is a major barrier to healthcare access and contributes to the disparities commonly seen in healthcare (Yearby et al., 2022). In addition, Medicaid expansion has been associated with decreased cardiovascular and renal mortalities (The Commonwealth Fund, 2020). Despite its benefits, not every state adopted the Medicaid expansion program. Many believe the lack of adoption is more related to politics and perhaps costs to the states than the health benefits for the population. As of March 2023, 40 states and DC have adopted the Medicaid expansion program, and 10 states have not adopted the expansion (Kaiser Family Foundation, 2023) (Table 7.1). Many

TABLE 7.1   Status of State Medicaid Expansion Decisions

Adopted	Not Adopted
Alaska	Alabama
Arizona	Florida
Arkansas	Georgia
California	Kansas
Colorado	Mississippi
Connecticut	South Carolina
Delaware	Tennessee
District of Columbia	Texas
Hawaii	Wisconsin
Idaho	Wyoming
Illinois	
Indiana	
Iowa	
Kentucky	
Louisiana	
Maine	
Maryland	
Massachusetts	
Michigan	
Minnesota	
Missouri	
Montana	
Nebraska	
Nevada	
New Hampshire	
New Jersey	
New Mexico	
New York	
North Carolina	
North Dakota	
Ohio	
Oklahoma	
Oregon	
Pennsylvania	
Rhode Island	
South Dakota	
Utah	
Vermont	
Virginia	
Washington	
West Virginia	

Source: Kaiser Family Foundation (KFF). (2023). *Status of State Action on the Medicaid Expansion Decision*. Retrieved from https://www.kff.org/medicaid/issue-brief/status-of-state-medicaid-expansion-decisions-interactive-map/ (Accessed on Feb 19, 2024).

states imposed a work requirement as an additional eligibility requirement for Medicaid populations (Yearby et al., 2022).

The ACA currently stands as law, not repealed under the Trump administration, but the law has survived many near-death experiences. Although the ACA underwent significant alterations under the Trump administration—cutbacks in Medicaid coverage, retrenching on ACA requirements for health insurance, defunding of prevention programs, and threats to contraceptive coverage—it remains standing (Berwick, 2018; Dawes, 2020). The ACA is considered safe under the Biden administration. Over 16 million people signed up for healthcare coverage in ACA marketplaces during the 2022–2023 year's open enrollment season, a record number (Centers for Medicare & Medicaid Service, 2023). The back-and-forth politics of the ACA is a clear example of the relationships among political views, policy, laws, and healthcare. Additionally, the Biden administration has made advancing health equity a priority through several legislative initiatives. The Biden initiatives not only focus on health (e.g., maternal health, access to quality care, survivors of violence, tribal health, rural health, and infectious diseases) but also include initiatives focused on what is traditionally considered outside the realm of healthcare, such as inequities in housing, education, workforce development, environmental justice, paid leave, and criminal justice reforms (The White House, 2023). Undoubtedly, laws governing healthcare can be determined by political ideology, and policies are born from those ideological beliefs. Thus politics and policies matter because both impact health.

THE INTERRELATEDNESS OF POLICY, POLITICS, AND HEALTH

If the SDOH are the drivers behind the inequities that create disparities, what drives the SDOH? The political determinants of health shape the SDOH (Mishori, 2019). Chapter 1 discussed how the SDOH extend beyond clinical care to shape health. For example, under the Fair Labor Standards Act, employers must abide by federal and state minimum wage laws. Minimum wage laws require employers to pay employees a specific wage designated by federal and state laws. The amount of the minimum wage has a powerful effect on the health status of individuals. Narain and Zimmerman (2019) found that increases in the minimum wage were positively associated with increased access to care and improved dietary quality. Komro and colleagues (2016) found that a $1 increase in the minimum wage above the federal level was associated with a 1–2% decrease in low birth weights and a 4% decrease in postneonatal mortality. There are other policies and political decisions that could be considered outside the healthcare domain but can shape health. These policies include laws governing immigration and women's reproductive health. For example, immigrants are excluded from participation in the ACA and most Medicaid expansion programs. These exclusionary laws contribute to poor immigrant health, with immigrants having decreased access to healthcare, lower healthcare utilization, and reduced health expenditures (Wilson & Stimpson, 2020). Policies that limit access to healthcare can have severe public health impacts, particularly considering the potential spread of infectious diseases such as coronavirus disease 2019 (COVID-19). The interrelatedness of laws and health includes decisions related to the COVID-19 pandemic, mandates to require face masks, and COVID-19 vaccines. While highly politicized, both mandates ultimately decreased the transmission of COVID-19 and reduced the threat of the pandemic.

The most famous court case related to women's reproductive health was the 1973 US Supreme Court decision in *Roe v. Wade*. The *Roe v. Wade* case challenged a Texas law that made abortion illegal unless conducted by a physician for life-saving purposes. With this ruling, the court recognized for the first time the constitutional right to privacy and that it was a woman's decision whether to terminate her pregnancy (Planned Parenthood, 2014). This case was, in effect, the case that legalized abortion nationwide (Planned Parenthood, 2014). Since *Roe v. Wade,* there have been several restrictive state laws related to protecting human life and disregarding women's reproductive health rights that influence maternal–child health. In 2021, Texas and Mississippi passed the most restrictive reproductive laws since the *Roe v. Wade* decision. However, in 2022, the Supreme Court, in the *Dobbs v. Jackson Women's Health Organization* case, overturned the constitutional right to abortion, unsettling a nearly 50-year decision and undermining constitutional freedom and equality for women (The National Constitution Center, 2022). Healthcare and politics are inextricably linked. Upstream political decisions can have downstream health effects, specifically on the health of certain marginalized populations.

HEALTH POLICY

To be influential in policy matters, nurses must first understand the basic terms. A policy is a governing principle for a specific action to achieve a given outcome. The CDC (2015) describes policy as a law, regulation, procedure, administrative action, incentive, or voluntary practice enacted by an organization. A policy is a planned course of activities to influence decisions, actions, and rules on matters. Policies guide behavior to address specific issues, and policy decisions are reflected in the distribution of goods and services and allocation of resources.

The WHO defines health policy as the specific decisions, plans, and actions undertaken to achieve health (WHO, n.d.). Health policy has also been defined as the "aggregate of principles, stated or unstated, that… characterize the distribution of resources, services, and political influences that impact the health of a population" (Shi, 2019, p. 19). Additionally, Shi (2019) adds that health policy is any legislation that may influence the social and physical environments, behavior, socioeconomic status, availability of healthcare services, and access to healthcare services. This broad definition of health policy reveals the extent to which policies influence health, directly or indirectly. Health policies are those specific actions taken to achieve healthcare goals and clarify what is valued in society via the allocation of resources.

"Healthy People 2030" uses evidence-based health policies to develop disease prevention and health promotion goals. One example is the policy that requires community water systems to use fluoridated water to improve the population's oral health. Health policies can critically impact the health of an individual, family, community, or population and, when evidence-based, can be used for risk reduction, disease prevention, and health promotion.

However, there is a clear distinction between health policy and healthcare policy. Health policy is directed toward improving the population's health. In contrast, healthcare policy refers to how healthcare is administered and accessed and aims to provide efficient, equitable access to high-quality healthcare services. Healthcare policy refers to a broad array of health-related services, including the financing, organization, and delivery of care, and practice laws—laws and codes related to electronic health records, administration of drugs and other therapeutics, scopes of practice for licensed healthcare professionals, and health insurance.

THE HEALTH IN ALL POLICIES APPROACH

In recent years, the concept of health in all policies (HiAP) has garnered national attention as a strategy to promote health equity. The HiAP approach does not describe a specific set of policies but refers to integrating health into all policymaking processes (Hall & Jacobson, 2018). The HiAP approach recognizes that the most critical factors that drive health outcomes—social, economic, and environmental—lie outside the domains of clinical care and public health departments. The WHO (n.d. a) defines the HiAP approach as a multisector collaborative approach to public policies that systematically considers the health implications of decisions, seeks synergies, and attempts to avoid harmful health impacts to improve population health and achieve health equity. The HiAP approach is branded as a method to achieve health equity, although there is no clear evidence that the approach produces a specific outcome. Despite the lack of clear evidence, there is practical value in working across sectors to address conditions that influence health.

Multisector and cross-sector engagement and collaboration are critical features of the HiAP approach. Multisector partnerships and cross-sector alliances are needed to address the built and lived environment, including environmental toxins, safe and adequate housing, availability of healthy foods and produce, and sufficient transportation infrastructures—all necessary for health. For example, cross-sector collaborations can be seen in municipalities where the local public health department might partner with the parks and recreation department to plan a walking path or bike trail for residents to engage in physical activity and exercise. Another example of collaboration is when the transportation department works with the parks and recreation department to add bike lanes to streets (Hall & Jacobson, 2018). Nurses can

bring expertise to these HiAP approaches by volunteering to serve on community and municipal boards. Although community and municipal boards are outside the traditional healthcare domain, the decisions made by these boards impact the health of residents and can improve population health.

Challenges associated with the collaborative nature of the HiAP approach include that multisector commitments and alliances depend on a high level of institutional integration and support beyond one's organization. Second, HiAP approaches require the engagement of high-level officials who have the power to initiate collaborations, make decisions, and follow through with implementing those decisions. Finally, the HiAP approach depends on the political ideology of elected officials, and as the ideological pendulum swings from liberal to conservative, so does support for the HiAP approach.

NURSES AND HEALTH POLICY

As the largest group of healthcare professionals, nurses can have a powerful voice and influence on policy-related matters. Nurses, as a collective, have untapped power to expedite public and perhaps political trust. Nurses, as policymakers, can be the voice of their constituents and initiate and champion legislation that will improve healthcare and advance the nursing profession (Curley, 2023). For example, Representative Lauren Underwood (D-IL), a nurse, introduced legislation to improve Black maternal health outcomes, the Black Maternal Health Momnibus Act of 2021 (https://www.congress.gov/bill/117th-congress/house-bill/959). Representative Underwood is one of three nurses in the US House of Representatives (Table 7.2).

Most nurses are not politically involved and see themselves as clinicians rather than politicians. The American Association of Colleges of Nursing's (AACN, 2021) document, "The Essentials: Core Competencies for Professional Nursing Education," identifies health policy as a concept for nursing practice. The document further relates that "Nurses play critical roles in advocating for policy that impacts patients, and the profession, especially when speaking with a united voice on issues that affect nursing practice and health outcomes" (AACN, 2021, p. 15). Therefore nurses should understand the political forces shaping individuals, families, communities, and health. Unfortunately, while nurses have been great in

TABLE 7.2 Nurse Legislators

Nurses Serving in Congress

Congresswoman Eddie Bernice Johnson (Democrat, TX)	Congresswoman Johnson was the first nurse to be elected to the US Congress. She began her nursing career as the Chief Psychiatric Nurse at the VA Hospital in Dallas, TX. She currently represents the 30th Congressional District of Texas in the US House of Representatives. First elected in 1992 and currently serving her 15th term. She is noted for being the first African American and the first female chair of the House Committee on Science, Space, and Technology. Her initiative, "A World of Women for World Peace," has gained national and international recognition.
Congresswoman Lauren Underwood (Democrat, IL)	Congresswoman Lauren Underwood was sworn into the 116th US Congress in 2019. She is the first woman, the first person of color, and the first millennial to represent her community in Congress. She is also the youngest African American woman to serve in the US House of Representatives. Congresswoman Underwood introduced the Momnibus bill, warning that the public health crisis surrounding Black maternal child health outcomes would not abate unless lawmakers acted.
Congresswoman Cori Bush (Democrat, MO)	Congresswoman Cori Bush was sworn into office in 2020. She is the first Black woman and first nurse to represent Missouri. Most recently she introduced the Drug Policy Reform Act to decriminalize drug possession and implement a health-centered approach.

From: American Nurses Association. (n.d.) *Nurses Serving in Congress*. Retrieved from https://www.nursingworld.org/practice-policy/advocacy/federal/nurses-serving-in-congress/.

advocating for patients and families, few of the nearly 4 million nurses in the United States get involved in the political world.

Several notable nurses have been actively involved in the policymaking process. Bethany Hall-Long is the Lieutenant Governor of Delaware, having been reelected in 2020. She previously served in the Delaware House of Representatives and the Delaware Senate. Marilyn Tavenner served as the Virginia Secretary for Health and Human Services, then an Administrator of the Centers for Medicare and Medicaid Services, an agency of the US Department of Health and Human Services. The current CEO of the National League of Nursing, Beverly Malone, served as the Deputy Assistant Secretary for Health in the Department of Health and Human Services during the Clinton administration. Mary Wakefield served in the Obama administration as the US Deputy Secretary of Health and Human Services, then as the head of the Health Resources and Services Administration. These are a few of several nurses who have served in important government leadership positions at local, state, or federal levels. While most nurses may not serve in high-ranking political offices, they should be involved in political processes. Their political activity may be as simple as voting in local school board elections or sharing research findings with a state legislator, or as complex as running for state office.

Nurses must attain the knowledge, skills, and abilities to understand the effects of the structures, systems, and policies that influence health, and design upstream, midstream, and downstream interventions to support population health. One way to do this is through political advocacy. Political advocacy is critical for nurses to serve as change agents in health and healthcare. However, King (2015) identified several reasons why nurses do not become involved in politics, including (1) lack of confidence in one's ability to clearly articulate the issues, (2) inability to communicate effectively with political leaders, (3) lack of knowledge of the political and policymaking process, (4) lack of mentorship in the policy arena, (5) lack of access to professional networks in the political arena, and (6) limited leadership development. Steps for nurses to learn more about politics, policy, and political advocacy are shown in Box 7.1.

Effectively addressing the SDOH requires upstream action. Upstream actions are described as the laws, policies, and regulations that create the conditions that support health at the level of the community downstream (Cropley et al., 2022).

BOX 7.1   Basic Steps to Get Involved in Political Advocacy

Basic Steps

1. Register to vote. Voting puts in place the legislators charged with the decision-making ability who can create and execute policy that affects all citizens, regardless of whether you have engaged in the political process. Voting ensures participation in American democracy.

2. Join a state- or national-level nurses' association. Your state chapter has a focus on state issues whereas the national association focuses on national issues. These associations advocate for political policies that promote nursing and health.

3. Become familiar with your state and federal legislators. Know where their political interests lie and what legislative initiatives they have sponsored or cosigned with other legislators.

4. Connect with your representatives. Visit their website. Send an email introducing yourself including your area of expertise. Extend an offer to share your expertise in needed areas. When you reach out and offer to assist your legislators, this action facilitates relationship building.

5. Commit to understanding the legislative process and political structures in your communities and at local, state, and federal levels.

Adapted from: Dawes, D. E. (2020). The political determinants of health. Johns Hopkins University Press and King C. A. (2015). Nursing advocacy 101: Start where you are to do what you can. Tarheel Nurse, 77(2 Spec. No.), 12–15.

THE POLICY DEVELOPMENT PROCESS: THE CDC POLICY ANALYTICAL FRAMEWORK

The CDC developed a five-step methodology for policy development. This methodology can be used to identify, analyze, and prioritize policies aimed at health improvement (Fig. 7.1).

Problem Identification

Policy development begins with the process of identifying the problem. This step starts with the awareness of a problem and a clear identification of the root cause, followed by an assessment of the scale and scope of the problem. Since health problems can be contextually based, stakeholder involvement at this point is essential. Stakeholders can be individuals, groups, or entities with a vested interest in the issue. Since policy decisions impact stakeholders, it is essential to identify stakeholders who can influence the policymaking process. Getting multiple perspectives from various stakeholders allows one to better understand the nature of the problem.

Policy Analysis

Policy analysis is identifying potential policy options to address the problem. All policy options should be compared to determine the most effective, efficient, and feasible option based on the best available evidence

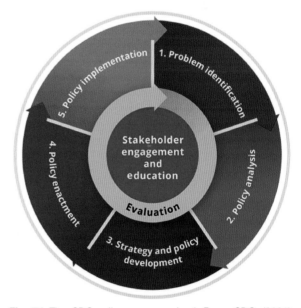

Fig. 7.1 The CDC policy process wheel. From: CDC. (2021). Office of the Associate Director for Policy and Strategy: Policy Process. Retrieved from https://www.cdc.gov/policy/polaris/policyprocess/index.html.

(CDC, 2021). This step involves thoroughly researching the options to assess possible policy solutions. What are the policy objectives? What would be the impact of each proposed option? What groups or populations would be impacted by each policy option? What are the social, cultural, and political contexts surrounding each option? What are the costs and benefits if the policy options are pursued? First, a cost-benefit analysis should be conducted for each policy option, followed by considerations of the feasibility of each option. What barriers exist to the implementation of each policy option? What would be the short-, intermediate-, and long-term gains from each option? Are there unintended consequences that could arise from the options? Finally, the proposed policy options should be prioritized and, when prioritized, the rationale and criteria for the prioritized ranking should be included.

Strategy and Policy Development

Strategy and policy development is the planning process that involves engaging stakeholders to create, draft, and make the policy an actionable item. Once the policy is drafted, there should be a plan to move the policy forward. A policy has a higher probability of enactment when the stakeholders are involved, when stakeholders are highly influential, and when stakeholders agree on the process of moving the policy forward. Therefore the involvement of stakeholders is critical at this stage in policy development.

Policy Enactment

Policy enactment is the official authorization to implement the new policy. The stakeholders involved in policy enactment depend on the type of policy and the governing body. Depending on the governing body, the official authorization can be from an institution or organization such as a school board, a governing authority such as a municipality within a city, a regulatory board such as a state board of nursing, or federal and state government agencies. It is important to understand that policy enactment can be iterative, slow, and multistep. As a result, it may take years before the actual enactment of the policy is realized.

Policy Implementation

Once the policy is implemented, more work is needed to ensure the highest likelihood that the policy will achieve the desired intent. The entity responsible for implementing the policy should embark on a public awareness and education campaign to ensure those affected by the policy are aware of it and how it will affect them. Be mindful of the resources needed to implement the new policy. Policy development is a continuous process. New policies should be reviewed periodically to see if they achieve the desired outcomes.

This five-step process—problem identification, policy analysis, strategy and policy development, policy enactment, and policy implementation—is a straightforward methodology for policy development. However, no matter how straightforward the process, it is essential to remember that politics greatly influence any policy outcome. Politics can influence the decision-making process that will ultimately determine the specific course of action. In most cases, the ability to influence decisions involves some aspect of power.

POWER

Power is the ability to influence the behavior of others to achieve a desired end. There are many types of power. Formal or legitimate power comes from a position or title within an organization or entity. Leaders who have legitimate power are also able to use coercive power. Coercive power is the ability to influence behavior through rewards or sanctions. Multiple sources of power can influence decisions related to a particular issue (Table 7.3). Often power is thought of as something held by an individual, yet social media platforms are becoming an increasing source of power.

Social media platforms empower citizens, groups, organizations, autocracies, and democracies. These platforms offer freedom of expression and can be a mobilizing and powerful force for persuasion and influence. For example, in the 2016 presidential election, social networks were deemed responsible for influencing election results through fake news. Fake news is information gathered and relayed among social network users that is unfiltered, not fact-checked, and has not undergone editorial oversight (Schleffer & Miller, 2021). Fake news is also intentional and verifiably false and could mislead others (Schleffer & Miller, 2021). It is essential to recognize that social media platforms can be used as a power source for propagating truth or rumors that can influence voting, political choices, and policy decisions.

Another form of influence and power is conformity. Conformity is when an individual behaves in a certain way, influenced by group behavior, yet the specific behavior does not result from a direct request by the group. Conformity is the tendency to behave according to the norms of a group. Conformity can result in behaviors not ordinarily done, but the individual joins in because the group engages in the behavior. For example, conformity could result when a group leader has

TABLE 7.3	Sources of Power
Source	**Description**
Legitimate	Legitimate power is vested in a formalized, organizational position and the stature associated with that position. The influence of power is granted and recognized by a hierarchical position. This person is in a higher-level position and often has direct control over others in the organization. Individuals comply because they accept the legitimacy of the person's power.
Coercive	Coercive power is based on compliance. The person holding this type of power can punish others for noncompliance or impose a sanction. The person complies with the request to avoid punishment or loss of privileges. The main objective of this form of power is compliance.
Expert	Expert power is based on the person's expertise, knowledge, skills, or abilities in a defined area, and this expertise sets the individual apart from others. The source of power is the respect earned through experience and knowledge.
Referent	Referent power is generated from being associated with an individual who is highly favored, highly likeable, and has strong interpersonal and charismatic skills that tend to attract others. Most often, referent power is bestowed on the individual by others. Referent power is associated with charisma, as people are attracted to them, desire to be like them, and desire to win their admiration.
Reward	Reward power is garnered from the ability to reward, incentivize, or provide favors such as perks. This influence is based on the ability to provide rewards to others in such a way as to motivate individuals.
Information	Information power is derived from the ability to possess and control information. In information power, the person has access to information that others do not have or cannot easily access. This information could be needed by others to complete a task.

Adapted from: Disch, J. (2020). Nursing leadership in policy formation. *Nursing Forum, 55,* 4–10 and Groenwald, S. L. (2019). Politics, power, and predictability of nursing care. *Nursing Forum, 55,* 16–22.

some power source and thereby induces the group to engage in a specific activity. The most notable example of the power of conformity was seen on January 6, 2021, known as Insurrection Day. On that day, joint sessions of Congress convened to certify Joe Biden's electoral vote win for the 2021 US presidency. The exiting President Trump had multiple sources of power (i.e., legitimate, coercive, reward, and referent) and rallied his supporters to protest the election of Joe Biden as the next president. The rally resulted in the storming of Capitol Hill, causing massive violence to break out and individuals engaged in behaviors that they may not have ordinarily done under different circumstances. Insurrection Day is a prime example of power and conformity and how they influence politics and behavior, causing people to engage in unethical and unlawful conduct.

FORCE FIELD ANALYSIS THEORY

Force field analysis theory is a theoretical framework that addresses factors that can drive or impede movement toward a specific goal or policy. Driving forces are those factors that favor the adoption of a particular policy, whereas restraining forces are those factors that impede the development of the policy. Force field

analysis is designed to enhance understanding of the probability of achieving a desired goal, policy, or change. This process encourages critical thinking and a deep dive into the issues that can drive or restrain the proposed policy.

To conduct a force field analysis, the person proposing the policy describes the desired policy in the middle of a chart or diagram (Fig. 7.2). Then, the forces for change or the driving factors are listed on the right side of the chart. Driving factors are the circumstances that support the need for the policy. Also listed is the relative strength of each driving force, including the relationship between and among the driving forces. The forces against the policy are listed as the restraining forces on the left side. What factors would impede the proposed policy? What is the relative strength of those factors? What are the relationships between and among the restraining factors? Next, the policy developer examines the driving and restraining forces to determine a course of action. Courses of action include strengthening and increasing the driving forces or decreasing the restraining forces. In either case, the policymaker examines both types of forces and develops strategies to influence the desired change or policy. During the analysis process, the relative strength of each force is estimated, and the

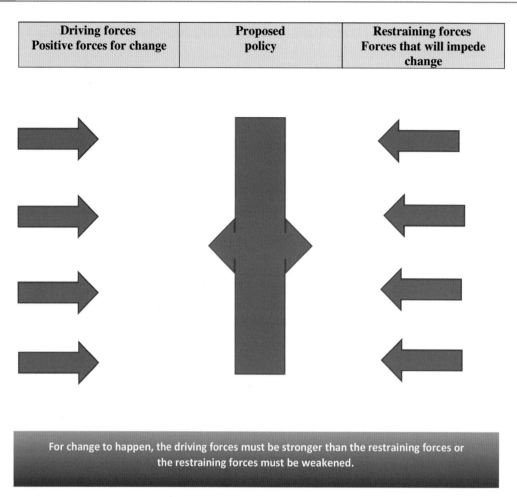

Driving forces Positive forces for change	Proposed policy	Restraining forces Forces that will impede change

For change to happen, the driving forces must be stronger than the restraining forces or the restraining forces must be weakened.

Fig. 7.2 Force field analysis theory.

most salient forces are noted and further analyzed. The next step is to list each force and develop strategies to strengthen each critical driving force or determine how to weaken the restraining forces. This level of analysis can provide a holistic understanding of the prevailing forces that can influence policy development and adoption and the factors that could impede that process.

Force field analysis provides opposing and diverging views on the issue at hand. It enables an understanding of the opposition and the type of support needed for the new policy or change in existing policy. Just as with the CDC's policy development process, stakeholders are involved in this process. Stakeholders are persons, groups, or organizations affected by a particular course of action or policy change and can be anyone or any group. Stakeholders include private citizens, special interest groups, congressional persons, lobbyists representing specific industries, professional organizations and associations, and advocacy groups with a vested interest in the outcome (Loversidge, 2019). Stakeholder engagement is essential and allows those developing a policy to consider the needs of those with a stake in the proposed policy. Oftentimes there are policy champions, individuals, or groups committed to making the policy change who offer their support for or against the change. The higher the champion's level within an organization or group, the more power and force they may bring to influence the policy change. One must always be aware of the political leanings of elected officials to determine whether the proposed policy is consistent with the ideology of those who have the power to adopt and implement the change. If the proposed policy is not aligned with their ideological views, chances are that the policy will not be adopted. Critics of the force field analysis theory emphasize that changes, goals, or proposed policies are often complex and nuanced and cannot readily be distilled into clear-cut driving or impeding forces.

STRATEGIES TO INFLUENCE POLICY

Voting

Voting is the most fundamental civic duty and is the simplest form of political and civic engagement. Voting puts in place the legislators with decision-making authority who have the power to create and execute policy that affects all, regardless of whether individuals are engaged explicitly in the political process (Dawes, 2020). Government entities are the structural mechanisms by which policymakers keep, enforce, or change policy at the local, state, regional, and national levels. Policies result from the finalized action by these entities.

When voting in local, state, and national elections is a straightforward way to make a difference. Voting is important and does matter. Voting can influence the distribution of power and resources that determine factors such as the minimum wage, employment conditions, social services, early childhood development resources, and education (Brown et al., 2020). Legislative actions determine health, and voting can send signals of support for or opposition to policies that can ultimately shape the SDOH.

When voting in campaigns, nurses should research the candidates up for election, visit their websites, and listen to their debates. Reviewing the candidate's background can help nurses understand which candidates align with their beliefs and values about health, healthcare, and nursing. First and foremost, nurses should be aware of the issues affecting nursing, health and healthcare, and patients. It is impossible to advocate for the profession and patients if nurses are uninformed. Most legislators do not have health backgrounds and therefore lack the necessary expertise in healthcare or nursing to make fully informed decisions about specific matters. When nurses do not regularly communicate with elected officials, elected officials listen to nonnursing individuals (Institute of Medicine [IOM], 2011). Nurses can help educate legislators, since there are very few legislators who have healthcare or nursing backgrounds. Legislators make decisions about healthcare,

scopes of practice, and healthcare insurance, among other things. Nurses are responsible for patient advocacy; therefore every nurse should know who represents them at the local, state, and federal levels. Additionally, the nurse should work with interprofessional colleagues to raise awareness and interest in policies that advance health and healthcare. Engagement in the electoral process also includes volunteering, campaigning for candidates, making campaign contributions, expressing your political voice and, most certainly, having knowledge and awareness of the issues that impact health (Brown et al., 2020).

Voter apathy occurs when there is a lack of interest or indifference to whether one votes in an election. Causes of voter apathy vary, but many individuals feel that the political systems do not work for them. Some voters may be indifferent because they think the election outcomes will have a limited effect on their daily lives. Thus they assume the effort of participation is not worth it, and become indifferent to the outcomes of the voting or election process. Other causes of voter apathy could include a disinterest in the candidates or the issues on the ballot. Finally, voter apathy could simply be due to a lack of information about how ballot issues may impact them. When larger numbers of people from underrepresented communities and groups vote, it translates into greater influence in determining the legislators who hold political power (Brown et al., 2020). Those legislators in power respond to the needs and demands of their constituents, shaping the social determinants of their health. Thus it is also important for nurses to educate the public about the relationship between voting and health (Brown et al., 2020).

Low voter turnout can have significant political and policy consequences, since government officials and entities have the power and authority to keep, change, or alter policy at local, state, and national levels. Voter turnout in presidential elections in the United States averages about 60%, and about 40% of the eligible voter population votes in the midterm elections. According to FairVote (2021), the 2020 presidential and 2018 midterm elections had the highest voter turnout in a century. Other factors that negatively impact voter turnout are stringent state voter registration laws, voter identification laws, elimination of early voting measures, and limiting polling place accessibility (FairVote, 2021).

Voter suppression is when laws make it more difficult for individuals to exercise their right to vote. A common form of voter suppression is restricting the registration requirements to vote. Many states have enacted laws that make it substantially more difficult for people of color, older adults, students, and people with disabilities to vote (American Civil Liberties Union [ACLU], 2021). For example, in 2011 the Kansas Secretary of State required proof of citizenship documents—a passport or a birth certificate, which most people did not have on hand—to register to vote. This action blocked the ability of 30,000 Kansans to register (ACLU, 2021a). The ACLU sued and defeated the law in 2018, only to have the Supreme Court and a 10th Circuit Court of Appeals affirm the ruling in 2020 (ACLU, 2021a). In addition, Georgia lawmakers made it a crime to provide nourishment such as food and water to voters standing in line at the polls (ACLU, 2021a). Felony disenfranchisement is another way to suppress voting rights. In 48 states, a felony conviction results in the loss of voting rights, although the period of disenfranchisement varies by state (The Sentencing Project, 2021). Because of racism in the criminal justice system, felony disenfranchisement laws most often affect people of color, since people of color face harsher sentences for committing the same offenses as White people (ACLU, 2021a). As a result of the privatization and profiteering of the prison systems with concordant expansion in the number of incarcerated individuals, in 2020, 5.2 million Americans were unable to vote due to state felony disenfranchisement policies (The Sentencing Project, 2021). States with the harshest disenfranchisement laws also have histories of suppressing the rights of Black people.

Gerrymandering is another form of voter suppression. Gerrymandering is when political parties reset district boundaries to give themselves an electoral advantage to predetermine the outcome of an election (ACLU, 2021b). Historically, gerrymandering first occurred when minorities were given the right to vote. Legislative bodies used gerrymandering to minimize the impact of minority voting. Redistricting most often disenfranchises people of color.

Opinion Pieces

An opinion piece is one way to raise public awareness about a specific policy issue. Opinion pieces are referred to as op-eds. The term *op-ed* was coined because the opinion piece originally appeared opposite the editorial page in a printed newspaper. Individuals, groups, associations, and organizations write op-eds because they have an opinion on a particular policy matter, are subject matter experts, and want to sway the public in a specific direction regarding the policy. The opening of the op-ed should be a hook that grabs the reader's attention and lays the foundation for the stated opinion. For example, after the 2021 Atlanta massage parlor shootings, there was an op-ed in the *Chicago Tribune* regarding the need for gun violence interventions. In the *Chicago Tribune* April 19, 2021, op-ed, the author writes, "What kind of example are we setting for the rest of the world?" "Must our flags always fly at half-mast?"

The op-ed should be relevant to the target audience. Op-eds begin with explaining the issue and a case or story that personalizes it. The author should ensure the piece is written for the appropriate audience, in plain language that is easily understood, and void of discipline-specific or technical jargon. The op-ed should be written in a conversational tone. The goal is for the public to understand the message conveyed in the op-ed. The concepts surrounding the policy or issue should be explained thoroughly to give the readers an understanding of the issue. For example, "While COVID-19 has dominated public health discussions over the last year, we have failed to address another deadly epidemic [gun violence]" (*Chicago Tribune*, 2021, para 1). Because op-eds are opinions, they should be backed by evidence-based research, statistics, facts, and figures that support a position on the policy; for example, "[Gun violence] has a fatality rate of approximately 30%" (*Chicago Tribune*, 2021, para 2). Op-eds should include the next steps that should be taken regarding the policy matter. The ending should summarize the main points, provide a memorable detail, and end with a call to action; for example, "Gun violence is a complicated and intractable epidemic … when dealing with a public health crisis, no measure is too small …. Understand that interventions take one step at a time" (*Chicago Tribune*, 2021, para 15 & 16).

The length of op-eds varies, but most are about 700–800 words. One crucial task is reading the newspaper submission guidelines. Op-eds often end with a conclusion that circles back to the original lead-in or hook that captured the reader's attention.

Policy Briefs

A policy brief is a concise summary of a specific policy with policy options that address an issue and offers recommendations for the best solutions. The purpose of the policy brief is fivefold: (1) to convince the target audience of the problem, (2) why it is critical, (3) why there is a need to consider a new policy solution, (4) to introduce preferred policy alternative options, and (5) to outline a recommended course of action (Community-Based Monitoring System Network Coordinating Team, n.d., paragraph 3). A policy brief targets officials who are developing a new policy or considering a change in an existing policy. While intended for political officials, policy briefs can be used by other audiences with a stake in the issue. Therefore the brief should be specific to the target audience and address the reader's stake in the matter.

Policy briefs provide policy advice and advocate for desired solutions to specific concerns; they are helpful to officials who have decision-making authority over a particular matter (DeMarco & Tufts, 2014). Policy briefs give context to the issue being addressed and contain evidence-based research using the best possible evidence available. Evidence-based health policies can help prevent disease and promote health (USDHHS, ODPHP, n.d.). For example, the establishment of smoke-free policies helped prevent smoking initiation and increased cigarette quit attempts (USDHHS, ODPHP, n.d.). The requirement for community water systems to provide fluoridated water improved the population's oral health (USDHHS, ODPHP, n.d.). Evidence-based policies are vital to improving population health (USDHHS, ODPHP, n.d.), and briefs are designed to facilitate policymaking. A policy brief can also be viewed as an advocacy document, since the purpose is to convince an audience or policymaker of the urgency of the current problem and the need to adopt an alternative course of action, ultimately serving as a call for action (epoc.cochrane.org, 2011).

According to the Community-Based Monitoring System Network Coordinating Team (n.d.), policy briefs have five main components:

1. Executive summary: The summary is a short synopsis or overview that describes the problem that needs to be addressed, states why the policy needs to be changed with other options, and recommends action.
2. A description of the context and importance of the problem: This section provides a clear and concise statement of the problem, the background or significance, the root causes, and a clear statement of the policy implications of the problem that establishes its importance and relevance. This section should include data, evidence, and references from science-based literature from well-respected, peer-reviewed, evidence-based sources (DeMarco & Tufts, 2014). This section should also include information from lay publications such as *The New York Times* or *The Washington Post* so that the reader understands that the issue is current and in the purview of the public (DeMarco & Tufts, 2014).
3. Critique of the existing policy: This section outlines the shortcomings of the current policy and provides an argument for why and how the current approach is failing. In this section, all opinions, including opposing ones, should be recognized; a balanced brief explains both sides of the issue, including the advantages and disadvantages of each proposed option, thus presenting a sense of fairness and balance in putting forth the proposed alternative (DeMarco & Tufts, 2014).
4. Outline of the policy recommendations: This section includes a listing of the steps that need to be taken and a summary statement reemphasizing the importance of action.
5. Appendices, if needed: If the argument for a specific policy needs further support or explanation, additional resources can be placed in an appendix.

A well-crafted policy brief can strongly influence policy and be an effective advocacy tool. The brief provides evidence for the proposed policy advice and links to the policy initiative or proposed changes. Additionally, the brief provides the policymaker with concrete recommendations that are evidence-based and derived from detailed and logical views.

Town Hall Meetings

Town hall meetings are held by elected officials, persons interested in running for an elected office, government officials, professional organizations and associations, and federations that may wish to gain feedback on a topic of interest or specific issue. Town hall meetings are a common way that policymakers connect with their constituents. These meetings provide policymakers with the opportunity to listen and learn from their constituents on matters related to the issue at hand. Constituents use town hall meetings to voice their opinions and ask questions. The meetings are generally open to the public, may include media representation, and can also be live streamed for later reference. Town hall meetings offered by politicians can be held in any venue, but the area is usually located in their constituency. There are two basic types of town hall meetings: general and specific. General meetings do not have a particular topic or focus area. These meetings are open forums where those in attendance are free to ask questions about various issues. Specific meetings focus on a particular topic, policy, or matter of concern.

If speaking at a town hall meeting, prepare using an elevator speech. Elevator speeches are short speeches delivered in the time that it takes to ride an elevator, usually between 30 and 60 seconds. When preparing the elevator speech for a legislator or policymaker at a town hall meeting, including the following seven components:
1. Your full name.
2. Your address which, if a legislator, allows them to know you are a constituent.
3. Your school or place of employment and any appropriate association you are representing, for example, "I'm Nurse Clark, an employee of XYZ Hospital, and I am here representing the Black Nurses Association." If you are not representing an organization, be sure to make that statement. For example, "I am an employee of XYZ Hospital, but I am not speaking on their behalf, nor am I authorized to speak on their behalf."
4. Identify the problem and the implications of the policy (its effect if implemented). The problem should be stated clearly and concisely, followed by persuasive facts that allow others to comprehend the issue at hand.
5. Inform the official of why you and others need the problem addressed.
6. Ask the official what their plan is to address the issue.
7. Thank the official for their time.

Practice the elevator speech repeatedly before you deliver it. Practice with your colleagues or friends. Practicing the speech will give you greater comfort and confidence before sharing your concerns with a larger audience. It is also good to type out the speech in bulleted form to leave with the official along with your contact information.

While there are no specific guidelines for town hall meetings, the expectation is that the discussions will be respectful and considerate of others with opposing views.

Meeting With Legislators

One way to influence the policymaking process is to meet the senators and representatives that serve your residential address. To do this, you must know the legislators representing you at the federal and state levels. To find your US representative, the https://www.house.gov/representatives/find-your-representative website allows you to enter your zip code, and your representative's name will be provided based on the information submitted (US House of Representatives, n.d. a). To find your US senator, you can follow this link: https://www.senate.gov/senators/senators-contact.htm and then put in the requested information (US Senate, n.d.). Once you have located your legislators' names, you can call or email them to request an appointment to either meet them in their home district office or at their congressional office in Washington, DC. Congressional member websites often have appointment requests available for online submission. You should follow up with a phone call once you have emailed.

It is important to identify yourself as a constituent. In the visit request, you should include your personal information, why you are requesting the visit, and the names of others who may be accompanying you. For example, you may schedule a meeting for a local professional organization to discuss nursing workforce development and national nursing shortage issues. Although you scheduled the appointment, the scheduling person will request the name of every member that will be attending the meeting with you. An example of an email request for a meeting is shown in Table 7.4. If you

TABLE 7.4   Sample Legislator Email Request for an Appointment
Dear Senator/Representative (insert name),
As a constituent and registered professional nurse, I am writing to request an appointment with you in your (insert location of the office) on (date and time) to discuss nursing workforce development funding.
Please let me know what time you or your legislative assistant might be available to meet. I will follow up with you or your assistant within the next week by phone or email to confirm the date and find out the time. I thank you in advance for considering this request.
Sincerely, Name with credentials Title Organization (if appropriate) Contact information

meet with the legislative assistant rather than the legislator, the assistant will report the topic and discussion points of the meeting to the legislator. It is important to note that legislative assistants know policy matters and usually have an educational background in political studies.

Social Media Platforms

Social media platforms are websites and applications that facilitate the sharing of ideas, thoughts, beliefs, and information through virtual networks and social communities (Dollarhide, 2021). Social media applications focus on the connection and exchange of information between users, user-based input, interaction, content sharing, and collaboration among nearly four billion users. The most popular social media platforms are Facebook, Instagram, Twitter, TikTok, YouTube, WhatsApp, Facebook Messenger, Reddit, and WeChat (Dollarhide, 2021). The advantages of social media include that you can discover what is happening worldwide in real time, have instant connections with large audiences and people worldwide, and have access to vast amounts of data and information at your fingertips. In addition, you can create content to share with others. The disadvantages of social media have been concerns about its addictive use, making users inattentive to environmental stimuli. It can also evoke user stress and anxiety. A major drawback is that the sites' contents lack oversight and fact-checking. Because communication does not occur face to face, people are sometimes more comfortable saying hurtful or mean things on online platforms. Social media can also diminish a person's ability to communicate face to face.

Social media sites have been responsible for skewing political views by filtering the information seen by individual users using algorithms. Algorithms can determine what a person likes or dislikes and, as a result, filter the data seen by the individual. This type of manipulation greatly influences what a person sees, since the person can unknowingly be inundated with certain kinds of information. Also of importance is the use of social media aggregators. Social network aggregation is the process of collecting content from multiple social network services into one unified presentation using a social media aggregator (Bojkov, 2021). Social media aggregators can influence politics by making information accessible from various sources in real time from supporters and influencers who back your cause for a specific policy.

Social Justice and Empowerment Movements

Community organizing is the process by which communities come together for a common cause or concern and act together on behalf of their shared interests (Wikipedia, n.d.). Community organizing is often directed at social change and can lead to changes in policies and laws. The Black Lives Matter (BLM) movement, which was energized and peaked after the death of George Floyd, is an example of how community organizing can lead to changes in policy, the allocation of resources, and the transformation of attitudes regarding particular social matters. The BLM movement was initially formed as a protest to raise awareness regarding the long-standing racial inequities in America (Race Equity Tools, 2020). This movement led to changes in laws regarding allocation of resources to police departments and led to the subsequent Defund the Police movement. The Defund the Police movement called for the divesture of funds from police departments and the reallocation of those funds to alternative forms of public safety, such as social services, youth services, housing and education, and additional community resources (Wikipedia, n.d. a). The Defund the Police movement significantly influenced politics and became a platform for both political parties, for and against the movement.

Similarly, the Me Too movement was focused on breaking the silence for victims of sexual assault (Wikipedia, n.d. b). These movements spread empathy and solidarity through mass numbers. In addition, they led to changes in policy and legislation such as updates in sexual harassment and other sexual policies and the removal of barriers requiring employees to sign nondisclosure agreements. Finally, they gave victims the ability to file complaints without fear of retaliation.

Advocacy

The WHO defines health advocacy as a combination of individual and social actions designed to gain political commitment, policy support, and social systems support for a particular goal or program (1998, p. 5). Promoting nurses' involvement in the advocacy process requires exposure to and an understanding of the policymaking process, an understanding of the nurse's responsibility to participate in the process, a sense of self-efficacy, and the development of leadership skills in terms of advocacy (Perry & Emory, 2017). Advocacy activities can include meetings with governmental officials, creating coalitions of individuals and organizations with a shared special interest, engaging in public mobilization activities, providing evidence-based research to advance a particular issue, and developing strategic messaging to increase awareness of the problem. Coalitions can be extremely effective in advocating for specific causes, including raising public awareness by alerting the media of a particular issue of concern (Table 7.5).

Most professional state nurse associations have what is known as Lobby Day, also known as Nurse Advocacy Day. Nurse Advocacy Day is intended to increase registered and student nurses' understanding of the political process. Moreover, state nurses' associations monitor legislation and provide testimony or offer their professional expertise on issues of concern related to nursing and health at the federal, state, and local levels of government, ensuring that nurses and nursing issues are adequately and effectively represented. State nurses' associations expect that nurses will lend their voices on healthcare matters to advance, protect, and promote the nursing profession. Their advocacy has been seen in scope-of-practice laws. In two reports on the future of nursing, "Leading Change and Advancing Health" (IOM, 2011) and "The Future of Nursing 2020–2030: Charting a Path to Achieve Health Equity" (National Academies of Sciences, Engineering, and Medicine [NASEM], 2021), recommendations were made for advanced-practice nurses to practice to the full extent of their licensure and education.

Recommendation 4: All organizations, including state and federal entities and employing organizations, should enable nurses to practice to the full extent of their education and training by removing barriers that prevent them from more fully addressing social needs and social determinants of health and improving health care access, quality, and value. These barriers include regulatory and public and private payment limitations; restrictive policies and practices; and other legal, professional, and commercial impediments (NASEM, 2021, p. 364).

The American Nurses Association (ANA) endorses advocacy as a pillar of nursing (ANA, n.d.). The ANA advocates for nurses by lobbying Congress and regulatory agencies on healthcare issues affecting nurses and the public. Additionally, the ANA educates and empowers nurses by providing education and training on advocacy, teaching them how to share their expertise and perspectives directly with their legislators (ANA, n.d.).

TABLE 7.5   Coalitions: Advantages and Disadvantages

Coalitions

Coalitions are where two or more organizations create an alliance to achieve a common goal. Coalitions can be formal and long-lasting or temporary. Longer-lasting coalitions meet periodically to determine issues and concerns worthy of advocacy that impact their causes. Coalitions strengthen advocacy work specifically for causes or goals that reach beyond the capacity of one organization. The goals of a coalition can be wide-ranging. Formal coalitions should have a clear mission and purpose, operating rules and regulations, and member roles and responsibilities. When coalitions form for a specific issue, it is usually a temporary alliance and revolves around a particular subject or concern.

Advantages	Disadvantages
Coalitions provide an enlarged base of support for the issue and bring credibility to the topic.	Coalitions can be bureaucratic and may require bylaws or operating procedures.
Coalitions can cover those who may wish not to act as individuals or single organizations.	One powerful organization can dominate coalitions and the other smaller organizations must acquiesce.
More significant gains can be realized through coalitions by pooling resources and eliminating duplication of services.	Large coalitions can slow the decision-making process because getting members to agree on issues of concern may be difficult.
Having a variety of individuals and organizations as part of the coalition brings perspective and cognitive diversity to the issue.	Member organizations can have their own aims and become unwilling to compromise.
Coalitions can provide members and organizations with networking opportunities, enhanced communication, and information sharing.	The coalition as a collective gets credit for the work as opposed to a single person or entity.

Data from World Animal Net. (2017). Managing a Coalition. Retrieved from https://worldanimal.net/managing-a-coalition.

For example, during the COVID-19 pandemic, ANA lobbied for increased availability of single-use personal protective equipment and engaged with the US Food and Drug Administration in developing evidence-based research on the effectiveness of decontamination methods to safeguard nurses as frontline workers.

Another strong advocacy group is comprised of the congressional Senate and House of Representatives nursing caucuses. A congressional caucus is a group of committee members committed to common themes or legislative objectives. The congressional nursing caucuses address policy issues that impact the nursing profession, the nursing workforce, and patient care, specifically, that patients have access to high-quality care. These caucuses may hold briefings, support legislation affecting the nursing profession, and ensure that nurses' voices are not lost in policy dialogues that impact health.

Another advocacy and engagement group is the Nursing Community Coalition (NCC). The NCC is a 64-member organization that represents a cross-section of the nursing profession and addresses education, practice, research, and regulation. This cross-section includes registered nurses, advanced-practice registered nurses, nurse leaders, students, faculty, and researchers. The NCC engages with political leaders to advance the health of the nation through the nursing lens (NCC, n.d.).

CONCLUSION

The purpose of this chapter was not to review all the legislation that impacts health but for nurses to understand how legislation is related to and influences health outcomes. Equally important is nurses' ability to recognize that if the SDOH are the drivers of the health inequities that lead to health disparities, then the political determinants of health (i.e., laws, policies, and structures) are the drivers of the SDOH. Because public and health policies have a major influence on health, nurses can promote health equity by bringing a health lens to bear on public policies and decision-making at the local, state, and federal levels (NASEM, 2021). In addition, nurses can use their health lens to inform policymakers about health disparities and SDOH, focusing on the challenges and solutions to addressing health (NASEM, 2021).

Upstream policies that reduce social disadvantage can reduce the health inequities that lead to health disparities. The history of nursing is grounded in social justice and health advocacy (NASEM, 2021). Moreover, The ANA Code of Ethics admonishes nurses to "integrate principles of social justice into nursing and health policy" (ANA, 2015, p. 15). Thus nurses have the responsibility to move beyond the downstream measures of engaging in clinical care and determining the patient's social needs, and to begin participating in upstream activities that facilitate progress toward health equity. Upstream activities call for addressing the political processes that influence health.

Upstream measures support policies that promote health and provide the greatest social good for marginalized populations. To engage in upstream activity, nurses must be knowledgeable about political processes and involved in undertakings that can influence health policy at the local, state, and national levels. Becoming involved in the policymaking process can be done in various ways, from the simple act of voting to more engaged strategies of attending town halls, writing policy briefs, and meeting with legislators. For example, engagement at the local or state levels could involve attending school board meetings and voting to locate more community health clinics in public schools. In addition, as an expert in a specialized field of nursing practice at the state level, the nurse could provide evidence-based research findings to a state senator (IOM, 2011).

Nurses must also engage with stakeholders outside of nursing to effectively implement upstream strategies that promote health equity. Most policies that improve health, such as those related to food, housing, transportation, and wages, lie outside the domain of health. Multisectoral approaches to achieve health equity can be seen in the HiAP approaches. In the "Future of Nursing 2020–2030" report, it states,

Nurses alone cannot solve the problems associated with upstream SDOH that exist outside of healthcare systems. However by engaging in efforts to change local, state, or federal policy with a "Health in All Policies" approach, they can address SDOH that underlie poor health…. Whether nurses engage in policymaking full time or work to inform policy part-time as a professional responsibility, their attention to policies that create or eliminate health inequities can improve the underlying conditions that frame people's health. Nurses can bring a health and social justice lens to public policies and decision-making at the community, state, and federal levels most effectively by serving in public- and private-sector leadership positions (NASEM, 2021, p. 139).

To improve the health of populations, students and nurses must become more involved in the political arena since nurses are the largest group of healthcare workers. Having a mentor who understands the policymaking process and politics and has expertise in political advocacy is one strategy to improve self-efficacy and ensure engagement in the political process.

STUDENT REFLECTION QUESTIONS

1. Writing an op-ed for a local newspaper can bring public health issues to the public's attention. When writing an op-ed, you should reach out to the targeted paper, introduce yourself, tell the editor you are interested in submitting an op-ed, and explain why the subject matter is important for the readership. You should explain what makes you an expert in the area. You should ask for and follow the submission guidelines. Most op-eds are submitted electronically via email. Select a public health issue such as gun control, reproductive health rights, voter suppression, the opioid crisis, COVID-19 mitigation strategies, or the legalization of marijuana to write an op-ed. Follow up with the editor in 1 week to confirm the op-ed was received.

2. Tweet about a position you have taken on a health policy. Find information on a relevant policy issue through a newsfeed aggregator such as the ANS Policy and Advocacy feed or Google Health Policy News Aggregator, which has curated news related to health from sources such as *The New York Times, The Washington Post,* and CNN (Nurse-Clarke, 2021).

3. Look up your state nurses' association. What health-related policies or nursing issues are they directing their advocacy efforts toward at this time? What are your thoughts about their stated issues and positions?

4. Visit the NCC website section on advocacy and engagement. Review the Coalition's advocacy and engagement activities for the last 2 years at https://www.thenursingcommunity.org/copy-of-2020-news-archive. How do their activities advance nursing?

ADDITIONAL STUDENT RESOURCES

1. To gain a deeper understanding of policy analysis, view the CDC Policy Analysis Key Questions and Policy Analysis websites at: https://www.cdc.gov/policy/analysis/process/docs/table1.pdf; https://www.cdc.gov/policy/analysis/process/docs/table2.pdf.

2. To understand how laws are made, visit the "Legislative Process on How Laws are Made" website at https://www.house.gov/the-house-explained/the-legislative-process.

3. US House of Representatives, n.d. b.

4. Learn about the Nurse in Washington Internship (NIWI) sponsored by the Nursing Organizations Alliance. The NIWI provides nurses the opportunity to learn how to influence healthcare through the legislative and regulatory processes. Nurses and nursing students are welcome to attend the internship program (https://tnoa.memberclicks.net/NIWI-Nurse-in-Washington-Internship; Nursing Organizations Alliance, 2019).

REFERENCES

American Association of Colleges of Nursing. (2021). *The essentials: Core competencies for professional nursing education.* https://www.aacnnursing.org/Education-Resources/AACN-Essentials.

American Civil Liberties Union. (2021). *Fighting voter suppression.* Retrieved from https://www.aclu.org/issues/voting-rights/fighting-voter-suppression.

American Civil Liberties Union. (2021a). *Block the vote. How politicians are trying to block voters from the ballot box.* Retrieved from https://www.aclu.org/news/civil-liberties/block-the-vote-voter-suppression-in-2020/.

American Civil Liberties Union. (2021b). *Gerrymandering.* Retrieved from https://www.aclu.org/issues/voting-rights/gerrymandering.

American Nurses Association. (n.d.). *Advocacy.* Retrieved from https://www.nursingworld.org/practice-policy/advocacy/

American Nurses Association. (2015). *Code of Ethics for Nurses.* American Nurses Association.

Berwick, D. M. (2018). Politics and health care. *Journal of the American Medical Association, 320*(14), 1437–1438.

Bojkov, N. (2021). Social media aggregator—Why do you need one in 2022? Retrieved from https://embedsocial.com/blog/social-media-aggregator/.

Brown, C. L., Raza, D., & Pinto, A. D. (2020). Voting, health and interventions in healthcare settings: A scoping review. *Public Health Reviews, 41*, 16. https://doi.org/10.1186/s40985-020-00133-6.

CDC. (2015). *Definition of policy.* Retrieved from https://www.cdc.gov/policy/analysis/process/docs/policyDefinition.pdf.

CDC. (2021). *Office of the Associate Director for Policy and Strategy: Policy Process.* Retrieved from https://www.cdc.gov/policy/polaris/policyprocess/index.html.

Center for American Progress. (2020). *10 ways the ACA has improved health care in the past decade.* Retrieved from https://www.americanprogress.org/article/10-ways-aca-improved-health-care-past-decade/.

Centers for Medicare & Medicaid Services. (2023). Biden-Harris administration announces record-breaking 16.3 million people signed up for health care coverage in ACA marketplaces during 2022–2023 open enrollment season. Retrieved from https://www.cms.gov/newsroom/press-releases/biden-harris-administration-announces-record-breaking-163-million-people-signed-health-care-coverage.

Au, Michelle. (2021). Op-ed: Fight gun violence like we fight cancer: One step at a time. *Chicago Tribune.* Retrieved from https://www.chicagotribune.com/opinion/commentary/ct-opinion-gun-violence-epidemic-fight-like-cancer-20210419-vybqo5wu5nawxalokn364em6qa-story.html.

The Commonwealth Fund. (2020). *The Affordable Care Act at 10 years: What's the effect on health care coverage and access.* Retrieved from https://www.commonwealthfund.org/publications/journal-article/2020/feb/aca-at-10-years-effect-health-care-coverage-access.

Community-Based Monitoring System Network Coordinating Team. (n.d.). *Guidelines for writing a policy brief.* Retrieved from https://www.pep-net.org/sites/pep-net.org/files/typo3doc/pdf/CBMS_country_proj_profiles/Philippines/CBMS_forms/Guidelines_for_Writing_a_Policy_Brief.pdf.

Cropley, S., Hughes, M., & Belcik, K. (2022). Engaging leadership competencies: Through population health policy advocacy: A review of the evidence. *Policy, Politics, & Nursing Practice*, 1–13. https://doi.10.1177/15271544221112893.

Curley, D. (2023). Powering policy. *American Nurse Journal, 18*(1), 30.

Dawes, D. E. (2018). The future of health equity in America: Addressing the legal and political determinants of health. *Journal of Law, Medicine, & Ethics 46*(4), 838–840.

Dawes, D. E. (2020). *The political determinants of health.* Johns Hopkins University Press.

DeMarco, R., & Tufts, K. A. (2014). The mechanics of writing a policy brief. *Nursing Outlook, 62*, 219–224. https://doi.org/10.1016/j.outlook.2014.04.002.

Dollarhide, M. (2021). *Social media.* Investopedia. Retrieved from https://www.investopedia.com/terms/s/social-media.asp.

Epoc.cochrane.org. (2011). *What is a policy brief?* Retrieved from https://epoc.cochrane.org/sites/epoc.cochrane.org/files/public/uploads/SURE-Guides-v2.1/Collectedfiles/source/01_getting_started/policy_brief.html.

FairVote. (2021). *Voter turnout 101.* Retrieved from https://www.fairvote.org/voter_turnout#voter_turnout_101.

Hall, R. L., & Jacobson, P. D. (2018). Examining whether the health-in-all-policies approach promotes health equity. *Health Affairs, 37*(3), 364–370.

Institute of Medicine. (2011). *The future of nursing: Leading change, advancing health.* The National Academies Press.

Kaiser Family Foundation. (2023). *Status of state Medicaid expansion decisions. Interactive map.* Retrieved from https://www.kff.org/medicaid/issue-brief/status-of-state-medicaid-expansion-decisions-interactive-map/.

King, C. A. (2015). Nursing advocacy 101: Start where you are to do what you can. *Tarheel Nurse, 77*(2 Spec. No.), 12–15.

Komro, K. A., Livingston, M. D., Markowitz, S., & Wagenaar, A. C. (2016). The effect of an increased minimum wage on infant mortality and birth weight. *American Journal of Public Health, 106*(8), 1514–1516. https://doi.org/10.2105/AJPH.2016.303268.

Loversidge, J. M. (2019). Policymaking processes and models. In Loversidge, J. M., & Zurmehly, J. (Eds.), *Evidence-informed health policy: Using EBP to transform policy in nursing and health care* (pp. 90–117). Sigma Theta Tau International.

Mishori, R. (2019). The social determinants of health? Time to focus on the political determinants of health! *Medical Care, 57*(7), 491–493.

Narain, K. D. C., & Zimmerman, F. J. (2019). Examining the association of changes in minimum wage with health across race/ethnicity and gender in the United States. *BMC Public Health, 19*(1069). https://doi.org/10.1186/s12889-019-7376-y.

National Academies of Sciences, Engineering, and Medicine. (2021). *The future of nursing 2020–2030: Charting a path to achieve health equity.* The National Academies Press. https://doi.org/10.17226/25982.

The National Constitution Center. (2022). *Dobbs versus Jackson Women's Health Organization.* Retrieved from https://constitutioncenter.org/the-constitution/supreme-court-case-library/dobbs-v-jackson-womens-health-organization.

Nurse-Clarke, N. (2021). Health Policy Newsfeed: An activity in current trends and issues. *The Journal of Nursing Education, 60*(11), 655. https://doi.org/10.3928/01484834-20210914-04.

Nursing Community Coalition. *About us.* Retrieved from https://131a058d-9186-c34a-b6f8-7f4cb1fce3f0.filesusr.com/ugd/148923_0f722f39035a4c1f98ec6f2e3c442e15.pdf.

Nursing Organizations Alliance. (2019). *Nurses In Washington Internship.* Retrieved from https://www.nursing-alliance.org/nurse-in-washington-internship.

Perry, C., & Emory, J. (2017). Advocacy through education. *Policy, Politics, and Nursing Practice, 18*(3), 158–165.

Planned Parenthood. (2014). *Roe v. Wade: Its history and impact.* Planned Parenthood Federation of America.

Pollitz, K., Long, M., Semanskee, A., & Kamal, R. (2018). *Understanding short-term limited duration health insurance.* Kaiser Family Foundation. Retrieved from https://www.kff.org/health-reform/issue-brief/understanding-short-term-limited-duration-health-insurance/.

Race Equity Tools. (2020). *Community organizing.* Retrieved from https://www.racialequitytools.org/resources/act/strategies/community-organizing.

Schleffer, G., & Miller, B. (2021). The political effects of social media platforms on different regime types. *Texas National Security Review, 4*(30), 76–103.

The Sentencing Project. (2021). *Fact sheet: Trends in US corrections.* The Sentencing Project.

Shi, L. (2019). *Introduction to health policy* (2nd ed.). Health Administration Press.

Silberman, P. (2020). Ten years with the Affordable Care Act in North Carolina. Retrieved from https://sph.unc.edu/sph-news/ten-years-with-the-affordable-care-act-in-north-carolina/.

US Department of Health and Human Services, Office of Disease Prevention and Health Promotion. (n.d.). *Healthy people 2030.* Health policy. Retrieved from https://health.gov/healthypeople/objectives-and-data/browse-objectives/health-policy.

US Department of Labor. (n.d.) *Break time for nursing mothers.* Retrieved from https://www.dol.gov/agencies/whd/nursing-mothers.

US Food and Drug Administration. (2018). *Summary: Food labeling: Nutrition labeling of standard menu items in restaurants and similar retail food establishments.* Retrieved from https://www.fda.gov/about-fda/economic-impact-analyses-fda-regulations/summary-food-labeling-nutrition-labeling-standard-menu-items-restaurants-and-similar-retail-food.

US House of Representatives (n.d.a) Finding your legislator. Retrieved from https://www.house.gov/representatives/find-your-representative.

US House of Representatives. (n.d.b) *The legislative process.* Retrieved from https://www.house.gov/the-house-explained/the-legislative-process.

US Senate. (n.d.). *Contacting your legislator.* Retrieved from https://www.senate.gov/senators/senators-contact.htm.

The White House. (2023). Fact sheet: President Biden's budget advances equity. Retrieved from https://www.whitehouse.gov/omb/briefing-room/2023/03/09/fact-sheet-president-bidens-budget-advances-equity/.

WHO. (n.d.) *Health inequities and their causes.* Retrieved from https://www.who.int/news-room/facts-in-pictures/detail/health-inequities-and-their-causes.

WHO. (n.d.a) *What you need to know about Health in All Policies.* Retrieved from https://www.who.int/social_determinants/publications/health-policies-manual/key-messages-en.pdf.

Wikipedia. (n.d.). *Community organizing.* Retrieved from https://en.m.wikipedia.org/wiki/Community_organizing.

Wikipedia. (n.d. a). *Defund the police.* Retrieved from https://en.wikipedia.org/wiki/Defund_the_police#:~:text=%22Defund%20the%20police%22%20is%20a,healthcare%20and%20other%20community%20resources.

Wikipedia. (n.d. b). *Me Too movement.* Retrieved from https://en.wikipedia.org/wiki/Me_Too_movement.

Wilson, F. A., & Stimpson, J. P. (2020). Federal and state policies affecting immigrant access to health care. *JAMA Health Forum, 4*, 1–3. https://doi.10.1001.jamahealthforum.2020.0271.

Yearby, R., Clark, B., & Figueroa, J. (2022). Structural racism in historical and modern US health care policy. *Health Affairs, 2*, 187–194. https://doi10.1037/hlthaff.2021.01466.

Social Justice and Health Equity

Lisa Anderson-Shaw, Lena Hatchett, and Mary Ann Lavin

Where justice is denied, where poverty is enforced, where ignorance prevails, and where any one class is made to feel that society is an organized conspiracy to oppress, rob, and degrade them, neither persons nor property will be safe.
—Frederick Douglas

CHAPTER OUTLINE

LEARNING OBJECTIVES

1. Review the principles of social justice in the context of the American Nurses Association's (ANA, 2015) *Code of Ethics for Nurses.*
2. Define structural competence as it relates to social justice in healthcare.
3. Discuss the concepts of moral distress and moral resilience.
4. Explore the concepts of social inclusion and exclusion as matters of social justice in healthcare.
5. Describe social justice advocacy activities for nurses and healthcare providers to drive systemic change.

SOCIAL JUSTICE

Social and health disparities have a long-standing history in human societies. Social mores and economic advantage, which underpinned one's place in life and society, were not based on equality but on class, wealth, privilege, and power, handed down from one generation to the next. It was not until the late 18th century that the idea of justice and "the pursuit and realization of social justice were inextricably linked to the preservation of individual liberty or freedom, the achievement of equality (of rights, opportunities, and outcomes), and the establishment of common bonds of all humanity" (Reisch, 2002, p. 343). Abu (2020)

defines social justice in a nursing context as the equitable distribution and redistribution of resources for positive health outcomes, recognition and removal of social and political barriers that impinge on health, and the promotion of parity for participation in decision-making regarding the allocation and utilization of health resources.

Contemporary philosophers and economists continue to debate what the term *social justice* means to the individual and society. John Rawls (1971), in his book, *A Theory of Justice*, wrote about two principles of justice. The first principle of justice states that "each person is to have an equal right to the most extensive scheme of equal basic liberties compatible with a similar scheme of liberties for others" (p. 53). The second principle of justice states that "social and economic inequalities are to be arranged so that they are both (a) reasonably expected to be to everyone's advantage, and (b) attached to positions and offices open to all" (p. 53). Further discussion indicates that the distribution of wealth and income does not have to be equal to all but that this distribution is to everyone's advantage. In addition, Rawls (1971) wrote that social values such as liberty, income, wealth, and self-respect are to be "distributed equally unless an unequal distribution of any, or all, of these values is to everyone's advantage" (p. 54), and that the definition of injustice simply means "inequalities that are not to the benefit of all" (p. 54). An example of an inequality that is not of benefit to all is positions of authority because not all people would benefit if everyone had the same authority. In other words, it is not to everyone's benefit if positions of authority are equally distributed. That does not mean that all people have the same rights and liberties but that a just society needs to have various levels of resources to function in fair and responsible ways.

Rawls further explained citizens' claims to social resources and primary goods in his 2001 book *Justice As Fairness.* "At least with regard to the constitutional essentials, and the all-purpose means needed for a fair opportunity to take advantage of our basic freedoms, justice as fairness rules out claims based on various wants and aims arising from people's different and incommensurable conceptions of the good" (Rawls, 2001, p. 151). What he means by this is that the distribution of goods should be fair, and fair is not necessarily going to be equal but must render what is "good" as defined by that society.

While Rawls' theory of justice is esteemed for its depth and applicability to decision-making within political structures, his theory did not directly address health justice (Kniess, 2021). Kniess, however, analyzed Rawls' principles and Rawls' potential contributions to health and healthcare justice over five decades. He recognizes that Rawls' theory (1) discusses competing values and their varying weights in our political system but does not resolve conflicts arising from competing interests, and (2) focuses on just political structures but not on the just behavior of individuals. However, this Rawlsian focus applies to health and healthcare in the following way: It reinforces the elucidation of the social determinants of health as upstream factors that play a direct role in the downstream health of individuals, families, and communities. It would seem, therefore, that Rawls was an upstream philosopher.

Kniess does discuss, however, Rawls' inclusion of social relations in his theory. More to the point, Rawls considers self-respect a primary good. It is difficult to maintain self-respect in a discriminatory school, healthcare institution, community, state, or nation. Thus from our perspective a societal and nursing focus on diversity, inclusion, and equity (DEI) may be made using Rawls' theory of justice and his specification of self-respect as a primary good.

The complexity of Rawls' theory is acknowledged by Rawls himself when he indicates that words are subject to varied interpretations and that ambiguities exist even in applying his principles. For Rawls, inequalities that are not to the benefit of all constitute injustice. This principle is ambiguous. The question is: Who are the "all"? On one hand, DEI is an acronym representing three elements aimed at correcting inequalities and inequities that do not benefit all where "all" means people of color plus White people together. This principle assumes that White people and people of color benefit when we live in a diverse, inclusive, and equitable society.

Social Movements

The 1960s was a turbulent time in the United States: war in Vietnam; social, political, and civil unrest; racial tension; and the Women's Rights Movement, among others. There was great interest in social justice reform in the political and academic arenas. Various social and political movements hoped to gain attention and power to make changes related to the social and economic constraints felt by many due to race, sex, and economic inequities in the United States. Social movements are often vehicles to get the attention of media and legislators focused on the needs of the oppressed. For example, in 1962, *The Other America,* by Michael Harrington, was published. The contemporary writer Allan Ornstein's review of this book said that Harrington's focus was on "the forgotten, overlooked, and invisible American, that is the poor who he claimed comprised one third of the US population" (Ornstein, 2017, p. 546). In support of Harrington's statistics, US census data indicated that 22% of all American households were below the poverty rate in 1959. The percentages are worse when the data are broken down by sex and race. When the male was the head of household, the White poverty rate was 9.8% and the non-White rate was 27%. The respective poverty rates for female heads of household were 35% and 60.2% (US Bureau of the Census, 1968). Harrington's main point was to draw attention to the fact that poverty was no longer transient or cyclical, but permanent. This book influenced then-President Kennedy and led to President Johnson's war on poverty and related legislation (Brauer, 1982).

The Department of Sociology at Washington University–St. Louis defines social movements as "collective efforts to produce political, economic, and/or cultural change" (https://sociology.wustl.edu/social-movements, para 1). Erica Chenoweth of Harvard's Kennedy School of Government, and speaking on behalf of the Carnegie Council for Ethics in International Affairs (2020), refers to social movements as mass mobilizations, with successful ones being characterized by:

- Numbers of diverse people involved
- An increasing number of defections from the central position when socioeconomic or political arguments become too strong to be ignored
- Tactical flexibility, that is, multiple types of mobilization campaigns
- Disciplined adherence to a movement's narrative even in the face of opposition/oppression (https://www.youtube.com/watch?v=_y62wT21nBs).

Social movements remain important agents of change, especially for social, justice, and political change (Fig. 8.1). Social movements facilitate change in important healthcare areas, including access to healthcare, financial assistance with healthcare services, levels of care needed in specific geographic areas, and privacy of personal healthcare information. Highly successful health-related social movements include antituberculosis campaigns, the March of Dimes and its antipolio crusade, and the water fluoridation campaign. Yet to be determined is the outcome of the current prochoice campaign for women's rights. It may be advantageous for its leaders, including nurses, to study Chenoweth's principles of successful mass mobilization in the international arena and apply them to the prochoice movement in the United States.

SOCIAL JUSTICE AND THE AMERICAN NURSES ASSOCIATION'S *CODE OF ETHICS*

Social justice can mean different things to different people. Ornstein (2017) identified 30 basic principles

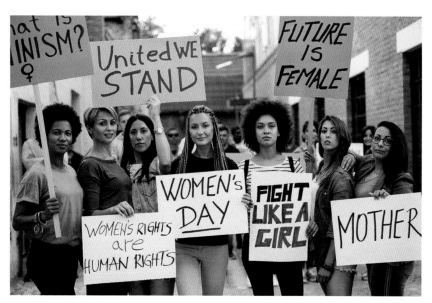

Fig. 8.1 Activist Protesting for Women's Rights. (From: iStock.com/Drazen Zigic.)

that help define his framework for social justice. Five of these basic principles are important to social justice and healthcare:

1. *In a just society, all lives have equal value, equal opportunity, and equal chances for success.*
2. *A socially just society cannot forget or ignore people in need, nor leave the majority of its people behind. It must put people first—neither property nor profits. It must be willing to examine its beliefs and philosophy on a regular basis.*
3. *Given a social contract, the government not only protects the people, but also provides revenue for building schools, roads, and bridges; it also provides safety nets and social programs for its disadvantaged populace, including the poor, sick, disabled, and elderly.*
4. *Although a dominant and subordinate group may exist in all societies, in a just society, the differences do not lead to institutional racism, class-consciousness, or economic warfare.*
5. *The idea is not to focus on the outcomes of inequality, but to address the reasons for inequality—and what can be done to improve the human condition (Ornstein, 2017, pp. 546–548).*

Social justice in health and healthcare services differs from its application in political philosophy, however. Healthcare providers abide by oaths or pledges of service in their profession upon graduation. Such oaths often include statements to serve and take care of poor and disadvantaged people in society. In addition, healthcare professionals abide by a code of ethics that provides normative and applied moral guidance as to what *ought* to be done when an ethical issue arises in their work. Rushton (2017) summarizes the following about the ANA's *Code of Ethics for Nurses* (ANA, 2015): first and foremost, nurses must be obligated to their patients and provide respectful, fair, and equal care to all people. In the most recent revision, there is special reinforcement of nurses' obligation to social justice and the profession's responsibility to integrate principles of justice into nursing and health policy. In today's environment, it is especially important that nurses be involved in the dialogue and policymaking process and offer an explicit and authentic voice in the policy decisions that will affect our nation.

The code includes nine provision statements that directly address social justice and healthcare issues upon which nurses can directly impact. In the following content, we elaborate upon the social justice–related provisions within the code that most directly address social justice issues.

Provision 1

Provision 1 of the code states: *"The nurse practices with compassion and respect for the inherent dignity, work, and unique attributes of every person"* (ANA, 2015, p. 1). The foundational principles of nursing practice are respect for all persons, that all persons who need care should receive it, and that nurses are change agents for public health and health policy. Nurses establish trusting relationships with those in their care and promote health and wellness. They respect age, racial identity, culture, religion, gender expression, lifestyle, and socioeconomic status. Respect for human dignity and recognition of patient rights are paramount in the care nurses provide to individuals, families, groups, and communities.

Respect is given to all persons with whom the nurse interacts, including other care providers, administrators, consultants, and all supportive staff. Nurses will collaborate with others in the care of individuals with the goal of "compassionate, transparent, and effective health services" (ANA, 2015, p. 4). The following three scenarios demonstrate the enactment of Provision 1 of the code of ethics.

A White student repeatedly asks monosyllabic questions of a polysyllabic Black patient. Change occurred when the instructor broke the silence. After several exchanges, the White instructor apologizes for interrupting, saying her curiosity got the best of her. She then asks the Black patient what university he attended. "Xavier," he said, "in New Orleans." "And your major?" she asked. "English literature." "You know," she said, "a couple of my friends and doctoral degree classmates were from Xavier. It is a great university." In this case, the White instructor's action is a downstream intervention in an outpatient setting. Change was apparent in the surprised eyes of the nursing student, in the smile of the patient, and in the returned smile of the instructor. Had silence not been broken, there would have been no change.

Change occurred similarly when a new Latinx nurse was taken aside by the Latinx director of clinical services serving immigrants. The director first asked the nurse if he had previously worked with patients who spoke indigenous languages. Since the answer was "no," she proceeded to caution the nurse to speak Spanish more slowly and more simply, as Spanish is *not* likely to be the primary language for the patient who was from rural Guatemala. Gently the director explained the patient's primary language was more likely to be Mayan or Garifuna and Xinca with Spanish as a second language. This same principle holds for some patients from Mexico, the director of clinical services continued. For example, people from the State of Oaxaca may speak any of multiple languages numbering in the double digits. For them, Spanish is an additional language, too. "So," she said, "at the outset, just be sure to assess the congruence between your Spanish and the patient's and adjust your Spanish accordingly. The patient will really appreciate that."

The third case is analogous to the first. A nurse practitioner said to an 80-year-old patient, "Your biopsy was benign, but the report includes a lot of big words, so I won't bother you with those." The patient, although feeling disrespected, responded without animosity and with a touch of humor. Chuckling, she said, "Actually, I have a doctorate from an Ivy League school, so I may be able to cope with the 'big words.'" The nurse practitioner breaks out laughing, obviously at herself. Apologizing, she says, "I didn't mean to be condescending." They both laugh, releasing tension. The nurse practitioner reviews the pathology report with the patient. The patient expresses her gratitude.

To recap, the clinical instructor in the first case and the patient in the third case interrupted and changed the narrative. In so doing they challenged the biases or unfounded assumptions that the student in the first case and the nurse practitioner in the third case were making. False or unfounded assumptions about another qualify as a definition of bias. Such assumptions affront the dignity of the patient, causing embarrassment or insult. In the second case, the clinical services director acted *a priori* to prevent provider–patient miscommunication and discomfort on the part of the patient. Such an action was based on prior experience insofar as some Spanish-speaking nurses may assume that Spanish is the primary language for all patients arriving from Mexico, Central America, or South America. If they act on that assumption and speak Spanish at their usual speed, they may make patients feel uncomfortable due to difficulty understanding what is being said. As a result, patients may say they understand when they do not, or they may feel inadequate for needing to ask the nurse to repeat a question or instruction.

Note, however, the gentleness used by the instructor, the director of clinical services, and even the patient in the third scenario. The moral is that there are no ethical grounds for affronting the dignity of students, nurses, or nurse practitioners when alerting them to interactions that may affront patient dignity. In the event their dignity is affronted, then it, too, must be restored. Provision 1 of the ANA *Code of Ethics* applies to all persons.

Note, too, that the race of the patient, student, and instructor was identified in the first case scenario. This was done intentionally to avoid normalizing the White race, which means assuming that White is the default race when the color of a person's complexion is not mentioned. In the third case, the race of the elderly patient and the race of the nurse practitioner were not noted. Did you, as the reader, assume each was White? If so, this is an example of the normalization of Whiteness. White people and perhaps some people of color, too, may be unaware of the assumptions made when writing or speaking of others. Be sensitive to assumptions, however, as they, too, reflect the dignity we extend to *all* others.

Provision 3

Provision 3 of the code states: *"The nurse promotes, advocates for, and protects the rights, health, and safety of the patient."*

In September 2020, Dawn Wooten, a licensed practical nurse, worked for the Immigration and Customs Enforcement (ICE) detention center in Irving County, Georgia. She broke her silence and blew the whistle on the center for a lack of coronavirus disease 2019 (COVID-19)-related safety, fabrication of records, and uninformed and unconsented reproductive sterilization surgeries performed on Latinx immigrants, primarily females from Mexico and Central America (https://projectsouth.org/wp-content/uploads/2020/09/OIG-ICDC-Complaint-1.pdf). Her whistle-blowing actions were supported by the following press releases/documents: (1) The *American College of Nurse-Midwives Regarding Complaints of Unwarranted Hysterectomies Performed without Consent at ICE Facilities* (American College of Nurse-Midwives, 2020), (2) the *American Nurses Association Response to High Rates of Hysterectomies on Immigrant Women under ICE Custody* (ANA, 2020), and (3) the *Association of Operating Room Nurses (AORN) Regarding Forced Hysterectomy Allegations* (AORN, 2020). In May 2021, the Government Accountability Project, the nonprofit agency representing Ms. Wooten, posted the following:

Today, Department of Homeland Security (DHS) Secretary Mayorkas directed Immigration and

Customs Enforcement (ICE) to sever its contracts with Irwin County Detention Center (ICDC) to stop detaining immigrants at that facility, stating in a memo to ICE Director Tae Johnson, "…we will not tolerate the mistreatment of individuals in civil immigration detention or substandard conditions of detention" (Sacchetti, 2021, para 6).

Ms. Wooten, a single mother of five, said the following in the same document.

When I saw the problems at Irwin, I simply could not stay silent. Today's decision to stop immigrants from being detained at Irwin shows that speaking truth can literally save lives. Blowing the whistle was the right thing to do, but it has come at the cost of my job and ability to find other employment. I am hopeful that the DHS OIG will issue a favorable decision soon into my whistleblower retaliation complaint not just for me, but to send a message to other whistleblowers that speaking up is essential and is a legal right that will be protected. (Project South, Institute for the Elimination of Poverty & Genocide, 2020, pp. 25–27).

As of September 9, 2021 all immigrant detainees have been removed from the Irving County, Georgia detention center. Furthermore, Dana Gold, who is Dawn Wooten's lead counsel and the lead senior counsel at the Government Accountability Project, indicates she is still hoping that Ms. Wooten will soon receive the justice she deserves for suffering reprisal for her whistle blowing (Government Accountability Project, 2021).

Ms. Wooten's public denunciation of the criminal medical malpractice being conducted at the Irving County, Georgia ICE detention center earned her the prestigious Hugh M. Hefner First Amendment Award, presented to her at the National Press Club in Washington, DC on September 15, 2022. Public recognition of her courage did not compensate for the loss of her job, going back on food stamps, and being ostracized, in the words of Ms. Wooten, by "Cinderella's evil sisters," the people of her town who had depended on the ICE facility for employment. Ian Herel, a communications associate for the Government Accountability Project, documented these facts in an October 3, 2022, interview with Ms. Wooten (https://whistleblower.org/blog/an-interview-with-dawn-wooten/). When asked by Mr. Herel what would be an appropriate ending to Cinderella's story, Ms. Wooten replied:

Cinderella gets retribution. She gets her RN degree, and then she gets to teach other nurses about ethics. Cinderella gets justice too—she gets to make the standards of practice so high at these facilities that nothing like this ever happens again. Ms. Wooten epitomizes the third provision of the ANA Code of Ethics.

For a more detailed biography of Ms. Wooten and the story of six other brave Americans, including two physicians, visit the Americans Who Tell the Truth website (https://americanswhotellthetruth.org/portraits/dawn-wooten/). For tips on the do's and don'ts of whistle blowing, refer to the ANA document, "Things to Know about Whistle Blowing" (ANA, n.d.).

Provision 5

Provision 5 states: "The nurse owes the same duties to self as to others, including the responsibility to promote health and safety, preserve wholeness of character and integrity, maintain competence, and continue personal and professional growth" (ANA, 2015, p. 19). The interpretation of this provision related to the principles of social justice includes the promotion of health and safety, integrity, competence in practice, and ongoing personal and professional growth.

During the COVID-19 era, health and safety duties to self and others included face masks, the use of other work-appropriate personal protective equipment, vaccinations, frequent handwashing, social distancing within limits imposed by the work environment, and air cleaners and heating, ventilation, and air conditioning (HVAC) filter systems. These are emotional and social, health, and safety issues.

Self- and other care are especially important when experiencing moral distress. Moral distress occurs when there is a moral conflict or when faced with moral challenges. Moral distress, first described by Andrew Jameton, occurs "in a given situation when a health professional knows, or believes they know, the ethically appropriate course of action to take but is unable to carry it out because of obstacles present" (Jameton, 1984, p. 6). When nurses take care of patients who may not have the resources to purchase their medications, who do not have transportation to their needed therapies, or who have no family/friends to help take care of them in their time of need, nurses may feel distressed. This distress is deeply associated with feelings of knowing what needs to be done for a patient but being unable to fulfill the need. In such situations nurses may feel helpless. Their inability to meet the patient's needs may leave them feeling that they have failed in performing their professional duty, leaving their professional integrity compromised.

Feelings of helplessness may also occur when faced with seemingly senseless deaths such as those of children like Trayvon Martin or any other child killed by gunshot wounds. They occur when a nurse witnesses an ICU death from COVID-19 in an unvaccinated young mother of two. They occur when a nurse in an under-resourced country witnesses the death of a 12-year-old from pulmonary tuberculosis disseminated to the brain and kidneys. Nurses also see daily the inequity in healthcare secondary to the educational, social, and financial inequities of our society.

The consequences of moral distress on a person may "include professional burnout, emotional exhaustion, and feelings of disengagement" (Rushton, 2017a, p. S11). Professional help may also be needed. This is because ongoing moral distress can cause serious negative effects on a person's health, happiness, and work life.

Notably, moral distress may become a "catalyst for positive outcomes, moral resilience, and growth" (Rushton, 2017a, p. S13). "Moral resiliency has been defined as the ability and willingness to speak and take right and good action in the face of an adversity that is moral/ethical in nature" (Lachman, 2016, p. 122). In addition, resiliency is the ability to sustain, restore, or "deepen (one's own) integrity in response to moral complexity, confusion, distress, or setbacks" (Schroeter, 2017, p. 290).

Courage is another positive outcome of moral distress. "The courage to advocate, whether within interpersonal, institutional, community-wide, national, or global spaces, may ultimately lead to action and to change, which may not have occurred otherwise" (Anderson-Shaw & Zar, 2020, p. 777). Advocacy moments break the silence. When nurses speak out against imminent health threats such as gun violence, their words do not stand alone. They align with someone who epitomized moral courage and resilience throughout much of the 20th and into the 21st century, the former US Representative and civil rights activist John Lewis. In a speech on the floor of the US House of Representatives in June 2016, following the Pulse nightclub mass shooting in Orlando, Florida, he called out gun violence stating, "The time for silence and patience is long gone" (The Government Publishing Office, 2016, paragraph 11). Although gun violence continues throughout the United States, his words were not in vain. They provide a lasting example of moral courage for others. The work of US Representative John Lewis in the US House of Representatives is an example of upstream interventions. So, too, are the works of Congresswoman Lauren Underwood. Representative Underwood is the youngest African American woman to serve as a US Representative in Congress. Her nursing-influenced upstream contributions are many. She is the cofounder and cochair of the Black Maternal Health Caucus, which focuses congressional attention on policy solutions to the Black maternal–child health crisis and ways to improve health outcomes and reduce and end health disparities.

Duties to self and others also include the provision of inclusive work or school spaces. This refers to the valuing of contributions made by a diverse workforce, student/faculty body, and neighborhood. In an *equitable* society or organization, access to societal/organizational benefits and the weight of its burdens are not skewed by sex, LGBTQ+ identity, race, religion, and so on. *Inclusivity* is a structural justice element highly important to emotional and social health and safety in a workplace or school. It is a welcoming space, an "I feel at-home" space, a microaggression-free space, a respectful space for people of all races, religions, genders, all LGBTQ+ identities, those with disabilities, breastfeeding mothers, immigrants, and any other group.

Provision 6

Provision 6 states that: "*The nurse through individual and collective effort, establishes, maintains, and improves the ethical environment of the work setting and conditions of employment that are conducive to safe, quality health care.*" A work setting that reflects an ethical environment manifests "beneficence or doing good; nonmaleficence or doing no harm; justice or treating people fairly; reparations or making amends for harm; fidelity, and respect for persons" expanding on how nurses can promote social justice in their practice obligations (ANA, 2015, p. 23). The bravery of a Navy nurse who spoke out about torture in Guantanamo is described next. His actions embody Provision 6 of the ANA *Code of Ethics.*

Article 5 of the 1948 Universal Declaration of Human Rights states: "No one shall be subjected to torture or to cruel, inhuman or degrading treatment or punishment" (University of Minnesota, Human Rights Library, n.d.). More specifically, the United Nations prohibits physicians and other healthcare personnel from participating in torture:

'Participation in torture' includes evaluating an individual's capacity to withstand ill-treatment; being present at, supervising or inflicting maltreatment; resuscitating individuals for the purposes of further maltreatment or providing medical treatment immediately before, during or after torture on the instructions of those likely to be responsible for it; providing professional knowledge or individuals' personal health information to torturers; and intentionally neglecting evidence and falsifying reports, such as autopsy reports and death certificates. The United Nations Principles also incorporate one of the fundamental rules of health-care ethics by emphasizing that the only ethical relationship between prisoners and health professionals is one designed to evaluate, protect and improve prisoners' health. Thus assessment of detainees' health in order to facilitate punishment or torture is clearly unethical.

(Office of the United Nations High Commission for Human Rights, Istanbul Protocol, 2004, p. 12).

Speaking out is sometimes insufficient. The appropriate ethical response in the event of orders that amount to torture is to speak out and refuse to obey. Some situations are less straightforward than outright torture. Take prison hunger strikes, for example. The prisoner makes a political decision to not eat while prison officials force-feed the prisoner because they oppose the prisoner's political decision, not for health reasons. Ethically nuanced choices for nurses caught up in such conflicts are difficult. Xenakis (2017) discusses the ethical dilemmas faced not only by healthcare professionals but also by judges. Reyes (1998) argues for protecting prisoner autonomy in the face of force-feeding prisoners to punish them and alter their behavior. These papers provide an ethical backdrop that directly supports the response of an unnamed Navy nurse lieutenant who refused to force-feed prisoners engaged in a hunger strike in Guantanamo.

Table 8.1 presents a brief chronology of the case. The *Miami Herald* was first to break the news. Hence the included statements are all *Miami Herald* (2015) headlines presenting, in effect, a chronology of events (Table 8.1). Why is this case pertinent in a chapter on social justice and health equity? It is pertinent because it illustrates the courage of a nurse and the primacy of a nurse's conscience over an unethical, oppressive, and sociopolitical order that inflicts pain and suffering. The case illustrates beneficence, doing no harm, and respect

TABLE 8.1 *Miami Herald* Headlines	
Timeline	Activity
July 15, 2014	Navy nurse refuses to force-feed Guantánamo captive.
August 8, 2014	Navy nurse who refused to force-feed still working at Guantánamo.
November 18, 2014	Top nursing group, the American Nurses Association (ANA), backs Navy nurse who wouldn't force-feed at Guantánamo.
May 13, 2015	Navy nurse who refused to force-feed at Guantanamo keeps his job.
July 22, 2015	Top nursing group (ANA) honors Navy nurse who wouldn't force-feed at Guantánamo.

for the prisoners involved and their conscience. The case exemplifies social justice in practice.

Provision 8

Provision 8 states that: *"The nurse collaborates with other health professionals and the public to protect human rights, promote health diplomacy, and reduce health disparities"* (ANA, 2015, p. 31). This provision attests to the principle that health is a universal right and that health includes economic, political, social, and cultural dimensions. Actions under this provision include the promotion of immunizations and collaboration with public agencies, schools, and other venues to promote basic healthcare such as reproductive health, nutrition, and health maintenance. In addition, collaboration with researchers and local public health agencies to provide information and assistance with basic human needs such as clean water, sanitation, healthy food, and basic healthcare in under-resourced areas also falls under this provision.

Consider the nurse's role in the COVID-19 pandemic. Nurses must be skilled in the communication of accurate health information. Health information of import includes infection risk, infection control, and health disparities, as well as case, hospitalization, and mortality rates. Communication is not the only answer. Public health, medical, and nursing leaders must have the knowledge and skill to plan and implement appropriate upstream, midstream, and downstream interventions. For example, the US government enlisted retail pharmacy corporate leaders to agree to the distribution, administration, and documentation of COVID-19 vaccines. This is an upstream action. Midstream action is when the actual vaccines are received by a regional center and, from there, distributed to local pharmacies. Downstream actions are when healthcare professionals, such as nurses, administer vaccines to individuals and then document results for local, state, and national public health data-collection purposes. Parallel to these actions, public health officials, nurses, and physicians use community development methods to enlist local community leaders and messengers to encourage people to be vaccinated. The same health professionals use ordinary, local community messengers to flood television, radio, and all forms of social media. This complex, well-organized, concerted effort is health diplomacy at work.

Provision 9

Provision 9 states that *all nurses must integrate principles of social justice into nursing and health policy* (ANA, 2015, p. 36). This provision addresses the actions of individual nurses at local and state nursing organization levels to "influence leaders, legislators, governmental agencies, non-governmental organizations, and international bodies in all related health affairs to address the social determinants of health" (ANA, 2015, p. 36). Nursing seeks to promote health, prevent illness, and alleviate pain and suffering. Such endeavors must be undertaken in a holistic and just manner that includes local, state, federal, and global responses.

This provision also addresses direct patient care. Nurses care for people from all walks of life, socioeconomic statuses, educational levels, and health statuses. They are the backbone of healthcare services and work in many different healthcare service lines. Nurses have many opportunities to witness vast disparities among people they interact with, including economic, social, and educational differences that influence how, where, and what kind of healthcare services they can access. It is within the scope of practice that nurses not only advocate for the patients they serve in important ways but also collaborate with communities in developing pilot programs and seeking funding. Such advocacy may include consultation with social workers, referrals to community services like Meals on Wheels and local food pantries, collaboration with local church and civic organizations that may assist patients in their home or neighborhood, and grant applications to foundation, state, or federal sources of funding for pilot projects.

Social justice in health and nursing care can be understood within several contexts. "The term refers to equitable distribution and redistribution of resources for positive health outcomes, recognition and removal of social and political barriers that impinge on health and promoting parity of participation in decision-making for the allocation and utilization of health resources" (Abu, 2020, paragraph 2). Social conditions, political issues, and financial issues in health policy can often create and "perpetuate poverty, unemployment, homelessness, discrimination, lack of education, among other social malaise" (Abu, 2020, paragraph 2). Nurses work in each of these contexts.

STRUCTURAL COMPETENCE AND SOCIAL JUSTICE

The term *structural competence* is a recent term in healthcare that is related to implicit biases that have been embedded in US health systems for many years. The term *structure* in this context "implies the buildings, energy networks, water, sewage, food and waste distribution systems, highways, airline, train and road complexes" (Metzl & Hansen, 2014, p. 5) and the electronic communications systems (local and global) that function together in our communities. Structure, however, does not have to be brick and mortar or cables. Structure can also be systemically embedded in social, human, and political ideas/values, prejudices, disparities, and belief systems. It is in these structures, physical and nonphysical, that bias occurs. Bias is a prejudice in favor of or against a thing, person, or group that may be held by an individual, group, or institution. Bias can lead to negative or positive outcomes. Bias can be explicit or implicit. Implicit and unconscious biases are stereotypes about certain groups of people that individuals form outside their conscious awareness.

A growing body of literature on implicit bias and the effects such biases have on healthcare has moved healthcare organizations and health professions education institutions to establish mandatory training and education in this area. The rationale for such training is perhaps best expressed by Metzl and colleagues (2018, p. 189). In explaining why he calls Whiteness a health risk; he states, "Racial disparities in health and healthcare reflect implicit biases embedded in the US healthcare system." Such disparities occur when healthcare providers make assumptions about a patient based on race, sex, ethnicity, income, and/or physical appearance that may lead to less informed decisions about the patient's care. Studies have shown in various healthcare settings that stigma and implicit bias have effects "not just in the attitudes of individual persons, but in actions of institutions, markets, and healthcare delivery systems" (Metzl & Hansen, 2014, p. 128).

Structural competency is a complex framework developed to understand and address implicit bias and the outcomes of such bias in healthcare-related social justice issues. This framework builds on cultural competency to assist healthcare providers in better understanding how "matters of race, social class, ability, sexual orientation, and other markers of difference shape interactions between" health providers and their patients (Metzl & Petty, 2017, p. 354). Structural competency programs show healthcare providers how their prejudgment of patients based on stereotypes perpetuates racial inequities in health, and to recognize how institutions and markets like insurance companies and industries and policy decisions lead to social, health, and financial imbalances. Nurses, physicians, technicians, administrators, and institutions, all whom interact with patients and systems, must have structural competence.

Structural competency is important not only when speaking with patients but also when documenting in the patient's electronic medical record. The US Food and Drug Administration (US FDA) has oversight of the 21st Century Cures Act (i.e., Cures Act). This act was signed into law on December 13, 2016, and is designed to help "accelerate medical product development and bring new innovations and advances to patients who need them faster and more efficiently" (US FDA, 2020). An important part of this legislation requires that healthcare institutions provide access to patients' information in their electronic medical records. This access includes notes clinicians write in electronic health records (EHRs). Patient access to EHR information regarding medications, diagnostic tests, and other information from different platforms has been available for years in many institutions. Many patients may not know what specific medical acronyms mean, such as SOB (shortness of breath). Other common assessment phrases include "history of drug abuse" (an emotionally sensitive issue) or "morbid obesity" (a knowledge gap and an emotionally sensitive issue). Patients may be uncomfortable about such information in their EHR, although the information is confidential and should only be shared with the patient themselves. McCarthy

and his team (2018) discuss the issues involved in full transparency in documentation and selective redaction, where some portions of the record may be withheld because of their sensitive nature.

How do health professionals view patient access to the EHR? A recent study of advanced practice nurses, physicians, registered nurses (RNs), physician assistants, and therapists reported their views and experiences sharing EHR clinical notes with patients. The results indicated that 74% viewed open notes as positive or a good idea; 74% were aware that their patients were reading their notes; and 37% reported they spent more time on documentation, with many respondents reporting "specific changes in the way they write their notes" (DesRoches et al., 2020, paragraph 5). In addition, many respondents noted that they encouraged their patients to read their notes. Interestingly, 14% of respondents reported that their patients contacted their office about their notes outside their regular office visits.

Structural competence is important for all providers in clinical areas. It shows respect and understanding that communicate verbally and in writing that each person we have the honor of taking care of has unique circumstances that play a major role in shaping their health.

SOCIAL JUSTICE AS PRAXIS IN ADDRESSING THE SOCIAL DETERMINANTS OF HEALTH

The social and structural determinants of health as discussed in Chapter 1 both complicate and constrain social justice in healthcare delivery and professional practice. Professional nurses can make a difference and improve social justice issues in healthcare by being aware of the barriers to healthcare services in their communities. Being aware of such barriers is the start of becoming a change agent for improving healthcare. One of the greatest challenges in healthcare has been and continues to be addressing the inequities that lead to health disparities.

As defined in Chapter 1, health inequities are the causes of disparities. For example, discrimination in access to healthcare services, limited or no health insurance, and biased treatment by healthcare providers based on an individual's social identity, such as race, ethnicity, sex, sexual orientation, or any other aspect of marginality leads to disparities. Those disparities can manifest in the provision of lower-quality healthcare services, longer delays in access to care, fewer treatment options, or later-stage diagnoses—all of which lead to poorer health outcomes.

"In the context of health disparities, social justice refers to the minimization of social and economic conditions that adversely affect the health of individuals and communities" (Dilworth-Anderson et al., 2012, p. 27). The word *justice* means fairness in that what one receives is what one is due, which is different from the meaning of *equal* which is that everyone receives the same no matter the need. This difference in terms is important when it comes to healthcare and health disparities. For example, justice in healthcare would be to render the individualized time needed for the provision of care rather than to allot each person who comes to the clinic the same amount of time despite individual needs and differences. Justice in healthcare has, however, assumed equality in the social realms of life as a starting point, but this assumption is an error. Even if it takes more time, equitable care therefore means addressing social determinants of health as important health-related factors that play a significant role in the health inequities that contribute to poorer health outcomes and disparity. The very act of documenting these in an electronic database (i.e., in the EHR) means they will be known by healthcare providers, including nurses, institutions, and healthcare systems who should address these determinants within the communities they serve and monitor the effects on patient outcomes.

Because social determinants seriously influence and determine individual health, "Healthy People 2030" has expanded its overarching focus for the next decade on social determinants of health with a focus on the five domains identified as having a great impact on a person's health over many years. These five domains, which are illustrated in the "Healthy People Framework" in Chapter 1, include economic stability, educational access and quality, healthcare access and quality, neighborhood and built environment, and social and community context.

Because nurses, physicians, and therapists—basically all disciplines in healthcare—see patients who represent various ethnic backgrounds, ages, health issues, professions, education, finances, and other personal characteristics, nurses must first care for the immediate healthcare needs, but nurses should be advocates for patient health. Healthcare providers see firsthand many of the health inequities present in patients' lives and families and, possibly, their neighborhoods. Nurses must be advocates for and leaders of change when inequity and disparity exist in patient populations. Berwick (2020) challenges those in healing professions to be morally guided to action when discrimination is seen or to act when human rights are being exploited (e.g., racism, child abuse, and exploitation of migrant workers and persons with disability) and to support ways to decrease harmful climate changes, hunger, and homelessness, and reform criminal justice and immigration laws. He states, "Healers are called to heal. When the fabric of communities upon which health depends is torn, then healers are called to mend it" (Berwick, 2020, p. 226).

There are several other ways to begin patient and community advocacy work. Look at local government activities and see what services are provided for senior citizens and persons with special needs. Inquire about the local school lunch programs and if there is a school nurse in the school district. These are just a few ideas to begin to learn about the social issues that affect local areas with the understanding that these issues are likely present in other area communities and the state.

Nurses must also advocate for important issues in our workplaces. According to the American Association of Colleges of Nursing (AACN), RNs are the largest workforce in healthcare in the United States with over 3.8 million RNs nationwide (AACN, 2019). Nurses work in all areas of healthcare services and touch most patients in their setting in one way or another. Many advanced practice nurses (APNs) work independently within their discipline area, providing primary care to many underrepresented patient populations in small and rural communities. Rural areas across the United States reflect diversity, as racial and ethnic minorities comprise about 22% of the US rural population (Rowlands & Love, 2021). A 2018 study, "Impact of nurse practitioner practice regulations on rural population health outcomes," showed that advanced registered nurse practitioners (APRNs) increased access and utilization of primary care services and reduced costs in the rural areas included in the study (Ortiz et al., 2018, p. 65).

Rushton (2017) writes that the nursing profession has an ethical obligation to social justice. "We are in a time of complex health care reform, and nurses are ideally situated to put real-life context to the decisions being made"; Rushton encourages nurses to:

- *Systematically document the impact of policy decisions on the people we serve. Nurses see firsthand the realities of decisions at the national level on the people affected at the point of care.*

Real life examples shift the dialogue from faceless policies to the stories of vulnerable Americans.

- *Constructively share observations and insights with nursing and organizational leaders, policy makers, and elected officials.*
- *Become involved and/or assume leadership positions in professional nursing organizations that have structures and mechanisms where our voices can be heard.*
- *Work in community agencies or organizations that focus on specialties and are already addressing issues of interest.*
- *Exercise our rights of citizenship by voting.*
- *Communicate and write letters to elected officials.*
- *Organize colleagues to think about specific strategies and messages we can employ in a constructive way (paras 4–10).*

Nurses are important contributors to the future of nursing and the future of healthcare. Nurses must identify and translate healthcare issues that are disruptive and destructive to healthcare services and be the change agents for solutions. All nurses should communicate with legislators to share information and policy ideas regarding the needs of patients being cared for and the staff caring for them.

Healthcare Access

Access to healthcare is just one of several factors that determine the health of a person over their life span. If access were the only social determinant addressed, many would live healthier and more productive lives, but while access is necessary to save lives and help people live healthier and more productive lives, it is not sufficient. More needs to happen. Marmot (2017) in his article "The health gap: The challenge of an unequal world" explained "that it is the social and economic factors of one's life that led to inequalities in the health of individuals and groups" (p. 1312). He described the social determinants of health as "the conditions in which people are born, grow, live, work, and age; and inequalities in power, money and resources that give rise to inequities in the conditions of daily life" (Marmot, 2017, p. 1312). He goes on to explain that it is these social determinants that lead to great inequalities in the health of people, from within and between countries. These inequalities form "the health gap." Within these determinant categories are related conditions such as early childhood experiences,

education, work experiences, issues of housing and transportation, security, and "a sense of community self-efficacy" (Berwick, 2020, p. 225). It is the wide gaps in these social determinants among and between individuals and groups that lead to inequities in health. Change can happen, even when the social determinants are daunting and fall outside the healthcare arena. Healthcare providers, institutions, and organizations—and citizens—must acknowledge the disparities in health outcomes and then work together diligently if there is to be a narrowing of the many gaps in the health of so many people.

In addition to the social determinants of health that create the inequities that lead to disparities, healthcare financing also challenges and constrains healthcare access and delivery systems. In the first half of 2020, according to the US Commonwealth Fund, 43.4% of adults (ages 19–64) were inadequately insured for healthcare services (Collins et al., 2020). Reasons for inadequate health insurance include unemployment without healthcare benefits, employment with no employer-based health insurance plans, and individuals unable to navigate insurance options online or in person.

"The Affordable Care Act (ACA), of 2010, was the most monumental change in US health care policy since the passage of Medicaid and Medicare in 1965" (Manchikanti et al., 2017, para 1). The ACA, passed during President Obama's administration, expanded insurance coverage by creating a state-specific marketplace where individuals could review, compare, and choose from a variety of health plans. The premise was to open the healthcare market, create competition, and allow consumers to pick the plan that best suited their healthcare and financial needs. The ACA also expanded government assistance for the purchase of a health plan and expanded eligibility to the current Medicaid program for individuals and families based on income. The ACA has had a great impact by significantly increasing the number of insured people in the United States since its inception. A 2018 study by McKenna and colleagues (2018) revealed that the ACA decreased financial strain "and improved access to and the utilization of health services for low- and middle-income adults who have traditionally not met income eligibility requirements for public insurance programs" (p. 1). Criticisms of the ACA include that most of the insurance expansion was in the Medicaid program and that access to healthcare services continues to be challenging for many people (Manchikanti et al., 2017).

MORAL DISTRESS AND MORAL RESILIENCE

There are many ethical challenges in nursing—taking care of patients in all settings can be difficult and may cause distress or feelings of helplessness. As mentioned earlier in this chapter, first described by Andrew Jameton in 1982, moral distress occurs "in a given situation when a health professional knows, or believes they know the ethically appropriate course of action to take but is unable to carry it out because of obstacles present" (Jameton, 1984, p. 6) (Fig. 8.2).

Nurses see the inequity in healthcare due to the educational, social, and financial inequities of our society. For example, you cared for Ms. A. for 2 weeks. She came in with a stroke that has left her right (dominant) side weak, and she is unable to take care of herself. She has no family support to help her upon discharge, and her insurance does not cover many of the supplies and services she needs when she goes home. You have worked with your unit social worker and discharge planner to get her all she needs at discharge; however, there are several serious gaps in her resources. The nurse feels emotionally helpless and morally distressed. The consequences of moral distress on a person "can include professional burnout, emotional exhaustion, and feelings of disengagement" (Rushton, 2017, p. S11). You decide to discuss the patient's needs with the nursing supervisor to see what else can be done for Ms. A. The action you are taking is best described as moral courage. "Moral courage supports nurses as advocates, both for themselves and their patients" (ANA, 2015, p. 21). After your discussion with the nursing supervisor, most of the resources

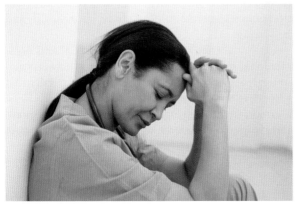

Fig. 8.2 Moral distress. (©Wavebreakmedia Ltd/Wavebreak Media/Thinkstock.)

Ms. A. needs will be taken care of through a benevolent fund. Although this example is rather simple, it shows how moral distress may prompt the courage to act to further advocate for a patient in need. The nurse's concern or distress in this case led to action, which may not have occurred otherwise (Anderson-Shaw & Zar, 2020).

Ongoing moral distress can cause serious negative effects on a person's health, happiness, and work life. However, there is evidence that moral distress may become a "catalyst for positive outcomes, moral resilience, and growth" (Rushton, 2017, p. S13). In addition, resiliency is the ability to sustain, restore, or "deepen integrity in response to moral complexity, confusion, distress, or setbacks" (Schroeter, 2017, p. 290). Nurses and the nursing profession are ones of resilience and healing.

SOCIAL INCLUSION AND EXCLUSION AS MATTERS OF SOCIAL JUSTICE

Social inclusion is a process that creates opportunities for resources, services, and rights. Social inclusion refers to an individual's or group's opportunities to participate in critical economic, social, and cultural areas (Killaspy et al., 2014). On the other hand with social exclusion, people cannot fully participate in economic, social, political, and cultural life (United Nations, 2016). Social exclusion goes beyond the lack of material possessions and encompasses the lack of agency, feelings of marginalization, and alienation usually associated with identity-based attributes such as race, ethnicity, sex, sexual orientation, migration status, or some other group ascription (Table 8.2). Social exclusion is what happens when marginalization occurs. Thus social inclusion is improving the conditions of individuals and groups to partake in the benefits and opportunities in society. Social inclusion is an action and a process; it is context based. Social inclusion and social exclusion are critical mechanisms by which the social determinants of health are compounded to negatively influence health (O'Donnell et al., 2018).

Social exclusion includes discrimination, stigma, and the experience of dehumanization (Wesselmann et al., 2019). The concept of unequal power in the definition of social exclusion reflects ever-changing, multidimensional processes driven by unequal power relationships characterized by unequal access to resources, capabilities, and rights, leading to health inequities (Popay et al., 2021). Two recent examples of social inequities are the disproportionate impact of COVID-19 on essential

TABLE 8.2 Social Inclusion and Exclusion

My Journey

I'm not a nurse! I wrote this chapter as an Executive Lead of a community-driven coalition working to advance racial and economic justice. Initially, I was excited to work on a book chapter about the social determinants of health. However, after reviewing the literature, I could not find my voice and my experiences of social justice action. I doubted whether I had something meaningful to say to nursing students. Is there a role for nursing students in community-driven coalitions?

My voice as a Black American is not in the literature, and every past academic failure came rushing to my mind as I sat down to write. Who am I to be writing a book chapter anyway? Book chapters seemed to be the voice of White editors informing White readers how to best include socially marginalized groups. I have privilege, but I represent the marginalized and I want to write from my authentic experience. Healthcare has somehow created an invisible shield that puts some social justice issues outside of healthcare, such as the police murders of Black people. While other social justice issues are viewed as inside of healthcare such as poor housing conditions.

The Black voice in my head created a sense of self-exclusion. I was taking away my opportunity to speak without giving myself a chance.

As I reflected on this journey, I found a way to speak my truth about the social determinants of health and balance this with the literature from other authors. Understanding social inclusion and social exclusion as a process that requires us to bring our wholes selves, not just our academic or clinical skills, but our authentic selves. Social justice action is about people with complex histories, everyday struggles, and the policies and systems that influence our health.

As a reader, I ask that you reflect on your personal experience of social inclusion and exclusion. What parts of social justice action remind you of your journey as a person and as a professional?

—Lena Hatchett, 2020

workers (Krieger, 2020) and the low-income Black and Latinx communities. Nursing students can explore the power dynamics that transform harmful policies into practical solutions. For example, Black doctors built a nonprofit consortium to provide mobile testing and vaccination services in the Black neighborhoods in Philadelphia most affected by COVID-19 (Persad et al., 2021). Understanding the ideas of social inclusion and exclusion can help nurses become more mindful of the emotional harms of living with complex, interrelated inequities. To create equity, nurses are asked to broaden their perspective to include power, policies, and systems as the root causes of health inequities and their own responsibility to address these causes. Laws, policies, and institutions can drive exclusion or mitigate its impacts.

SYSTEMS CHANGE AND ACTION

Nursing students are a powerful bridge to connect the individual experience of inequities to systems change in healthcare. Students acting through in-class projects and service-learning opportunities can advance systems-level change. The "Six Conditions of Systems Change" is a framework developed by Kania and colleagues (2018) that unpacks key leverage points

in a system so readers can better understand where change is possible (Table 8.3). Some levers are explicit and others are implicit. The latter makes the ability to change more obscure. The framework is described across three levels: structural, relational, and transformative change (Fig. 8.3). Structural changes represent those that address governmental and institutional policies and practices that shape and reshape regulations and activities. The process of how people, finances, and information resources flow is a critical structural change component. Students can investigate how specific policies operate to promote or harm health and well-being.

Relational change describes the personal and organizational relationships and connections between and among partners and the existing power dynamics that affect development and social justice action.

Transformative change refers to the thoughts, beliefs, and assumptions underlying decisions. Transformation may occur at an individual, group, institutional, system, and societal level to the extent that undergirding thoughts, beliefs, and assumptions change for the better.

Where are the opportunities for students to partner in systems change? Nursing students may explore the structural change conditions in coursework and

TABLE 8.3	**Systems Change Conditions: Definitions**		
Structural change	Policies	Governmental, institutional, and organizational rules, regulations, and priorities that guide the entity's and others' actions.
	Practices	Espoused activities of institutions, coalitions, networks, and other entities targeted to improving social and environmental progress; within the entity, the procedures, guidelines, or informal shared habits that comprise their work.
	Resource flows	How money, people, knowledge, information, and other assets such as infrastructure are allocated and distributed.
Relational change	Relationships and connections	Quality of connections and communication occurring among actors in the system, especially among those with differing histories and viewpoints.
	Power dynamics	The distribution of decision-making power, authority, and both formal and informal influence among individuals and organizations.
Transformative change	Mental models	Habits of thought—deeply held beliefs and assumptions and taken-for-granted ways of operating that influence how we think, what we do, and how we talk.

Adapted from: Kania, Kramer, & Senge (2018). *The Water of Systems Change*. FSG. Retrieved from http://efc.issuelab.org/resources/30855/30855.pdf.

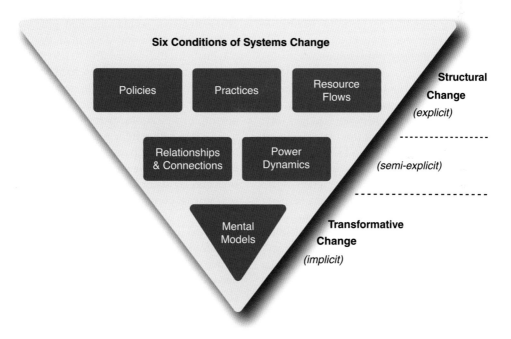

Fig. 8.3 Six conditions of systems change. (Adapted from: Kania, Kramer, & Senge (2018). *The Water of Systems Change*. FSG. Retrieved from http://efc.issuelab.org/resources/30855/30855.pdf.)

service-learning projects to recognize individual patients' social needs and understand the systems and policies that create health inequities. The complex, interrelated social determinants of health include institutional racism and community disinvestment (Woolf, 2017). Williams and colleagues describe the nurse advocacy role in improving social policy in early childhood education, job security, educational attainment, and housing stability (Williams et al., 2018).

Advocacy and action for relational change can represent relationships, connections, and the power dynamics between nurses and communities that experience health inequities. Students can be innovators and change agents to advance social justice action (Cusson et al., 2020).

The social unrest of 2020 requires all to learn the skills to build trust and balance power at the individual and organizational levels (Butterfoss & Kegler, 2002). At the societal level, the country has yet to confront the context of historical oppression that perpetuates and maintains structural racism. In a qualitative study, Burnette and Sanders (2014) outlined transparency and reciprocity to help students practice trust-building.

There are several new partnership roles for nurses that help build relationships and connections and balance the power dynamics faced by disenfranchised and oppressed communities and coalitions. For example, Gregg and colleagues (2018) introduced the *nurse policy entrepreneur* role. In this capacity, the nurse policy entrepreneur is a catalyst to identify social and political concerns to generate collaborative solutions in rural health (Gregg et al., 2018). Other work describes the practice of culturally responsive care as a decolonizing and antioppressive approach to care for excluded populations (Jakubec & Bearskin, 2020). Nursing students will face social, cultural, and political challenges with community members across different power bases, values, and privileges. Students can take individual and collective action on the power dynamics at play and explore solutions in partnership with other stakeholders. The first step is to take time and prioritize listening and learning from people closest to inequity. There are opportunities to learn from community wisdom, knowledge, and existing solutions about institutional racism, segregation, and immigrant rights that best promote inclusion. Nursing students can explore their roles as change agents (Rafferty, 2018), encourage discussions of improving equity and reducing structural racism for Black Americans (Nardi et al., 2020), and improve power differences for American Indian/Alaska Native populations (Pool & Stauber, 2020).

The ANA states: "Nursing can be described as both an art and a science; a heart and a mind" (ANA, 2015, paragraph 3). Student nurses are pivotal as bridge builders to connect neighborhoods of concentrated poverty with policymakers and to create a platform for effective communication. Effective social justice action requires nurses to reflect on their personal beliefs and values about systems change as they listen and learn from others.

CONCLUSION

This chapter reviewed concepts related to social justice and health equity in healthcare. These concepts include the principles of social justice and how these principles apply to healthcare, structural competence in healthcare, social inclusion and exclusion related to social justice, and how nurses can advocate for social justice, health equity, and safe patient care. Being a social justice advocate is an opportunity to look beyond superficial approaches to healthcare to something deeper that gets to the heart of the issue and can potentially improve the experiences of many. Advocates focus on questioning protocols, laws, regulations, and practices in systems and organizations that perpetuate or sustain unequal playing fields that cause harm to people.

Upstream activities may include becoming an active member in local and state professional organizations, such as the state nurses' association and affiliated state nursing organizations; participating in local town hall meetings to gather information on healthcare programs in the area; and meeting local politicians or municipality officials and reviewing the local town committee persons and legislators social media and public records to see on what committees they serve, their areas of political interest, and their track record related to healthcare and social justice issues. Midstream interventions might include volunteering at local homeless shelters, warming centers, or food pantries to better understand individual needs; seeking out local charities that aid women and children; or teaching in an after school program. Downstream interventions include the provision of services to those in need, such as taking care of patients who are impoverished, malnourished, and homeless.

▋ STUDENT LEARNING AND REFLECTION ACTIVITIES

1. Student social justice action: Participate in community-driven coalition approaches.

   Action for transformative change: One form of transformative change is building community power, which is the ability of the communities most impacted by structural inequity to develop, sustain, and grow (Speer et al., 2020). Transformative change allows the lever of beliefs and assumptions to bend toward social justice. Individuals living in poverty are perceived to have individual problems such as low skills and limited income.

However, awareness of power and privilege allows students to see the policies and systems that create poverty and the opportunity to work upstream toward solutions. The anchor institutional approach is one effective upstream solution. "Anchor institutions"—universities, hospitals, and other large, place-based organizations—invest in their communities as a way of doing business" (Koh et al., 2020, p. 309). Students can reimagine solutions for the social determinants of health by exploring the anchor institutions' roles in partnership with communities. For example, Weston and colleagues (2020) describe collaboration with anchor institutions that advances workforce development initiatives in neighborhoods with concentrated poverty; wealth attainment for immigrant groups (Vallejo & Keister, 2019); and a diverse workforce program in nursing with racial and ethnic minority groups (Williams et al., 2018). Anchor institutions leverage current business practices to create inclusive policies for hiring and workforce development, purchasing, and investments to develop disenfranchised communities. Nurses can act by joining the Healthcare Anchor Network and be a pathway of communication and understanding between communities and institutions.

2. Student social justice action: Participate in anchor institution approaches.

Experiential exercise: "Community of Solutions Framework for Equity" (100 million lives) is a reflection and action tool that students can use to develop critical-thinking skills to take on the role of change agent in collaborative projects to advance health, well-being, and equity.

Review the four questions from the "Community of Solutions Framework for Equity":

1. Leading from within: What areas of personal reflection and self-awareness would you need to build to promote equity in partnership with others? What identities do you claim in relationship to individuals and the community? Where in the relationship are you included or excluded? Where in the relationship do you include or exclude others?

2. Leading together: How would you collaborate with a community partner to promote equity? Students should explore the power dynamics between themselves and community partners. How could you use personal and professional skills to support the partnership?

3. Leading for outcomes: How would you measure success that benefits all partners? How would you collaborate to create plans and evaluation tools?

4. Leading for sustainability: How would you design a sustainable plan? How would you fund the initiative long-term?

REFERENCES

Abu, V. K. (2020). Let us be unequivocal about social justice in nursing. *Nurse Education in Practice, 47*, 102849. https://doi.org/10.1016/j.nepr.2020.102849.

American Association of Colleges of Nursing. (2019). Nursing fact sheet. Retrieved from: AACN Fact Sheet–Nursing, aacnnursing.org.

American College of Nurse-Midwives. (2020). Statement from the American College of Nurse-Midwives regarding complaints of unwarranted hysterectomies performed without consent at ICE facilities. Retrieved from https://www.midwife.org/statement-from-the-american-college-of-nurse-midwives-regarding-complaints-of-unwarranted-hysterectomies-performed-without-consent-at-ice-facilities.

American Nurses Association. (n.d.). Things to know about whistleblowing. Retrieved from www.nursingworld.org/practice-policy/workforce/things-to-know-about-whistle-blowing/.

American Nurses Association. (2015). What is nursing? Retrieved from https://www.nursingworld.org/practice-policy/workforce/what-is-nursing/#:~:text=Nursing%20can%20be%20described%20as,form%20of%20rigorous%20core%20learning.

American Nurses Association. (2020). ANA responds to high rates of hysterectomies on immigrant women under ICE custody. Retrieved from https://www.nursingworld.org/news/news-releases/2020/american-nurses-association-responds-to-high-rates-of-hysterectomies–on-immigrant-women-under-ice-custody/#:~:text=ANA%20Responds%20to%20High%20Rates%20of%20Hysterectomies%20on%20Immigrant%20Women%20Under%20ICE%20Custody,-Sep%2016th%202020&text=ANA%20advocates%20for%20the%20provision,investigation%20into%20these%20troubling%20allegations.

Anderson-Shaw, L., & Zar, F. (2020). COVID-19, moral conflict, distress, and dying alone. *Journal of Bioethical Inquiry, 17*(4), 777–782. https://doi:10.1007/s11673-020-10040-9.

Association of Operating Room Nurses. (2020). AORN statement regarding forced hysterectomy allegations. Retrieved from https://www.aorn.org/about-aorn/aorn-newsroom/aorn-statement-regarding-forced-hysterectomy-allegations.

Berwick, D. M. (2020). The moral determinants of health. *JAMA, 324*(3), 225–226. https://doi.org/10.1001/jama.2020.11129.

Brauer, C. (1982). Kennedy, Johnson, and the war on poverty. *The Journal of American History, 69*(1), 98–119. http://doi:10.2307/1887754.

Burnette, C. E., & Sanders, S. (2014). Trust development in research with indigenous communities in the United States. *Qualitative Report, 19*(44), 1–19.

Butterfoss, F. D., & Kegler, M. C. (2002). Toward a comprehensive understanding of community coalitions: Moving from theory to practice. In DiClemente, R. J., Crosby, R. A., & Kegler, M. C. (Eds.), *Emerging theories in health promotion practice and research: Strategies for improving public health* (1st ed., pp. 157–193). Jossey Bass.

Carnegie Council for Ethics in International Affairs. (2020). Erica Chenoweth: Organizing a Successful Social Movement [video]. You Tube. https://www.youtube.com/watch?v=_y62wT21nBs.

Collins, S. R., Gunja, M. Z., & Aboulafia, G. N. (2020). U.S. health insurance coverage in 2020: A looming crisis in affordability. The Commonwealth Fund. Retrieved from https://www.commonwealthfund.org/publications/issue-briefs/2020/aug/looming-crisis-health-coverage-2020-biennial.

Cusson, R. M., Meehan, C., Bourgault, A., & Kelley, T. (2020). Educating the next generation of nurses to be innovators and change agents. *Journal of Professional Nursing, 36*(2), 13–19.

DesRoches, C. M., Leveille, S., Bell, S. K., Dong, Z. J., Elmore, J. G., Fernandez, L., Harcourt, K., Fitzgerald, P., Payne, T. H., Stametz, R., Delbanco, T., & Walker, J. (2020). The views and experiences of clinicians sharing medical record notes with patients. *JAMA network open, 3*(3), e201753. https://doi.org/10.1001/jamanetworkopen.2020.1753.

Dilworth-Anderson, P., Pierre, G., & Hilliard, T. S. (2012). Social justice, health disparities, and culture in the care of the elderly. *The Journal of Law, Medicine & Ethics, 40*, 26–32. https://doi.org/10.1111/j.1748-720X.2012.00642.x.

Government Accountability Project. (2021). Press statement: One year after Dawn Wooten's disclosures of immigrant abuse, Irwin County Detention Center finally moves out all detained immigrants. Retrieved from Press Statement: One Year After Dawn Wooten's Disclosures of Immigrant Abuse, Irwin County Detention Center Finally Moves Out All Detained Immigrants. whistleblower.org.

Gregg, J., Miller, J., & Tennant, K. F. (2018). Nurse policy entrepreneurship in a rural community: A multiple streams framework approach. *Online Journal of Issues in Nursing, 23*(3), 1–11.

Harrington, M. (1962). *The other America*. Simon & Schuster.

Jakubec, S. L., & Bearskin, R. L. B. (2020). Decolonizing and anti-oppressive nursing practice: Awareness, allyship, and action. In L. McCleary & T. McParland (Eds.), *Ross-Kerr &*

Woods Canadian Nursing: Issues and perspectives (6th ed., pp. 243–268). Elsevier.

Jameton, A. (1984). *Nursing practice: The ethical issues.* Prentice-Hall.

Kania, J., Kramer, M., & Senge, P. (2018). *The water of systems change.* FSG Reimaging social change. Retrieved from http://efc.issuelab.org/resources/30855/30855.pdf.

Killaspy, H., White, S., Lalvani, N., Berg, R., Thachil, A., Kallumpuram, S., Nasiruddin, O., Wright, C., & Mezey, G. (2014). The impact of psychosis on social inclusion and associated factors. *The International Journal of Social Psychiatry, 60*(2), 148–154. https://doi.org/10.1177/0020764012471918.

Koh, H. K., Bantham, A., Geller, A. C., Rukavina, M. A., Emmons, K. M., Yatsko, P., & Restuccia, R. (2020). Anchor institutions: Best practices to address social needs and social determinants of health. *American Journal of Public Health, 110*(3), 309–316. https://doi.org/10.2105/AJPH.2019.305472.

Kniess, J. (2021). Health Justice and Rawls's Theory at Fifty: Will new thinking about health and inequality influence the most influential account of justice? *The Hastings Center Report, 51*(6), 44. https://doi-org.ezp.slu.edu/10.1002/hast.1277.

Krieger, N. (2020). ENOUGH: COVID-19, structural racism, police brutality, plutocracy, climate change—and time for health justice, democratic governance, and an equitable, sustainable future. *American Journal of Public Health, 110*(11), 1620–1623. https://doi.org/10.2105/AJPH.2020.305886.

Lachman, V. D. (2016). Moral resilience: Managing and preventing moral distress and moral residue. *MEDSURG Nursing, 25*(2), 121–124.

Manchikanti, L., Helm, I. S., Benyamin, R. M., & Hirsch, J. A. (2017). A critical analysis of Obamacare: Affordable care or insurance for many and coverage for few? *Pain Physician, 20*(3), 111–138.

Marmot, M. (2017). The health gap: The challenge of an unequal world: The argument. *International Journal of Epidemiology, 46*(4), 1312–1318. https://doi.org/10.1093/ije/dyx163.

McCarthy, C., Garets, D., & Eastman, D. (2018). *Effective strategies for change.* New York: HIMSS Publishing.

McKenna, R. M., Langellier, B. A., Alcalá, H. E., Roby, D. H., Grande, D. T., & Ortega, A. N. (2018). The Affordable Care Act attenuates financial strain according to poverty level. *Inquiry, 55*, 46958018790164. https://doi.org/10.1177/0046958018790164.

Metzl, J. M., & Hansen, H. (2014). Structural competency: Theorizing a new medical engagement with stigma and inequality. *Social Science & Medicine, 103*, 126–133. https://doi.org/10.1016/j.socscimed.2013.06.032.

Metzl, J. M., & Petty, J. (2017). Integrating and assessing structural competency in an innovative prehealth curriculum at

Vanderbilt University. *Academic Medicine, 92*(3), 354–359. https://doi.org/10.1097/ACM.0000000000001477.

Metzl, J. M., Petty, J., & Olowojoba, O. V. (2018). Using a structural competency framework to teach structural racism in pre-health education. *Social Science & Medicine, 199*, 189–201. https://doi.org/10.1016/j.socscimed.2017.06.029.

Miami Herald. (2015). Nursing group honors navy nurse who wouldn't force feed Guantanamo prisoners. Retrieved from https://www.miamiherald.com/news/nation-world/.

Nardi, D., Waite, R., Nowak, M., Hatcher, B., Hines-Martin, V., & Stacciarini, J. R. (2020). Achieving health equity through eradicating structural racism in the United States: A call to action for nursing leadership. *Journal of Nursing Scholarship, 52*(6), 696–704.

O'Donnell, P., O'Donovan, D., & Elmusharaf, K. (2018). Measuring social exclusion in healthcare settings: A scoping review. *International Journal for Equity in Health, 17*(1), 1–16.

Office of the United Nations High Commission for Human Rights, Geneva, Professional Training Series No. 8/Rev.1, *Istanbul Protocol.* (2004). Retrieved from https://www.ohchr.org/documents/publications/training8rev1en.pdf.

Ornstein, A. C. (2017). Social justice: History, purpose and meaning. *Social Science and Public Policy, 54*, 541–548. https://doi.org/10.1007/s12115-017-0188-8.

Ortiz, J., Hofler, R., Bushy, A., Lin, Y. L., Khanijahani, A., & Bitney, A. (2018). Impact of nurse practitioner practice regulations on rural population health outcomes. *Healthcare, 6*(2), 65. https://doi.org/10.3390/healthcare6020065.

Persad, G., Emanuel, E. J., Sangenito, S., Glickman, A., Phillips, S., & Largent, E. A. (2021). Public perspectives on COVID-19 vaccine prioritization. *JAMA Network Open, 4*(4), 1–12, e217943. https://doi.org/10.1001/jamanetworkopen.2021.7943.

Pool, N. M., & Stauber, L. S. (2020). Tangled pasts, healthier futures: Nursing strategies to improve American Indian/Alaskan native health equity. *Nursing Inquiry, 27*(4), e12367.

Popay, J., Whitehead, M., Ponsford, R., Egan, M., & Mead, R. (2021). Power, control, communities and health inequalities I: Theories, concepts and analytical frameworks. *Health Promotion International, 36*(5), 1253–1263.

Rafferty, A. M. (2018). Nurses as change agents for a better future in health care: The politics of drift and dilution. *Health Economics, Policy, and Law, 13*(3–4), 475–491.

Project South, Institute for the Elimination of Poverty & Genocide. (2020). Re: Lack of Medical Care, Unsafe work practices, and absence of adequate protection against Covid-19 for detained immigrants and employees alike at the Irwin County Detention Center. Retrieved from www.projectsouth.org.

Rawls, J. (1971). *A theory of justice.* Harvard University Press.

Rawls, J. (2001). *Justice as fairness.* Harvard University Press.

Reisch, M. (2002). Defining social justice in a socially unjust world. *Families in society: The Journal of Contemporary Human Services, 83*(4), 343–354.

Rowlands, D. W., & Love, H. (2021). Brookings: The avenue, mapping rural America's diversity and demographic change. Retrieved from https://www.brookings.edu/blog/the-avenue/2021/09/28/mapping-rural-americas-diversity-and-demographic-change/.

Reyes, H. (1998). Medical and ethical aspects of hunger strikes in custody and the issue of torture. In Maltreatment and Torture in the series Research in Legal Medicine – Volume 19/ Rechtsmedizinische Forschungsergebnisse - Band 19. M. Oehmichen, ed., Verlag Schmidt-Römhild, Lübeck, 1998. https://www.icrc.org/en/doc/resources/documents/article/other/health-article-010198.htm.

Rushton, C. (2017). Our ethical obligation to social justice: On the pulse. *Johns Hopkins Nursing Magazine.* Retrieved from https://magazine.nursing.jhu.edu/2017/05/our-ethical-obligation-to-social-justice/.

Rushton, C. (2017a). Cultivating moral resilience. *American Journal of Nursing, 117*(2), S1–S15. https://doi:10.1097/01.NAJ.0000512205.93596.00.

Sacchetti, M. (2021). *The Washington Post.* ICE to stop detaining immigrants at two controversial county jails in Georgia and Massachusetts.

Schroeter, K. (2017). Ethics in practice: From moral distress to moral resilience. *Journal of Trauma Nursing, 24*(5), 290–291.

Speer, P. W., Gupta, J., Haapanen, K., Balmer, B., Wiley, K. T., & Bachelder, A. (2020). *Developing community power for health equity: A landscape analysis of current research and theory.* Robert Wood Johnson Foundation. Retrieved from https://static1.squarespace.com/static/5ee2c6c3c085f746bd-33f80e/t/5f89f1325e27a51436c97b74/1602875699695/Landscape±-±Developing±Community±Power±-for±Health±Equity±%281%29.pdf.

The Government Publishing Office. (2016). Commonsense gun control. Retrieved from Congressional Record, *162*(100). www.govinfo.gov.

United Nations. (2016). Identifying social inclusion and exclusion. Retrieved from https://www.un.org/esa/socdev/rwss/2016/chapter1.pdf.

University of Minnesota, Human Rights Library. (n.d.). Universal declaration of human rights, G.A., res. 217A (III), U.N. Doc A/810 at 71 (1948). Retrieved from Universal Declaration of Human Rights, G.A. res. 217A (III), U.N. Doc A/810 at 71 (1948). www.umn.edu.

US Food and Drug Administration. (2020). 21st Century Cures Act. Retrieved from https://www.fda.gov/regulatory-information/selected-amendments-fdc-act/21st-century-cures-act.

US Census Bureau. (1968). Statistical abstract of the United States. Retrieved from https://www.census.gov/library/publications/1968/compendia/statab/89ed.html.

Vallejo, J. A., & Keister, L. A. (2019). Immigrants and wealth attainment: Migration, inequality, and integration. *Journal of Ethnic and Migration Studies, 46*(18), 3745–3761.

Wesselmann, E. D., Michels, C., & Slaughter, A. (2019). *Understanding common and diverse forms of social exclusion*. In S. Rudert, R. Greifeneder, & K. Williams (Eds.), *Current Directions in Ostracism, Social Exclusion, and Rejection Research*. Routledge.

Weston, M. J., Pham, B. H., & Zuckerman, D. (2020). Building community well-being by leveraging the economic impact of health systems. *Nursing Administration Quarterly, 44*(3), 215–220.

Williams, S., Phillips, J., & Koyama, K. (2018). Nurse advocacy: Adopting a health in all policies approach. *Online Journal of Issues in Nursing, 23*(3). https://ojin.nursingworld.org/table-of-contents/volume-23-2018/number-3-september-2018/adopting-health-in-all-policies-approach/.

Woolf, S. H. (2017). Progress in achieving health equity requires attention to root causes. *Health Affairs, 36*(6), 984–991.

Xenakis, S. N. (2017). Ethics dilemmas in managing hunger strikes. *The Journal of the American Academy of Psychiatry and the Law, 45*(3), 311–315.

Culture and Health Equity

Priscilla Limbo Sagar, Teri A. Murray

Public health is a powerful tool to level that playing field, to bend the arc of our country away from distrust and disparities and back towards equity and justice.
—*Leana S. Wen, Lifelines: A Doctor's Journey in the Fight for Public Health*

CHAPTER OUTLINE

LEARNING OBJECTIVES

1. Analyze the role of culture in achieving health equity.
2. Discuss the intersectionality of cultural diversity and health.
3. Reflect on the importance of cultural awareness, the need for culturally congruent care, and being a culturally humble healthcare provider.
4. Describe strategies that lead to the provision of culturally responsive care.

UNDERSTANDING CULTURE AND WHY IT MATTERS IN ACHIEVING HEALTH EQUITY

In 2021, the largest racial or ethnic group in the United States was White (non-Hispanic), which accounted for 59.3% of the population, down from 63.8% in 2010 (US Census Bureau, 2023). The Hispanic/Latino population has shown the most significant growth in the last decade, from 16.4% in 2010 to 18.9% in 2021 (US Census Bureau, 2023). Black (non-Hispanic), American Indian/Alaskan Native, and Native Hawaiian and other Pacific Islander (non-Hispanic) populations have remained relatively flat in terms of growth between 2010 and 2021, from 12.3% to 12.6%, 0.7% to 0.7%, and 0.2% to 0.2%, respectively (US Census Bureau, 2023). During that same 11-year period, multiracial groups, defined as two or more races, grew from 1.8% to 2.3% (US Census Bureau, 2023). Projections indicate that the White non-Hispanic population will become the minority by 2045, as population estimates show White (non-Hispanic) losses and racial and ethnic minority gains (US Census Bureau, 2018).

Concomitant with the growing racial and ethnic diversity is the expansive diversity in gender identities, lifestyle practices, socioeconomic statuses, and geographical locations. In 2019, nearly 68 million people in the United States did not speak English at home (Dietrich & Hernandez, 2022) (Fig. 9.1). The five most spoken languages in the United States other than English are Spanish (61.6%), Chinese (5.2%), Tagalog (2.6%), Vietnamese (2.3%), and Arabic (1.9%) (Dietrich & Hernandez, 2022). The increasing racial and ethnic diversity and language variance challenge healthcare professionals to provide culturally and linguistically congruent care to the populations they serve (Sagar, 2014). This wide variation in cultural backgrounds, linguistic styles, religious and political affiliations, and sexual orientations brings to the forefront the need for students to learn to function in diverse, multicultural contexts.

Disparities in access, quality, and care delivery exist for minoritized, vulnerable, impoverished patients, including those with limited language proficiency (Okoniewski et al., 2022). These disparities can be associated with age, sex, religion, socioeconomic status, sexual orientation, gender identification, disability, and other social identities, including stigmatized diagnoses such as HIV, obesity, mental health disorders, and substance use disorders (Narayan, 2019). Becoming culturally conscious is critical given the increasing diversity in the US population and the adverse health outcomes frequently seen in minoritized populations, including populations whose primary language is not English. Okoniewski and colleagues (2022) acknowledge that providing care specific to the cultural needs of individuals, families, and communities can help address health disparities and promote health equity.

THE SOCIAL DETERMINANTS OF HEALTH

The WHO (2023) emphatically states:

The social determinants of health (SDOH) are the non-medical factors that influence health outcomes. They are the conditions in which people are born, grow, work, live, and age, and the wider set of forces and systems shaping the conditions of daily life. These forces and systems include economic policies and systems, development agendas, social norms, social policies, and political systems (paragraph 1).

The tremendous effects of SDOH on health inequities, estimated to be approximately 30% to 55%, are unfair and avoidable yet cause glaring disparities in health status among people within and between nations (WHO, 2023). People at the lowest socioeconomic level manifest the worst health outcomes. Socially and economically disadvantaged populations are unlikely to be healthy, less likely to access quality healthcare, and prone to have a shorter life span (Williams et al., 2018).

Lacking documentation are the effects of structural determinants, the "formal and informal rules of the institution, policies, culture, and values which include structural discrimination such as classism, racism, sexism, … xenophobia, and homophobia" on health equity (Solar et al., 2023, p. 2). The National Center for Chronic Disease Prevention (National Center for

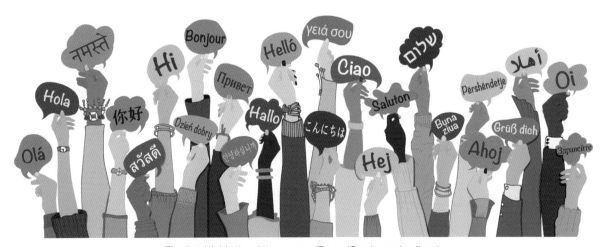

Fig. 9.1 Multicultural languages. (From: iStock.com/melitas.)

Chronic Disease Prevention and Health Promotion [NCCDP], 2022) at the CDC acknowledged that inequitable and undue differences in SDOH contribute to chronic disease disparities in the United States among racial, ethnic, and socioeconomic groups. The NCCDP (2022, 2022a) recognizes that rightfully addressing differences in SDOH and moving toward health equity, "a state in which every person has the fair and just opportunity to attain their highest level of health" (paragraph 2) could be achieved through collaborating with partners; planning, developing, and disseminating accurate, timely, and respectful communication; engaging with communities; and focusing on workforce improvement.

Tackling SDOH—which requires action by entire sectors of society—is essential to advancing health and eliminating disparities. The contribution to health outcomes from outside sectors surpasses the contribution from the health sector (WHO, 2023). Delivering health services alone is inadequate in fostering health equity since clinical services do not address the SDOH (Drevdahl, 2018; Pacquaio, 2019).

DIVERSITY AND CULTURE

Diversity can be described as the various ways individuals and groups differ. These differences, referred to as social identities, are the distinct characteristics that encompass a set of broad attributes inclusive of but not limited to, race, ethnicity, national origin, immigration status, linguistic characteristics, sex, gender identification, sexual orientation, religious tradition, age, socioeconomic status, ability, and veteran status (American Association of Colleges of Nursing [AACN], 2017). Most individuals occupy several social identities, given that social identities are dynamic and complex. For example, an individual can be racially Black, of Hispanic origin, identify as a homosexual male, middle-aged, and Catholic. He is a man. His race is Black. He is of Hispanic origin. He is homosexual. He is a middle-aged adult. His religious affiliation is Catholic. As such, his social identity combines many intersecting identities such as race, ethnicity, sexual orientation, age, and religion.

Intersectionality

Intersectionality is a term used to describe the multiple social identities a person may occupy throughout the life course. Intersectionality is a theoretical framework coined by Kimberle Crenshaw that explains the experiences of privilege and oppression at the individual level based on the multiple and complex aspects of the individual's identity. Intersectionality disrupts the idea of social identities acting in isolation (Fitzgerald & Campinha-Bacote, 2019). Intersectionality holds that marginalized groups suffer from forms of oppression within society such as racism, sexism, classism, ableism, homophobia, transphobia, xenophobia, and other belief-based bigotry, and the impacts of this oppression do not function independently of each other but have a multiplier effect in terms of oppression beyond simply adding together the marginalization experienced by each group (Mandelbaum, 2020). Marginality refers to groups that are said to exist on the lower or outer limits of social desirability, most often determined by one's race, ethnicity, sex, sexual orientation, socioeconomic status, and religion (Sue & Sue, 2016). One example of intersectionality is the high rate of mortality during childbirth and postpartum among Black women. The two marginalized identities (female and Black) highlight the oppression Black women face from both the sexism and racism deeply embedded within society and healthcare.

Sociocultural identities are important areas to assess to enlighten providers about their patient's history of trauma, discrimination, and oppression. These are vital in developing strategies to empower and inspire the client and essential in planning, implementing, and evaluating culturally and linguistically congruent care. Intersectionality addresses multiple identities and how they affect a person's experience (Bi et al., 2020). Those of multiple minoritized statuses may be confronted with an intersecting system of oppression, perpetuating discrimination based on race, sex, sexual orientation, and gender identity. Healthcare professionals must use intersectional lenses to view individuals and plan care for positive healthcare outcomes. Person-centered care is of utmost importance in every patient interaction. Self-reflection, recognizing one's biases, and genuine empathy for everyone are essential. It is important to recognize the complexity of individuals and their histories as central to person-centered care (Broom et al., 2020).

Why Do Diversity and Understanding Cultural Context Matter?

The integrated patterns of behavior among individuals who identify with specific social groups have been described as *culture* (Office of Minority Health [OMH], US Department of Health and Human Services [USDHHS] (OMH, 2019) (Fig. 9.2). Culture represents the shared values, norms, and codes that collectively shape a group's beliefs, attitudes, and behavior. Considered lifeways, culture is learned, shared, and transmitted from generation to generation (Leininger, 1995) (Figs. 9.3–9.5). Culture determines how an individual might view and interact with others and how those interactions are shaped by each person's background, attitudes, values, and beliefs. The following story exemplifies how cultures, values, and beliefs differ; the story depicts how two gentlemen had different cultural practices:

Two gentlemen went to the cemetery to pay respect to their late wives. The first, an American, had a bouquet of roses; the second, a Nigerian, had a pot of soup. As they knelt side by side in front of their wives' graves, the American asked the Nigerian, "When do you expect your wife to eat the soup?" The Nigerian responded, "As soon as your wife begins to smell the roses."

This anecdote exemplifies two cultural values practiced by two men from two different cultures. Neither practice had any practical significance for the beneficiary. However, both practices have such profound cultural value that the practical irrelevance to the foreign eye is unimportant. The study of culture is a study of ideas and values. No one culture is more important than the another, just different (Airhihenbuwa, 2007, p. 3).

Understanding the cultural contexts of others is important to avoid ethnocentrism or the belief that one's way of life and view of the world is the "right" way. Healthcare providers are expected to provide services that are respective and responsive to diverse

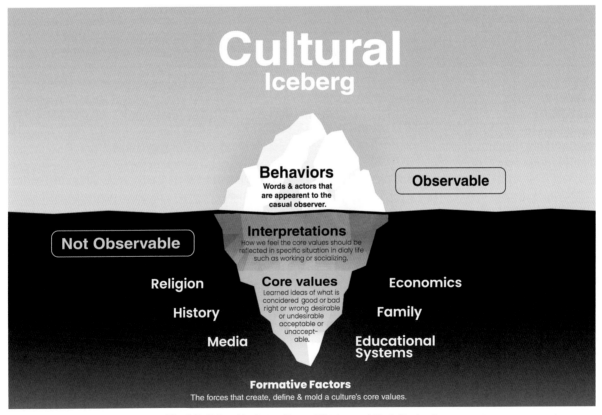

Fig. 9.2 Cultural iceberg. (From: iStock.com/WhaleDesign.)

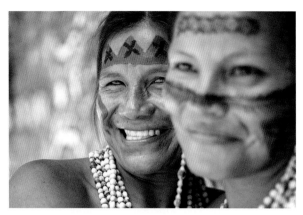

Fig. 9.3 Cultural practices among various cultures (indigenous tribe). (From: iStock.com/filipefrazao.)

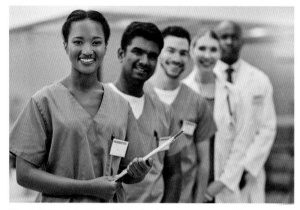

Fig. 9.6 Racially and ethnically diverse nurse workforce. (From iStock.com/MoyoStudio.)

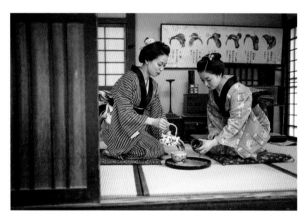

Fig. 9.4 Cultural practices among various cultures. Two Japanese women wearing a kimono are drinking tea indoors in the tea room. (From: iStock.com/AzmanL.)

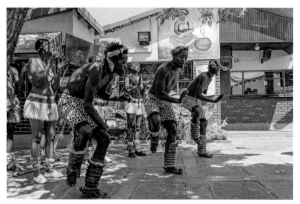

Fig. 9.5 Cultural practices among various cultures. African Zulu traditional dancing. (From: iStock.com/THEGIFT777.)

populations' health beliefs, practices, and needs (OMH, USDHHS, 2019). As the country continues to become more and more diverse, now more than ever, there is a pressing need to have a workforce that can deliver efficient, effective, high-quality care that is responsive to the diverse cultural and linguistic needs of patients (OMH, USDHHS, 2019) (Fig. 9.6).

Cultural and linguistic competencies allow nurses to become more aware of patients' varying perspectives and their own personal attitudes, beliefs, values, biases, and behaviors that can impact care (OMH, 2013). The American Nurses Association (ANA) developed a set of standards, *The Scope and Standards of Practice,* to guide nurses in all aspects of practice. One standard, Standard Eight, was specifically designed to ensure nurses were prepared to care for patients from diverse backgrounds in ways that are appropriate to the patient's cultural needs, and not merely through the Eurocentric lens of the nurse (ANA, 2015). The Standard states, "The registered nurse practices in a manner that is congruent with cultural diversity and inclusion principles" (ANA, 2015, p. 4). While cultural diversity describes a person's social identities, inclusion means the nurse embraces the differences intentionally and not just with acceptance or tolerance (AACN, 2017). The eighth standard sets forth a mandate for nurses to provide care consistent with the healthcare recipient's preferred values, beliefs, worldviews, and practices.

It is incumbent upon nursing education programs to prepare a nursing workforce that can provide healthcare services that are responsive to and consistent with the needs of any given population. Because students will engage with patients from various backgrounds and cultures, students must recognize the influence of culture on the individual's health, health-seeking behaviors, and healthcare practices. To provide culturally congruent care, students should have a general understanding of the person's culture. At one point, the prevailing wisdom was for the nurse to gather as much information as possible about the typical behaviors and beliefs of the patient's cultural group. For example, if the nurse were assigned to a patient from Nigeria, the nurse would gather as much information about the Nigerian culture as possible and use this information to guide nursing care. This would enable the nurse to provide culturally specific care, using the newly gained knowledge as a strategy to bridge cultural differences. Awareness of various cultures is appropriate, but one should be cautioned against believing that all members of a certain race, ethnicity, or cultural group behave in a certain way or espouse the same beliefs and practices. The assumption that all members of a specific group behave similarly and hold the same beliefs and practices can lead to stereotyping. A closely related concept to stereotyping is *essentialism*. Essentialism is when people believe other groups have natural, cultural characteristics or tendencies without variation (OMH, 2013). For example, the belief that all African Americans have rhythm or what is referred to as "soul" and can dance can be considered stereotypical. The assumptions made about a group's behavior are often based on limited information and interaction with the group. It is important to recognize how stereotypes influence one's behavior. Stereotypes are characterizations of groups of people belonging to specific social groups. The following examples are stereotypical beliefs and behaviors: (1) a person encounters a young Mexican male and automatically assumes he is an illegal immigrant; (2) a young African American male walks down the street toward a person and the person places a tighter grip on their purse; and (3) an obese person is eager to go to lunch and it is assumed the person eats excessively. These false beliefs are often based on limited encounters with groups, misinformation, or media descriptions. When a healthcare provider engages in behaviors based on stereotypes, the behavior can have untoward effects when rendering patient care. The case study that follows exemplifies how cultural norms, values, and the poor care received when a nurse generalized traits and assigned stereotypical beliefs to all members of a specific ethnic group:

An African American nurse was caring for a middle-aged Latina woman several hours after the patient had undergone surgery. A Latino physician on call approached the bedside and noted, the moaning patient. He commented to the nurse that the patient appeared to be in a great deal of post-operative pain. The nurse dismissed his perception, informing him that she took a course in nursing school on cross cultural care and "knew" that Hispanic patients over-expressed pain…The nurse's notion of her own expertise actually stereotyped the patient's experience and ignored cues of the patient's pain (Tervalon & Murray-Garcia, 1998, pp. 188–189).

Although cultural knowledge requires an understanding of the norms, values, and beliefs of a specific group, it is important to focus on the individual rather than assumptions about the group's typical behaviors. Focusing on the individual will allow the nurse to gain an understanding of the person's culture that is grounded in the individual's real-life experiences.

Cultural Dimensions

Cultural competence is defined as the capacity to respond respectfully and effectively to people of all cultures, languages, classes, races, ethnic backgrounds, religions, spiritual traditions, immigration status, and other factors in a manner that recognizes, affirms, values, and preserves their dignity (Danso, 2018). Individuals with intersecting identities often display attributes of more than one identity or culture. Thus, ascribed identities can be meaningful or meaningless since there are no fixed scripts and, most importantly, individuals determine the extent to which their identities influence their behavior. The use of the term *cultural competence* has been an issue of debate, since it is impossible to become competent or expert in knowing about the multitude of cultures and identities that exist in the population (Danso, 2018). Therefore, it is critical that cultural competence be viewed as a continuous process of learning, understanding, and engaging with others whose cultural backgrounds differ from one's own.

Cultural humility has been used as a replacement or complement to cultural competence (Fitzgerald & Campinha-Bacote, 2019). Cultural humility describes a person's ability to have an open attitude toward others in relation to aspects of their cultural identity (Tervalon & Murray-Garcia, 1998). A crucial component of cultural humility is self-awareness because it enables one to examine one's own cultural identity, biases, patterns of thought, and behaviors that might interfere with the ability to interact with others who are different. When a person displays culturally humble behavior, the individual displays the following characteristics:

1) Looks within self to examine his or her biases and stereotypes.
2) Opens up to learning more about the other person's culture, perspectives, beliefs, values, and worldview. The provider is in learning mode, attempting to understand rather than being an expert in another culture (Tervalon & Garcia, 1998).
3) Prioritizes the person's beliefs.
4) Acknowledges limitations and gaps in their cultural knowledge, freeing them to approach the person as a learner rather than an expert.

5) Commits to learning more, self-reflection, growing, and developing over time (OMH, 2013).

Promoting cultural humility is central to the ethical underpinning of the nursing profession (Hughes et al., 2020). A culturally humble person is willing to acknowledge their limitations, express curiosity, and ask questions when uncertain rather than make assumptions based on stereotypes. Cultural humility allows for mutual empowerment through openness, self-awareness, and self-reflection when interacting with individuals from different backgrounds (Foronda et al., 2016). Additionally, cultural humility addresses the healthcare provider/patient/population dynamic imbalances and is deigned to develop relationships and partnerships that are mutually beneficial to individuals, communities, and populations (Ellis et al., 2023).

Although many terms describe cultural interactions, the goal is to appreciate and respect the varying understandings and values that people from different cultures bring to bear in any situation or circumstance (Table 9.1). While some people prefer cultural humility

TABLE 9.1	Culture and Cultural Dimensions
Culture	• The integration of the thought patterns, communication, beliefs, values, and actions associated with a group. From: Office of Minority Health, US Department of Health and Human Services, 2013.
Cultural agility	• The capacity that enables one to operate capably in any environment and appreciate the varying understandings and values that people from different cultures bring to an issue or situation. From: Aoun, 2017.
Cultural competence	• The ability to respond respectfully and effectively to people from all cultures, languages, classes, races, ethnic backgrounds, religions, spiritual traditions, immigration status, and other factors in a manner that recognizes, affirms, values, and preserves their dignity. From: Danso, 2018.
Cultural congruence	• Culturally congruent practice describes nursing care that agrees with the preferred values, beliefs, worldviews, and practices of the healthcare recipient. From: American Nurses Association, 2015.
Cultural dimensions	• Race and ethnicity • Language and linguistic characteristics • Religion, faith, and spirituality • Biological traits and features • Geographical characteristics and boundaries • Sociological characteristics and traits From: Office of Minority Health, US Department of Health and Human Services, 2019a.
Cultural humility	• The lifelong process of self-reflection and self-critique whereby the individual not only learns about another's culture but starts with an examination of his/her own beliefs and cultural identities. From: Yeager & Baurer-Wu, 2013.
Cultural incongruence	• A lack of cultural similarities or understanding between two or more people. From: Ong-Flatherty, 2016.
Cultural sensitivity	• Having an appreciation for the inherent worth of different cultural groups, being aware of one's background, values, and beliefs, and how one's social conditioning influences the view of others. From: Danso, 2018. • Delivering care within the context of appropriate healthcare provider knowledge, understanding, and appreciation of cultural distinctions (Kibakaya, 2022).

over cultural competence, some believe those concepts are not either-or but both. Campinha-Bacote proposed a synergistic integration of cultural competence and cultural humility, creating the word *competemility* (Fitzgerald & Campinha-Bacote, 2019). Fernandez (2020) proposed using cultural humility along with culturally congruent care. Sagar (2014) viewed cultural competence as without an endpoint but rather as a lifelong journey and preferred to use culturally and linguistically congruent care along with cultural humility, empathy, and compassion in all interactions, collaborations, and partnerships with individuals, groups, and communities.

Along with self-critique and reflection, Tervalon and Murray (1998) noted the need to address power imbalances and partner with others who advocate for the poor and marginalized in society. Power is the ability to exert or leverage influence over another. Power can play out in the relationship between patients and providers and can often be viewed as an imbalance, with the healthcare provider having more power than the patient. These imbalances can often put patients in awkward positions such that the patient may not question how they are being treated, or even the treatment plan. Power differentials are thought to be magnified when the individuals involved are from different backgrounds. Small actions such as greeting the patient, calling the patient by name, and treating all patients with respect and dignity can help overcome any actual or perceived power imbalance. Patients should be viewed as equal partners in the provider–patient relationship. All patients have a right to expect excellent-quality care not compromised by the healthcare provider's implicit or explicit biases.

CULTURAL FRAMEWORKS

Leininger: Theory of Culture Care Diversity and Universality

Leininger (2002), widely regarded as the mother of transcultural nursing, defined culture as "learned and shared beliefs, values, and lifeways of a …particular group that are transmitted intergenerationally and influence one's thinking and action modes" (p. 9). Culture influences thinking and action; it impacts how health is perceived, what healers are used, when help is sought from healthcare professionals and preferences

for treatment. Leininger spent decades refining the Theory of Culture Care Diversity and Universality (CCDU) for use in nursing and related healthcare fields (Fig. 9.7). The CCDU fans into eight sun rays of factors that influence individuals, families, groups, organizations, and communities in health and illness: Cultural values, beliefs, and lifeways; biological, kinship and social; political and legal; religious, spiritual, and philosophical; economic, technological, and educational (Leininger, 2002). Situated between generic and folk care and professional care, integrative care practices could effectively bridge them; nursing can be most impactful in assessing, planning, implementing, and evaluating culturally and linguistically congruent care (Sagar, 2014). Leininger specified three modes of care decisions and actions: preservation and/or maintenance, accommodation and/or negotiation, and repatterning and/or restructuring (Leininger, 2002). Leininger's Sunrise Enabler model illustrates the need to approach cultural care with sensitivity and receptivity to various cultural beliefs, practices, and values. The model is consistent with a holistic approach to care, illustrating how healthcare goes beyond treatment and includes the cultural meanings attached to health, illness, and healing, and considering the social, spiritual, and emotional aspects of providing care. The model depicts how nurses should approach healthcare with a deep understanding of culture's role in health and healing.

Leininger envisioned a field of transcultural nursing that brings the study of culture and caring together globally (McFarland & Wehbe-Alamah, 2018). In her work in transcultural nursing and culturally congruent care, Leininger did not advocate for an endpoint of competence but viewed the process as lifelong learning. Leininger, as cited in Pacquiao (2008), advocated examining similarities and differences across cultures as fundamental to culturally congruent care (Pacquiao, 2008). Leininger was a visionary, and her CCDU was ahead of its time in considering factors impacting health and illness.

Pacquiao: Framework for Culturally Competent Health Care

Pacquiao (2018) advocated for a Framework for Culturally Competent Health Care linking cultural competence and ethics in promoting individual and population health

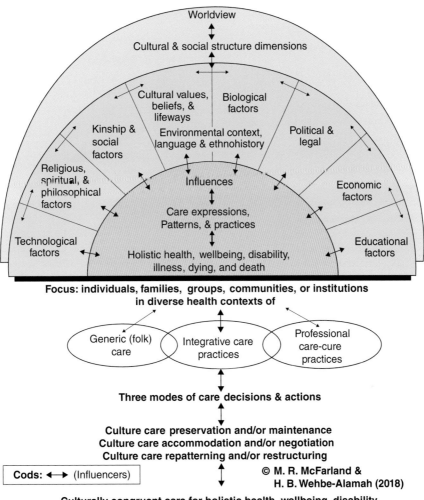

Fig. 9.7 Leininger Theory of Culture Care Diversity & Universality. (From: McFarland, M., & Wehbe-Alamah, H. (2018). *Transcultural nursing concepts, theories, research, & practice.* (4th ed., p. 47). McGraw-Hill Education. https://www.researchgate.net/figure/Leiningers-Sunrise-Enabler-to-Discover-Culture-Care-McFarland-and-Wehbe-Alamah-2018_fig2_358900167.)

(Fig. 9.8). At the top of the model is advocacy for social justice and the human rights of others who have been marginalized, deemed vulnerable or powerless, and reliant on others to address their needs. Advocacy for social justice and human rights must be informed by the cultural context of people and their situated environments, and culturally appropriate care happens when healthcare providers are committed to both principles (Pacquiao, 2008). Compassion is at the base of the model. Compassion compels one to act on behalf of others and distinguishes the disadvantaged from the powerful. Compassion arises from an empathetic identification with others and a commitment to promote their health and healing (Pacquiao, 2008). Pacquiao further describes compassion as the commitment

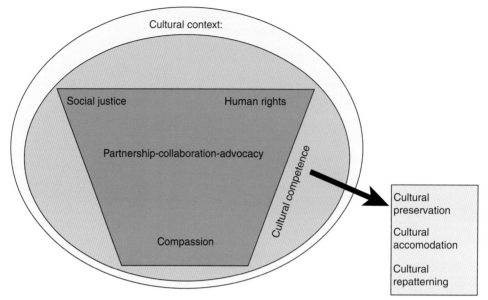

Fig. 9.8 Pacquiano Framework for Culturally Competent Care. (From: Pacquiao, D. F. (2008). Nursing care for vulnerable populations using a framework of cultural competence, social justice and human rights. *Contemporary Nurse, 28*(1–2), 189–197.)

to move beyond one's perspective. This compassion ignites healthcare providers to act on behalf of others to promote health equity. Pacquiao (2008) uses cultural competence analogous to culturally appropriate care, as one can never be competent in a culture that is not their own.

Modes of action for culturally appropriate care are embedded in cultural preservation, accommodation, and repatterning. Preservation allows for maintaining core values, beliefs, and practices significant to the cultural group. Accommodation allows cultural groups to negotiate differences and find meaningful existence in cultural lifeways with others. Repatterning helps individuals and groups change ways of life to achieve health and well-being in a way that is meaningful to them (Pacquiao, 2008). When a person's cultural preference goes against the prevailing standard of care, the nurse should include the patient's preference to the extent possible. However, accommodating patient preferences should never violate the standard of care. The nurse should seek to understand the underlying reasons behind the specific patient preferences and see if those reasons can be addressed with other options. For example, a Hmong family wanted to take their placenta home after birth due to the belief that one's soul may not rest in peace unless it is united with their afterbirth in death (Pacquiao, 2008). Due to infection control concerns, accommodation

occurred when the public health nurses taught the family how to dispose of the placenta in the home environment according to public health guidelines (Pacquiao, 2008). Repatterning occurred when the family adjusted their practices to meet public health concerns but maintained their tradition (Pacquaio, 2008).

The framework aims for social justice and the protection of human rights through culturally competent collaboration, partnerships, and advocacy for vulnerable populations. Additionally, Pacquaio's framework is designed to attain health equity—especially for vulnerable groups who tend to be most afflicted by SDOH resulting in disparities. Health promotion should be grounded in appreciating the social pathways to poor health as consequences of people's living and working conditions (Pacquaio, 2018). Preserving human rights and administering justice to those needing it the most is central to health and health equity.

Choi: Theory of Cultural Marginality

The Theory of Cultural Marginality (TCM) was developed to guide the plan for culturally relevant care for immigrants straddling two cultures (Choi, 2023). Choi was optimistic that the TCM would contribute to the culturally congruent care of immigrants. While the TCM was conceived for the care of immigrants, the theory may apply to caring for individuals with backgrounds such as being indigenous and those of two or more races.

Three concepts contribute to the development of the TCM: acculturation, acculturative stress, and marginality (Choi, 2013, 2023). Acculturation is a multidimensional process—whether the individual gives up one's culture or maintains different cultural identities—of learning and integrating the values, beliefs, language, and customs of a new country. Acculturation is a broad concept and was earlier defined as when groups of individuals from a different culture interact with another cultural group and subsequently change their original cultural pattern (Choi, 2001). Additionally, individuals can be selective across cultural domains and maintain two cultural identities simultaneously (Choi, 2001). More recently, the term has come to mean a process of cultural exchange by which a person modifies their attributes, beliefs, cultural norms, values, or behaviors due to interaction with a different culture than one's own (Choi, 2001). *Acculturation* is an umbrella term that embodies two concepts: acculturative stress and cultural marginality.

Acculturative stress is considered a byproduct of acculturation. It is associated with the personal exposure of individuals to social situations and environments that challenge them to adjust, either in their behavior or their concept of themselves (Choi, 2001). Acculturative stress highlights the connection between acculturation and mental health consequences (Choi, 2023). Acculturative stress has been associated with mental health issues in acculturating adolescents.

Marginality theory originated with Park (1928), as cited in Choi (2013), and describes an individual experiencing a divided, restless self, alternating between old and new selves and between two cultures. Hall and colleagues (1994), as cited in Choi (2013), referred to marginality as the peripheral existence from mainstream society because of racial, gender, political, and economic oppression. Choi (2001) viewed the concept of marginality from a cultural-societal perspective and saw marginality as a transition from one cultural society to another or "situations and feelings of passive betweenness when people exist between two different cultures and do not perceive themselves as centrally belonging to either one" (p. 198).

Cultural marginality occurs when individuals have continuous contact with distinct cultures, engaging with both cultures with distinct value systems and accompanying expectations, yet are forced to make difficult choices (Choi, 2001). For example, a 15-year-old Korean adolescent had to choose between attending a party with new American friends or helping her mom prepare food for the Chinese New Year celebration. The events were on the same day. The adolescent understood both how meaningful it was to meet new friends and her family's cultural customs and traditions (Choi, 2001).

Fig. 9.9 highlights the components of cultural marginality. According to Choi (2023), cross-cultural recognition is when the individual begins to understand differences between two contradicting cultural values, customs, behaviors, and norms in the culture of origin and the new culture. To ease the cultural tension, the individual employs one of four adjustment responses that are not mutually exclusive: Assimilation, reconstructed return, poise, and integration. In assimilation, the person is absorbed into the new culture. However, the person may return to his former culture (reconstructed return) or maintain a tentative fit between the two (poise) (Choi, 2023). Integration is when the individual merges the former and new culture, gaining access to multiple cultural worlds (Choi, 2023). Contextual factors include the individual's and receiving culture's tolerance for diversity and available resources and supports.

Campinha-Bacote: Cultural Competemility

Evolving from a cultural humility workgroup, Ansari (2017) developed the five Rs model for learning cultural competemility: reflection, respect, regard, relevance, and resiliency. This model focuses on individual and organizational bias to enable open-mindedness. Cultural humility puts the healthcare professional on a level playing field with no authority figure (Ansari, 2017). Cultural competemility, a concept coined by Campinha-Bacote (2020), is defined as a process, whereas the five components or constructs of cultural competence (awareness, knowledge, skill, desire, and encounters) are coupled with all aspects of cultural humility. This synergistic combination of competence with humility demands that healthcare providers become competent while humble, noting that competence has no endpoint.

Delving into the five constructs and their integration with cultural humility will provide a better understanding of cultural competemility. Awareness involves introspection, the self-reflection of one's biases, prejudices, and beliefs, and knowledge about the historical injustices often suffered by specific cultural groups. (Campinha-Bacote, 2020; Downey, 2021). This also

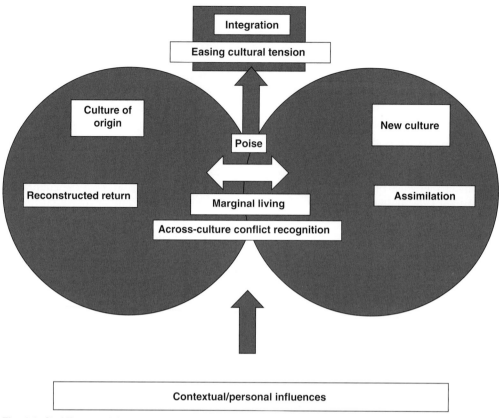

Fig. 9.9 Choi Theory of Cultural Marginality. (From: Choi, H. (2013). Theory of cultural marginality. In M. J. Smith & P. Liehr, (Eds.), *Middle range theory for nursing* (3rd ed., pp. 289–307). Springer Publishing Company.)

includes understanding traumatic experiences faced because of one or more of their social identities. Knowledge is understanding a specific cultural group relative to their healthcare rituals, beliefs, traditions, and values, including the incidence and prevalence of diseases in the cultural group, along with the customary treatment plan and its efficacy (Campinha-Bacote, 2020; Downey, 2021). Skill concerns the nurse's ability to collect relevant assessment data (Campinha-Bacote, 2020; Downey, 2021). Cultural encounters involve direct interactions with individuals from different backgrounds and considering their beliefs about the specific culture to counteract possible stereotyping (Fitzgerald & Campinha-Bacote, 2019). Cultural desire is the healthcare provider's willingness to become more culturally aware, knowledgeable, and skillful (Campinha-Bacote, 2020; Downey, 2021; Fitzgerald & Campinha-Bacote, 2019). All five components require engaging with individuals or communities in a culturally humble way (Fitzgerald & Campinha-Bacote, 2019).

As cited in Fitzgerald and Campinha-Bacote (2019), Chang and colleagues (2012) and Hook and coworkers (2013) suggest that healthcare providers continually consider how they would like to be treated if they were in the person's place and what may make their exchanges with the person more respectful. Just as becoming culturally humble is a lifelong process, so is cultural competemility, and both are integrated with social justice concepts.

THE CORONAVIRUS DISEASE 2019 PANDEMIC EXPOSED STARK REALITIES OF HEALTH INEQUITIES AMONG VARIOUS CULTURAL AND ETHNIC GROUPS

Coronavirus disease 2019 (COVID-19) was one of the largest and longest-lasting pandemics in the history of the world (Lin et al., 2022). According to Solar (2023), the WHO estimates 50.4 million COVID-19 cases were confirmed globally, with 6.3 million deaths. However, these figures may be underreported due to a lack of testing and a dearth of accurate system reporting of mortality data and cause of death. COVID-19 amplified and laid bare the inequities resulting in higher morbidity and mortality rates among communities of color. The disproportionate toll on minoritized populations emphasized the importance of examining health inequities (Solar et al., 2023).

In the United States, disasters and public health emergencies tend to affect disadvantaged racial and ethnic communities disproportionately (Golden et al., 2021). There were inequitable COVID-19 rates related to access to treatment, infection, and increased morbidity and mortality among vulnerable and marginalized populations (Solar et al., 2023). COVID-19 infection and death rates were distinctively associated with overcrowded areas, greater body mass index, and low incomes—characteristics prevalent in Hispanic and Black communities (Lin et al., 2022). This is consistent with the findings of Lundberg and colleagues (2023) that as COVID-19 initially overcame public health systems, the major effects were on American Indians, Alaskan Natives, Blacks, Hispanics, and Pacific Islander populations.

Rural communities also faced chronic disparities in healthcare related to COVID-19. Rural Americans had a mortality rate twice as high as those living in urban areas (Grome et al., 2022). Using provisional data from the National Center for Health Statistics, Lundberg and colleagues (2023) posited that the substantial COVID-19 mortality impact observed in rural areas—especially for Black, Hispanic, and American Indians and Alaska natives—could suggest that rural health systems lacked preparedness to respond to the pandemic; public health measures including lockdowns and required masking had fewer effects in these communities; and lower vaccination rates were observed among these racial and ethnic groups.

One underlying reason for the disproportionate representation of COVID-19 morbidity and mortality rates among communities of color and rural communities is that these communities often lack regular healthcare access, leading to delayed diagnosis and treatment. Additionally, these communities bear a high chronic disease burden; live in segregated and overcrowded housing, which increases the risk of transmission; and are less able to maintain social distancing measures. Low-wage earners often have frontline jobs as essential workers. Essential workers were at risk since these jobs could not be done from home during the national shutdown. Lastly, vaccine access and hesitancy among minoritized communities influenced the impact of COVID-19 on these communities. Vaccine hesitancy was due to the long-standing historical mistrust of and mistreatment by the healthcare systems among minoritized populations, lack of confidence in the vaccine development process, misinformation and issues around culturally accessible information, skepticism about effectiveness, and structural barriers to vaccine access (Shearn & Krockow, 2023).

CULTURALLY AND LINGUISTICALLY APPROPRIATE SERVICES

In 2000, the OMH (2013), USDHHS developed culturally and linguistically appropriate services (CLAS), drawing on three primary sources: public comments, a National Project Advisory Committee, and a systematic literature review. CLAS "refers to services that are respectful and responsive to individual cultural health beliefs, practices, preferred languages, health literacy levels, and communication needs" (paragraph 1). The CLAS was designed to be effective in various settings: ambulatory care centers (e.g., federally qualified health centers, hospitals, behavioral health settings, and public health agencies (Davis et al., 2018). Initially, the standards were designated as guidelines, and only language access services were mandatory (OMH, 2013). The 15 enhanced CLAS standards are equally important in advancing health equity, improving quality, and eliminating health disparities (OMH, 2013, 2021) (Box 9.1). Healthcare organizations must ensure that healthcare providers with language proficiency or interpreters are available.

A study conducted by Terlizzi and colleagues (2019) conveyed that patients are more likely to trust, adhere to therapeutic regimens, and be more satisfied with care from providers who share the same race, ethnicity, and language or have similar values and beliefs. Racial and ethnic minorities verbalized more satisfaction with providers sharing or understanding their culture but admitted they see few of these types of providers (Terlizzi et al., 2019). Unfortunately, individuals from minoritized racial and ethnic groups continue to face systemic barriers that impede their ability to access, persist, and thrive in science, technology, engineering, and math higher education and the workforce (National Academies of Sciences, Engineering, & Medicine [NASEM], 2023).

BOX 9.1   National CLAS Standards

The National CLAS Standards are Intended to Advance Health Equity, Improve Quality, and Help Eliminate Healthcare Disparities by Establishing a Blueprint for Health and Healthcare Organizations to:

Principal Standard

1. Provide effective, equitable, understandable, and respectful quality care and services that are responsive to diverse cultural health beliefs and practices, preferred languages, health literacy, and other communication needs.

Governance, Leadership and Workforce

2. Advance and sustain organizational governance and leadership that promotes CLAS and health equity through policy, practices, and allocated resources.
3. Recruit, promote, and support culturally and linguistically diverse governance, leadership, and workforce that are responsive to the population in the service area.
4. Educate and train governance, leadership, and workforce in culturally and linguistically appropriate policies and practices on an ongoing basis.

Communication and Language Assistance

5. Offer language assistance to individuals who have limited English proficiency and/or other communication needs, at no cost to facilitate timely access to all healthcare and services.
6. Inform all individuals of the availability of language assistance services clearly and in their preferred language, verbally and in writing.
7. Ensure the competence of individuals providing language assistance, recognizing that the use of untrained individuals and/or minors as interpreters should be avoided.
8. Provide easy-to-understand print and multimedia materials and signage in the languages commonly used by the populations in the service area.

Engagement, Continuous Improvement, and Accountability

9. Establish culturally and linguistically appropriate goals, policies, and management accountability, and infuse them throughout the organization's planning and operations.
10. Conduct ongoing assessments of the organization's CLAS-related activities and integrate CLAS-related measures into measurement and continuous quality improvement activities.
11. Collect and maintain accurate and reliable demographic data to monitor and evaluate the impact of CLAS on health equity and outcomes and to inform service delivery.
12. Conduct regular assessments of community health assets and needs and use the results to plan and implement services that respond to the cultural and linguistic diversity of populations in the service area.
13. Partner with the community to design, implement, and evaluate policies, practices, and services to ensure cultural and linguistic appropriateness.
14. Create conflict and grievance resolution processes that are culturally and linguistically appropriate to identify, prevent, and resolve conflicts or complaints.
15. Communicate the organization's progress in implementing and sustaining CLAS to all stakeholders, constituents, and the general public.

Office of Minority Health. (2021). Think cultural health: The national CLAS standards. https://thinkculturalhealth.hhs.gov/clas/standards.

Cultures clashed—between healthcare providers at a small county hospital in California and a Laotian refugee family—in the care of Lia Lee, their daughter with severe epilepsy, resulting in a tragedy. This was eloquently narrated in the widely acclaimed and disturbing book *The Spirit Catches You and You Fall Down* (Fadiman, 2012). Both sides aimed for what was best for Lia but did not understand each other's culture. Fadiman, a gifted storyteller, evoked compassion, reflection, and empathy. This tragic story is a prime example of how CLAS standards could eliminate health inequities and disparities (Box 9.1).

For more than two decades, two landmark publications, *Crossing the Quality Chasm* (Institute of Medicine [IOM], 2001) and *Unequal Treatment: Confronting Racial and Ethnic Disparities in Health Care* (IOM, 2003), have called for the provision of culturally sensitive care to reduce racial and ethnic healthcare disparities. Nevertheless, decades later, disparities prevail, primarily due to a lack of focus on structural inequities and race-related biases (Bailey et al., 2021). Among the reasons for disparate outcomes is clinicians' implicit or explicit bias toward marginalized patients. Narayan (2019) identified four major effects of clinician bias, incomplete or inadequate patient assessments, misdiagnosis, and inappropriate treatment decisions based on viewing race as a causative factor of disease despite the 2003 Genome Project revealing that racial categories were inconsistent with biological explanations of disease (Bailey et al., 2021; Duello et al., 2021), spending less time with patients with different backgrounds and discharging patients without the requisite follow-up. It is well documented that racism is a major public health concern and a factor in the morbidity and mortality of people of color (American Public Health Association, 2023; Centers for Disease Control, 2023). Structural racism, provider biases, and mistrust in healthcare organizations due to historical and contemporary mistreatment have contributed to the genesis and perpetuation of health disparities.

BIAS

All people are exposed to a social conditioning process that imbues them with prejudices, stereotypes, and beliefs that lie outside their awareness (Sue & Sue, 2016) (Fig. 9.10). Biases operate primarily in the subconscious and can influence how others are seen and treated, even when a person believes they are fair and objective (White & Stubblefield-Tave, 2017). Healthcare providers have been found to harbor stereotypes and biases (favorable and unfavorable) toward patients and even colleagues whose backgrounds are similar or different from their own (White & Stubblefield-Tave, 2017). Biases can be microaggressions, prejudices, and "isms." Implicit biases are the attitudes or stereotypes that affect our understanding, actions, and decisions in an unconscious manner (Staats, 2016). When nurses and other healthcare professionals harbor implicit biases, they contribute to the disparities commonly seen in minoritized groups (Narayan, 2019). The fact that healthcare providers hold implicit biases contributing to healthcare disparities is difficult for many people to understand. However, these automatic biases can influence the healthcare provider's actions and decisions. During stressful situations, as when working in a busy healthcare environment, there is a tendency to default to implicit biases because there is less time and energy to work through situations to determine whether the initial impression of a person is correct (Narayan, 2019). Unfortunately, implicit bias impacts the equitable delivery of evidence-based interventions and, ultimately, patient outcomes, leading to healthcare disparities. Thirsk and colleagues (2022) concluded in their scoping review that, given the serious impact of bias on nurses' clinical judgment and, thereby, patient outcomes, there is a need to identify and test debiasing strategies in the nursing profession. Examples of debriefing strategies include learning about other cultural norms and practices, having simulated practice experiences followed by debriefing, increasing interactions with different cultural groups, listening to lived experiences, and perspective-taking. These strategies could help realize the first principle of the ANA *Code of Ethics,* where nurses are charged to practice with compassion and respect and value the inherent dignity, worth, and unique attributes of all persons (ANA, 2015).

One way to become more aware of one's beliefs and attitudes is to take the free implicit association (bias) test, which can be found at https://implicit.harvard.edu/implicit/ (Harvard University, n.d.) These types of assessment tools and tests can help one learn about his or her assumptions, biases, and stereotypes. However, the validity of the Implicit Association Test and its use as a metric to determine bias has been called into question (Oswald et al., 2013; Sukhera et al., 2020). To counteract unconscious bias, self-awareness, introspection, authenticity, humility, and a willingness to change are critical (White & Stubblefield-Tave, 2017). Narayan (2019) identified strategies for managing implicit bias and ways to self-regulate against implicit bias (Table 9.2).

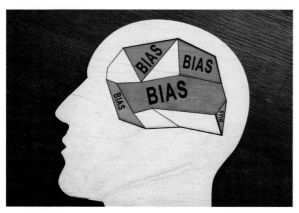

Fig. 9.10 Bias. (From: iStock.com/designer491.)

TABLE 9.2   Strategies for Self-Regulation Against Implicit Biases

Strategies	
Counter imaging	A conscious choice to identify members of the same social group who do not represent the stereotypical image of the group, replacing the person with the image of the nonrepresentative person.
Emotional regulation	The ability to identify the "feelings" associated with the stereotypical person, such as anxiety, fear of the unknown, distrust, or dislike, and making a conscious effort to practice empathy and compassion toward the person.
Habit replacement	The attempt to replace negative thoughts and actions toward a person of a specific group with positive thoughts.
Increased frequency of contact	Attempts to increase contact with members of a certain group may counter the stereotypical beliefs held about that group.
Individuation	The ability to see the person as an individual and not a member of a marginalized or stereotypical group.
Mindfulness	Initiation of mindfulness techniques such as deep breathing, calm thoughts, introspection, and calm feelings toward a person to help elicit compassion and empathy. Mindfulness can prevent the triggering of automatic stereotypical reactions.
Copartnering with the patient	The ability to establish a therapeutic collaborative relationship with the person.
Perspective-taking	The ability to examine the situation from the patient's point of view.
Stereotype replacement	The ability to reflect on negative thoughts regarding a person belonging to a specific social group and attempt to replace these thoughts with compassion and empathy (similar to counter imaging).

Adapted from Narayan, M. C. (2019). CE: Addressing implicit bias in nursing: A review. *The American Journal of Nursing, 119*(7), 36–43. https://doi.org/10.1097/01.NAJ.0000569340.27659.5a.

Implicit biases can also shape the healthcare provider's behavior when working with members of the LGBTQ+ community. These biases can be in the form of prejudices, stereotypes, or discrimination (differential treatment). Healthcare provider's implicit or explicit biases can lead to lower-quality healthcare and poor health outcomes. According to Reich and colleagues (2022), more than 50% of adult gender and sexual minorities (GSMs) experience some form of discrimination in healthcare, and for those who identify as transgender or gender nonconforming, the percentage increases to 70%. A direct correlation between healthcare provider discrimination and bias and the perpetuation of health disparities in the LBGTQ+ community exists, specifically causing individuals in the community to either delay care or not seek care at all. GSMs have a high risk for chronic health conditions due to delaying care for fear of bias and discrimination in disclosing gender identity and sexual orientation, further adding to the burden of health disparities.

Moreover, Reich and colleagues (2022) and Bell (2019) identified the need for nurses to have additional education and training related to this population. Oftentimes, the heteronormative perspective restricts sexual and gender categories from being recognized, and the

fear of bias prohibits members of the LGBTQ+ community from coming forward with their identity. To promote inclusivity, nurses should render nonjudgmental care using one of the cultural care frameworks identified in this chapter and the bias-mitigating strategies found in Table 9.2. It is important to recognize that disparities result from structural inequities and clinician bias in the treatment and management of various cultural groups.

Microaggressions are the subtle everyday slights, insults, disregard, dismissals, ignoring, and other indignities often directed at people who are from marginalized groups (Sue & Spanierman, 2020). Microaggressions are mainly covert but can be overt. Overt behaviors are generally manifested in "isms" and can take the form of prejudice or discrimination. Unfortunately, microaggressions often go unacknowledged because the slights create discomfort for the recipient, the bystander who witnessed the event, and often the offender if pointed out (Sue & Spanierman, 2020). Thus, conversations about these tension-filled interactions are usually avoided and, because of this avoidance, the behavior continues unchecked. Acts of microaggression can have harmful psychological consequences for the recipient, and the cumulative effects of repeated offenses can be devastating (Sue & Spanierman, 2020).

Bias in Clinical Decision-Making

Highly publicized is the fact that racial and ethnic cultural groups suffer bias at the hands of clinicians. Black women with the highest level of education, income, and social status have far worse health outcomes than White women in impoverished states (Agrawal & Enekwechi, 2020). Additionally, as a cultural group, women were found to have less accurate diagnoses, presented with fewer treatment options, and received less effective pain management than men (Agrawal & Enekwechi, 2020). To remedy bias in the healthcare workforce, all healthcare practitioners should receive bias education to learn skills and techniques to mitigate bias prior to interacting with cultural groups.

Assessment algorithms that embed racial corrections in clinical decision-making are equally relevant to clinician bias. Race is a social rather than biological construct. These race-based algorithms have come under increased scrutiny because of the harm inflicted on certain cultural and racial/ethnic groups. For example, Fawzy and colleagues (2022) found that underperformance of the pulse oximeters in dark-skinned individuals led to false norms in oxygen saturation, causing delayed COVID-19 treatments. Williams and colleagues (2021) called for reconsidering race in calculating glomerular filtration rates (eGFR) because it inflates the eGFR, which could lead to unnecessary delays in treatment for kidney disease, including transplants. The US FRAX calculator, a test used to measure the risk of osteoporosis in women, returns a much lower fracture risk for Black than Asian or Hispanic women, which could cause delays in providing therapeutic treatment for osteoporosis (Kanis et al., 2020). Additionally, there is a call to end race correction in pulmonary spirometry, citing the lack of empiric evidence and the failure to consider contextual assessment parameters such as previous smoking history, childhood respiratory diseases, obesity, exposure to environmental pollutants, and socioeconomic status as factors that contribute to lung function (Bonner & Wakeam, 2022). Race-based adjusted algorithms guide clinical decisions in ways that potentially direct more resources to White patients than to members of racial and ethnic cultural groups (Vyas et al., 2020). Structural inequities inherent in clinical decision-making tools founded on race have the potential to perpetuate health disparities in minoritized patients.

UPSTREAM AND DOWNSTREAM THINKING

The widely told River Story in public health has been attributed to various authors, especially Irving Zola (McKinlay, 2019). In the telling, the story—as most stories go—became modified and evolved. Essentially, a person downstream exhaustively saves drowning victims from the dangerous river. In this version, a woman kept diving into the raging waters to save drowning children one at a time, performing cardiopulmonary resuscitation on each child as needed. In the brief lull after saving the last one, a man came to help her. After thanking the man, the woman bravely proceeded upstream to find out who was throwing the children into the river.

The analogy between this story and the present US healthcare system is powerful. Most of its resources are concentrated in downstream, short-term efforts to treat illnesses (McKinlay, 2019; NASEM, 2019). Upstream thinking analyzes the core of the problem and looks at conditions affecting physical, mental, and emotional well-being, such as safe housing, nutritious foods, and reliable transportation. Improvement in health metrics presumably depends on attention to the SDOH, incentivizing prevention and improved outcomes versus delivery of care alone (Connolly et al., 2021; NASEM, 2019). Tasked by the "Future of Nursing 2020–2030" report on health equity initiatives, nurses must integrate SDOH and structural determinants of healthcare into nursing education, practice, leadership, and policymaking (NASEM, 2021).

Upstream efforts deal with root causes, such as actively participating in policymaking. Ackerman-Barger (2022) coined the term "equity-minded nurses" as those nurses possessing knowledge, skills, and a desire to advance health equity. These nurses are poised strategically to influence policymaking in practice, research, education, and local, regional, national, and international arenas. Nurses have unique expertise to lead the nation in policy agenda concerning upstream SDOH (Sharpnack, 2022). How prepared are nurses to advocate and influence policy for health equity? In their study, Thomas and colleagues (2019) found that nursing students possess values and beginning experiences necessary for competency and engagement in health policy. They provided useful suggestions for faculty to foster understanding, engagement, and leading policy efforts by providing opportunities aligned with the AACN's *Essential Core Competencies for Professional Nursing Education* (AACN, 2021). Most nursing curricula do not provide classroom and clinical experiences in policymaking (Sagar,

2023). Sharpnack (2022) recommended four strategies to impact policy: (a) prioritize nurse well-being, (b) encourage membership in community boards, (c) increase the diversity of the nursing workforce, and (d) expand academic-practice partnerships.

Involving students in marginalized, underserved communities exposes them to SDOH and the process of multisectoral collaborations (Pacquaio et al., 2023). To promote health, the Ottawa Charter (1986), as cited in Pacquaio and Douglas (2019), highlighted three major strategies: (a) advocacy for resources that are advantageous to health; (b) empowerment of persons and groups, thus controlling their social determinants and attaining their utmost quality of life; and (c) mediation using governmental, organizational, and community multisectoral and multilevel collaborations. Engaging students in these activities at different stages of their education promotes the capacity for advocacy and empowerment. Affording students the opportunity to attend policy meetings affecting the community increases awareness and skill in navigating the process (Pacquaio, 2019).

Other collaborative examples include a university in an underserved community partnering with the local health department to increase vaccination rates by bringing vaccines where people live, work, and interact with other community members (Nickitas et al., 2022). Neighborhood clinics and mobile healthcare vans are effective. When vulnerable populations lack the means to access services—perhaps due to a lack of belongingness, communication, knowledge, or transportation—services should be delivered to them (Sagar, 2014).

CONCLUSION

Culture has been defined in many ways but generally refers to the shared values, norms, and codes that collectively shape a group's beliefs, attitudes, and behavior through interaction in and with their environment. The first step in delivering culturally appropriate care is to become self-aware and assess your behaviors, beliefs, and biases. When caring for patients from different backgrounds, the expected outcome is to provide nursing care that agrees with the healthcare recipient's preferred values, beliefs, worldviews, and practices. Before becoming nurses, students must learn to function within multicultural groups as the United States becomes more diverse (Aoun, 2017).

This chapter provided an analysis of culture and its relation to health equity. Culturally and linguistically congruent care and the attitude of humility are essential in working with multicultural, marginalized, and disadvantaged populations. There are over 4 million nurses in the United States and they comprise the largest group of healthcare professionals. Gallup polls have shown nursing to be the most trusted and ethical profession for 21 years, from 2002 to 2023 (Brenan, 2023) and in 1999 and 2000. In 2001, firefighters received this honor for their heroism during the September 11th attacks on the United States. With public trust, nurses are at such a vantage point to lead health equity initiatives (Sagar, 2023; Sagar et al., 2014). Working collaboratively, nurses have tremendous power in reforming the nation's healthcare system. They are strategically positioned to influence policy by engaging in the policy process, including interpretation, evaluation, and leading policy change in work settings, boardrooms, and at local, state, and federal levels (AACN, 2021; Sagar, 2023; Sharpnack, 2022).

With their unique strength in numbers and public trust, nurses can play a pivotal role in planning, implementing, and evaluating health equity strategies. Much is needed in nursing education, practice, leadership, research, and policymaking to enable nurses to contribute to health equity in their practice settings. The focus of care must shift from downstream and midstream thinking to upstream problem-solving. Nurses must impact the underlying cause of health outcomes deeply entrenched in political, educational, cultural, and other structures. Nurses must lead and work with interprofessional teams in multilevel collaborations with government, nongovernment organizations, and community agencies in partnering with communities.

The ANA *Code of Ethics* (2015) affirms respect for the dignity and rights of all human beings in accordance with the United Nations, the International Council of Nurses (ICN), and other treaties on human rights. The ANA embraces health as a universal human right and calls upon nurses to collaborate with other professionals to advance health, reduce disparities, and integrate social justice principles into nursing and health policy. Nursing leadership is vital in altering systemic structures that negatively influence the health of individuals and communities (ANA, 2015). Additionally, practice guidelines that are evidence based can limit the untoward effects of clinician bias by leaving little room for subjectivity in the interpretation of findings. Moreover, all patients, regardless of race and ethnicity, are entitled to receive patient-centered healthcare services that reflect their cultural distinctions and differences.

STUDENT REFLECTION QUESTIONS

1. You are trying to differentiate upstream, midstream, and downstream factors when caring for individuals and populations. Can you identify examples from this chapter's Upstream and Downstream Thinking section?

2. Your clinical instructor accompanies your group to the State Capitol for Lobby Day. Before meeting with a legislator, you are preparing for a group discussion on maternal-child health. Explain why this is an upstream-thinking, problem-solving activity.

CASE STUDY WITH QUESTIONS

A Vietnamese American recently gave birth to a baby girl who is now 6 weeks old. When she returned to the clinic for her follow-up visit, she appeared quiet and withdrawn and shared with the nurse that she had been "feeling down." The first nurse suspected the patient could be experiencing postpartum depression. The initial nurse who greeted the patient decided to consult with another nurse. When conferring with her colleague about the case, the second nurse stated, "All Asian women are quiet and submissive; it is their culture. She is probably cheerier at home, although she may feel ashamed that she has not lost much weight since delivery. Asian women are usually thin, so the weight could be the problem."

1. Was the second nurse's comment about the patient stereotypical? Why or why not?
2. Do you perceive bias in this situation? Why or why not?
3. What would have been a better approach to elicit more conversation from the patient?

REFERENCES

Ackerman-Barger, K. (2022). *Advancing health-equity: The rise of equity minded nurses.* Campaign for action. https://campaignforaction.org/the-rise-of-equity-minded-nurses/.

Agrawal, S., & Enekwechi, A. (2020). It's time to address the role of implicit bias within health care delivery. *Health Affairs Blog.* doi:10.1377/hblog2020108.34515.

Airhihenbuwa, C. (2007). *Healing our differences: The crisis of global health and the politics of identity.* Rowman & Littlefield Publishers, Inc.

American Association of Colleges of Nursing (AACN). (2017). *AACN Position Statement on Diversity, Inclusion, & Equity in Academic Nursing.* https://www.aacnnursing.org/Portals/42/Diversity/AACN-Position-Statement-Diversity-Inclusion.pdf.

American Association of Colleges of Nursing (AACN). (2021). *The essentials: Core competencies for professional nursing education.* American Association of Colleges of Nursing.

American Nurses Association (ANA). (2015). *ANA Scope & Standards of Practice* (3rd ed.). American Nurses Association.

American Public Health Association. (2023). Racism is a public health crisis. https://apha.org/Topics-and-Issues/Racial-Equity/Racism-Declarations.

Ansari, A. (2017). Battling biases with the 5Rs of cultural humility. *The Hospitalist.* https://www.the-hospitalist. org/hospitalist/article/136529/leadership-training/battling-biases-5-rs-cultural-humility.

Aoun, J. (2017). *Robot-proof: Higher education in the age of artificial intelligence.* The MIT Press.

Bailey, Z. D., Feldman, J. M., & Bassett, M. T. (2021). How structural racism works—Racist policies as a root cause of U.S. racial health inequities. *The New England Journal of Medicine, 384*(8), 768–773. https://doi.org/10.1056/NEJMms2025396.

Bell, K. (2019). Part of the solution to address sexual and gender minority health and health care disparities: Inclusive professional education. *Delaware Journal of Public Health, 5*(3), 56–62. https://doi.org/10.32481/djph.2019.06.010.

Bi, S., Vela, M. B., Nathan, A. G., Gunter, K. E., Cook, S. C., López, F. Y., Nocon, R. S., & Chin, M. H. (2020). Teaching intersectionality of sexual orientation, gender identity, and race/ethnicity in a health disparities course. *MedEdPORTAL: The Journal of Teaching and Learning Resources, 16,* 10970. https://doi.org/10.15766/mep_2374-8265.10970.

Bonner, S. N., & Wakeam, E. (2022). the end of race correction in spirometry for pulmonary function testing and surgical implications. *Annals of Surgery, 276*(1), e3–e5. https://doi.org/10.1097/SLA.0000000000005431.

Brenan, M. (2023). *Nurses retain top ethics rating in U.S., but below 2020 high.* https://news.gallup.com/poll/467804/nurses-retain-top-ethics-rating-below-2020-high.aspx.

Broom, A., Kirby, E., Kokanović, R., Woodland, L., Wyld, D., DeSouza, P., Eng-Siew, K., & Lwin, Z. (2020).

Individualising difference, negotiating culture: Intersections of culture and care. *Health: An Interdisciplinary Journal for the Study of Health, Illness, and Medicine, 24*(5), 552–571. doi:10.1177/1363459319829192.

Campinha-Bacote, J. (2020). *The process of cultural competemility in the delivery healthcare services: Unremitting encounters* (6th ed.). Braughler Books LLC.

Centers for Disease Control (2023). Impact of racism on our nation's health. https://www.cdc.gov/minorityhealth/racism-disparities/impact-of-racism.html.

Chang, E. S., Simon, M., & Dong, X. (2012). Integrating cultural humility into health care professional education and training. *Advances in Health Sciences Education: Theory and Practice, 17*(2), 269–278. https://doi.org/10.1007/s10459-010-9264-1.

Choi, H. (2001). Cultural marginality: A concept analysis with implications for immigrant adolescents. *Issues in Comprehensive Pediatric Nursing, 24*, 193–206.

Choi, H. (2013). Theory of cultural marginality. In Smith, M. J., & Liehr, P. (Eds.), *Middle range theory for nursing* (3rd ed., pp. 289–307). Springer Publishing Company.

Choi, H. (2023). Theory of cultural marginality. In Smith, M. J., Liehr, P., & Carpenter, R. D. (Eds.), *Middle range theory for nursing* (5th ed., pp. 257–272). Springer Publishing Company, LLC. doi:10.1891/9780826139276.

Connolly, M., Selling, M. K., Cook, S., Williams, J. S., Chin, M. H., & Umscheid, C. A. (2021). Development, implementation, and use of an "equity lens" integrated into an institutional quality scorecard. *Journal of the American Medical Association Informatics Association, 28*(8), 1785–1790. doi:10.1093/jamia/ocab082.

Danso, R. (2018). Cultural competence and cultural humility: A critical reflection on key cultural diversity concepts. *Journal of Social Work, 18*(4), 410–430.

Davis, L. M., Martin, L. T., Fremont, A., Weech-Maldonado, R., Williams, M. V., & Kim, A. (2018). Development of a long-term evaluation framework for the national standards for culturally and linguistically appropriate services (CLAS) in health and health care. https://www.minorityhealth.hhs.gov/omh/browse.aspx?lvl=2&lvlid=11.

Dietrich, S., & Hernandez, E. (2022). *Nearly 68 million people spoke a language other than English at home in 2019.* https://www.census.gov/library/stories/2022/12/languages-we-speak-in-united-states.html.

Downey, N. (2021). The importance of culture in treating substance use disorder: Example application with indigenous people. *Journal of Psychosocial Nursing and Mental Health Services, 59*(6), 7–12. https://doi.org/10.3928/02793695-20210512-02.

Drevdahl, D. J. (2018). Culture shifts: From cultural to structural theorizing in nursing. *Nursing Research, 57*(2), 146–160. doi:10.1097/NNR.000000000000026.

Duello, T. M., Rivedal, S., Wickland, C., & Weller, A. (2021). Race and genetics versus 'race' in genetics: A systematic review of the use of African ancestry in genetic studies. *Evolution, Medicine, and Public Health, 9*(1), 232–245. https://doi.org/10.1093/emph/eoab018.

Ellis, A., Pappadis, M. R., Li, C., Rojas, J., & Washington, J. S. (2023). Interprofessional perceptions of diversity, equity, inclusion, cultural competence, and humility among students and faculty: A mixed-methods study. *Journal of Allied Health, 52*(2), 89–96.

Fadiman, A. (2012). *The spirit catches you and you fall down: A Hmong child, her American doctors, and the collision of two cultures.* Farrar, Straus, and Giroux.

Fawzy, A., Wu, T. D., Wang, K., Robinson, M. L., Farha, J., Bradke, A., Golden, S. H., Xu, Y., & Garibaldi, B. T. (2022). Racial and ethnic discrepancy in pulse oximetry and delayed identification of treatment eligibility among patients with COVID-19. *JAMA Internal Medicine, 182*(7), 730–738. https://doi.org/10.1001/jamainternmed.2022.1906.

Fernandez, K. R. (2020). Developing cultural humility during short-term study abroad immersion. *Internal Journal of Studies in Nursing, 5*(3), 48–53.

Fitzgerald, E., & Campinha-Bacote, J. (2019). An intersectionality approach to the process of culture competemility–Part II. *The Online Journal of Nursing, 24*(2), 1–12.

Foronda, C., Reinholdt, M. M., & Ousman, K. (2016). Cultural humility: A concept analysis. *Journal of Transcultural Nursing, 27*(3), 210–217.

Golden, S. H., Galiatsatos, P., Wilson, C., Page, K. R., Jones, V., Tolson, T., Lugo, A., McCann, N., Wilson, A., & Hill-Briggs, F. (2021). Approaching the COVID-19 pandemic response with a health equity lens: A framework for academic health systems. *Academic Medicine, 96*(11), 1546–1552. doi:10.1097/ACM.0000000000003999.

Grome, H. N., Raman, R., Katz, B. D., Fill, M., Jones, T., Schaffner, W., & Dunn, J. (2022). Disparities in COVID-19 mortality rates: Implications for rural health policy and preparedness. *Journal of Public Health Management and Practice, 28*(5), 478–485. doi:10.1097/PHH.0000000000001507.

Hall, J. M., Stevens, P. E., & Meleis, A. I. (1994). Marginalization: A guiding concept for valuing diversity in nursing knowledge development. *Advances in Nursing Science, 16*(4), 23–41. https://doi.org/10.1097/00012272-199406000-00005.

Harvard University (n.d.). Project Implicit. https://implicit.harvard.edu/implicit/.

Hook, J. N., Davis, D. E., Owen, J., Worthington, E. L., & Utsey, S. O. (2013). Cultural humility: Measuring openness to culturally diverse clients. *Journal of Counseling Psychology, 60*(3), 353–366. https://doi.org/10.1037/a0032595.

Hughes, V., Delva, S., Nkimbeng, M., Spaulding, E., Turcson-Orcman, R., Cudjoe, J., Ford, A., Rushton, C., D'Aoust, R., & Han, H. (2020). Not missing the opportunity—Strategies to promote cultural humility among future nursing faculty. *Journal of Professional Nursing, 36*, 28–33.

Institute of Medicine (IOM), & (US) Committee on Quality of Health Care in America. (2001). *Crossing the Quality Chasm: A New Health System for the 21st Century*. National Academies Press.

Institute of Medicine (IOM), & (US) Committee on Understanding and Eliminating Racial and Ethnic Disparities in Health Care (2003). In Smedley, B. D., Stith, A. Y., & Nelson, A. R. (Eds.), *Unequal Treatment: Confronting Racial and Ethnic Disparities in Health Care*. National Academies Press.

Kanis, J. A., Cooper, C., Dawson-Hughes, B., Harvey, N. C., Johansson, H., Lorentzon, M., McCloskey, E. V., Reginster, J. Y., Rizzoli, R, & International Osteoporosis Foundation. (2020). FRAX and ethnicity. *Osteoporosis International, 31*(11), 2063–2067. https://doi.org/10.1007/s00198-020-05631-6.

Kibakaya, E. C., & Oyeku, S. O. (2022). Cultural humility: A critical step in achieving health equity. *Pediatrics, 149*(2), e2021052883. https://doi.org/10.1542/peds.2021-052883.

Leininger, M. M. (1995). *Transcultural nursing: Concepts, theories, and practices* (2nd ed.). McGraw-Hill.

Leininger, M. M. (2002). Transcultural nursing and globalization of health care: Importance, focus, and historical aspects. In Leininger, M. M., & McFarland, M. R. (Eds.), *Transcultural nursing: Concepts, theories, research, and practice* (3rd ed., pp. 1–43). McGraw Hill Companies, Inc.

Lin, S., Deng, X., Ryan, I., Zhang, K., Zhang, W., Oghaghare, E., Gayle, D. B., & Shaw, B. (2022). COVID-19 symptoms and deaths among healthcare workers, United States. *Emerging Infectious Disease, 28*(8), 1624–1641. doi:10.3201/eid2808.212200.

Lundberg, D. J., Cho, A., Raquib, R., Nsoesie, E. O., Wrigley-Field, E., & Stokes, A. (2023). Geographic and temporal patterns in COVID-19 mortality by race and ethnicity in the United States from March 2020 to February 2022. Retrieved March 30, 2023, from https://pubmed.ncbi.nlm.nih.gov/35898347/.

Mandelbaum, J. (2020). Advancing health equity by integrating intersectionality into epidemiological research: Applications and challenges. *Journal of Epidemiology and Community Health, 74*(9), 761–762.

McFarland, M., & Wehbe-Alamah, H. (2018). *Leininger's transcultural nursing: Concepts, theories, research, & practice.* (4th ed.). McGraw-Hill Education.

McKinlay, J. B. (2019). A case for refocusing upstream: The political economy of illnesses. *Interdisciplinary Association for Population Health Science, 1*, 1–10.

Narayan, M. C. (2019). CE: Addressing implicit bias in nursing: A review. *The American Journal of Nursing, 119*(7), 36–43. https://doi.org/10.1097/01.NAJ.0000569340.27659.5a.

National Academies of Sciences, Engineering, & Medicine. (2019). *Integrating social care into the delivery of health care: Moving upstream to improve the nation's health*. National Academies Press. doi:10.17226/25467. https://pubmed.ncbi.nlm.nih.gov/31940159/.

National Academies of Sciences, Engineering, and Medicine (NASEM). (2023). *Advancing antiracism, diversity, equity, and inclusion in STEMM organizations: Beyond broadening participation*. The National Academies Press. https://doi.org/10.17226/26803.

National Academies of Sciences, Engineering, & Medicine. (2021). *The future of nursing report: 2020–2030: Charting a path to health equity*. https://www.nationalacademies.org/our-work/the-future-of-nursing-2020-2030.

National Center for Chronic Disease Prevention and Health Promotion (NCCDP). (2022). Equitably addressing social determinants of health and chronic diseases. https://www.cdc.gov/chronicdisease/healthequity/social-determinants-of-health-and-chronic-disease.html.

National Center for Chronic Disease Prevention and Health Promotion (NCCDP). (2022a). *Global public health equity guiding principles for communication*. https://www.cdc.gov/globalhealth/equity/guide/cultural-humility.html.

Nickitas, D. M., Emmons, K. R., & Ackerman-Barger, K. (2022). A policy pathway: Nursing's role in advancing diversity and health equity. *Nursing Outlook, 70*(6S1), S38S47.

Office of Minority Health. (2013). *National Standards for Culturally and Linguistically Appropriate Services (CLAS) in Health and Health Care*. US Department of Health and Human Services, Office of Minority Health.

Office of Minority Health (OMH), US Department of Health and Human Services (USDHHS). (2019). *Culturally competent nursing care: A cornerstone of caring*. https://ccnm.thinkculturalhealth.hhs.gov/default.asp?ErrorMessage=Your+session+has+been+timed+out%2E+Please+log+in+to+access+the+site%2E&fromURL=%2FContent%2FIntroduction%2FIntroduction1%2Easp%3F.

Office of Minority Health (OMH), US Department of Health and Human Services (USDHHS). (2019a). *Think cultural health*. https://thinkculturalhealth.hhs.gov/education/behavioral-health.

Office of Minority Health. (2021). *Think cultural health: The national CLAS standards*. https://thinkculturalhealth.hhs.gov/clas/standards.

Okoniewski, W., Sundaram, M., Chaves-Gnecco, D., McAnany, K., Cowden, J. D., & Ragavan, M. (2022). Culturally sensitive interventions in pediatric primary care settings: A systematic review. *Pediatrics, 149*(2), e2021052162. https://doi.org/10.1542/peds.2021-052162.

Ong-Flaherty, C. (2016). Cultural incongruence in nursing education. *American Journal of Nursing, 116*(11), 11.

Oswald, F. L., Mitchell, G., Blanton, H., Jaccard, J., & Tetlock, P. E. (2013). Predicting ethnic and racial discrimination: A meta-analysis of IAT criterion studies. *Journal of Personality and Social Psychology, 105*(2), 171–192. https://doi.org/10.1037/a0032734.

Ottawa Chapter for Health Promotion. (1986) The 1st international conference on health promotion, https://www.who.int/teams/health-promotion/enhanced-wellbeing/first-global-conference.

Pacquiao, D. F. (2008). Nursing care of vulnerable populations using a framework of cultural competence, social justice, and human rights. *Contemporary Nurse, 28*(1–2), 189–197.

Pacquiao, D. F. (2018). Framework for culturally competent health care. In Douglas, M. M., Pacquiao, D. F., & Purnell, L. D. (Eds.), *Global applications of culturally competent health care: Guidelines for practice* (pp. 1–30). Springer International Publishing AG.

Pacquiao, D. F. (2019). "Place" and health. In Pacquiao, D. F., & Douglas, M. M. (Eds.), *Social pathways to health vulnerability: Implications for health professionals* (pp. 3–22). Springer International Publishing.

Pacquiao, D. F., & Douglas, M. M. (Eds.). (2019). *Social pathways to health vulnerability: Implications for health professionals*. Springer International Publishing.

Pacquiao, D. F., Maxwell, J. B., Ludwig-Beymer, P., Stievano, A., Sagar, P. L., Purnell, L., Daub, K., & Halabi, J. O. (2023). Integration of population health, social determinants, and social justice in transcultural nursing and culturally competent care. *Journal of Transcultural Nursing, 34*(3), 1–3.

Park, R. E. (1928). Human migration and the marginal man. *American Journal of Sociology, 33*(6), 881–893.

Reich, A. J., Perez, S., Fleming, J., Gazarian, P., Manful, A., Ladin, K., Tjia, J., Semco, R., Prigerson, H., Weissman, J. S., & Candrian, C. (2022). Advance care planning experiences among sexual and gender minority people. *JAMA Network Open, 5*(7), e2222993. https://doi.org/10.1001/jamanetworkopen.2022.22993.

Ruth, T. (2019). *Tony Ruth for 2019 design in tech report.* https://www.slideshare.net/GabrielGaldamez/tony-ruths-equity-series-2019-247617994.

Sagar, P. L. (2014). *Transcultural nursing education strategies.* Springer Publishing Company.

Sagar, P. L., Camuñas, C., & Melli, S. O. (2014). Then, now, and beyond: Quo vadis, TCN? In Sagar, P. L. (Ed.), *Transcultural nursing education strategies* (pp. 341–353). Springer Publishing Company.

Sagar, P. L. (2023). TCN scholars: How prepared are nurses in advocacy and influencing policy for health equity? *Journal of Transcultural Nursing, 34*(3), 174.

Sharpnack, P. A. (2022). Overview and summary: Nurses' impact on advocacy and policy. *OJIN: The Online Journal of Issues in Nursing, 27*(2). https://ojin.nursingworld.org/table-of-contents/volume-27-2022/number-2-may-2022/nurses-impact-on-advocacy-and-policy/.

Shearn, C., & Krockow, E. M. (2023). Reasons for COVID-19 vaccine hesitancy in ethnic minority groups: A systematic review and thematic synthesis of initial attitudes in qualitative research. *SSM. Qualitative Research in Health, 3*, 100210. https://doi.org/10.1016/j.ssmqr.2022.100210.

Solar, O., Valentine, N., Castedo, A., Brandt, G. S., Sathyandran, J., Ahmed, Z., Cheh, P., Callon, E., Porritt, F., Espinosa, I., Fortune, K., Kubota, S., Elliott, E., David, A. J., Bigdeli, M., Hachri, H., Bodenmann, P., Morisod, K., Biehl, M., Nambiar, D., & Rasanathan, K. (2023). Action on the social determinants for advancing health equity in the time of COVID-19: Perspectives of actors engaged in a WHO Special Initiative. *International journal for equity in health, 21*(Suppl. 3), 193. https://doi.org/10.1186/s12939-022-01798-y.

Staats, C. (2016). Understanding implicit bias: What educators should know. *American Educator, 39*(4), 29–33.

Sue, D. W., & Sue, D. (2016). *Counseling the culturally diverse* (7th ed.). Wiley.

Sue, D. W., & Spanierman, L. B. (2020). *Microaggressions in everyday life* (2nd ed.). Wiley.

Sukhera, J., Watling, C. J., & Gonzalez, C. M. (2020). Implicit bias in health professions: From recognition to transformation. *Academic, 95*(5), 717–723. https://doi.org/10.1097/ACM.0000000000003173.

Terlizzi, E. P., Connor, E. M., Zelaya, C. E., Ji, A. M., & Bakos, A. D. (2019). Reported importance and access to health care providers who understand or share cultural characteristics with their patients among adults, by race and ethnicity. *National Health Statistics Reports, 130*, 1–12.

Tervalon, M., & Murray-Garcia, J. (1998). Cultural humility versus cultural competence: A critical distinction in defining physician training outcomes in multicultural education. *Journal of Health Care for the Poor and Underserved, 9*(2), 117–125.

Thirsk, L. M., Panchuk, J. T., Stahlke, S., & Hagtvedt, R. (2022). Cognitive and implicit biases in nurses' judgment and decision-making: A scoping review. *International Journal of Nursing Studies, 133*, 104284. https://doi.org/10.1016/j.ijnurstu.2022.104284.

Thomas, T., Martsolf, G., & Puskar, K. (2019). How to engage nursing students in health policy: Results of a survey assessing students' competencies, experiences, interests, and values. *Policy, Politics, & Nursing Practice, 21*(1), 12–20. https://journals.sagepub.com/action/showCitFormats?doi=10.1177%2F1527154419891129&mobileUi=0.

US Census Bureau. (2023). USA Facts. How has the racial and ethnic makeup of the US changed? https://usafacts.org/data/topics/people-society/population-and-demographics/our-changing-population/?utm_source=google&utm_medium=cpc&utm_campaign=ND-Dem-Pop&gclid=EAIaIQobChMI-amL3Iqn_wIVdSnUAR2B-fAYrEAAYASAAEgLhjvD_BwE

US Census Bureau. (2018). *U. S. Census Bureau Quick Facts.* https://www.census.gov/quickfacts/fact/table/US/RHI725218.

Vyas, D. A., Eisenstein, L. G., & Jones, D. S. (2020). Hidden in plain sight—Reconsidering the use of race correction in clinical algorithms. *The New England Journal of Medicine, 383*(9), 874–882. doi:10.1056/NEJMms2004740.

White, A. A., & Stubblefield-Tave, B. (2017). Some advice for physicians and other clinicians treating minorities, women, and other patients at risk of receiving health care disparities. *Journal of Racial and Ethnic Health Disparities, 4*(3), 472–479.

Williams, S. D., Phillips, J. M., & Koyama, K. (2018). Nurse advocacy: Adopting a health in all policies approach. *OJIN: The Online Journal of Issues in Nursing, 23*(3). https://ojin.nursingworld.org/MainMenuCategories/ANAMarketplace/ANAPeriodicals/OJIN/TableofContents/Vol-23-2018/No3-Sept-2018/Policy-Advocacy.html.

Williams, W. W., Hogan, J. W., & Ingelfinger, J. R. (2021). Time to eliminate health care disparities in the estimation of kidney function. *The New England Journal of Medicine, 385*(19), 1804–1806. doi:10.1056/NEJMe2114918.

WHO. (2023). *Social determinants of health.* https://www.who.int/health-topics/social-determinants-of-health#tab=tab_1.

Yeager, K. A., & Bauer-Wu, S. (2013). Cultural humility: Essential foundation for clinical researchers. *Applied Nursing Research, 26*(4), 251–252.

Community Engagement and Action-Oriented Models of Community Research

Vetta L. Sanders Thompson

Real, sustainable community change requires the initiative and engagement of community members.
—Helene D. Gayles. MD, President and CEO of the Chicago Community Trust

CHAPTER OUTLINE

LEARNING OBJECTIVES

1. Discuss the history and principles important to community collaborations and CBPR and its role in addressing health inequity.
2. Identify and describe the continuum of community engagement in research, beginning with outreach and education and ending with the development of community partnerships.
3. Develop the skills to identify and engage the appropriate community representatives and build community relationships and trust.
4. Describe the use of planning tools and logic models to effectively implement community-engaged research.
5. Outline steps and strategies to facilitate community capacity to engage in research.

INTRODUCTION

Community engagement can be defined as:

> "... The process of working collaboratively with and through groups of people affiliated by geographic proximity, special interest, or similar situations to address issues affecting the well-being of those people. It is a powerful vehicle for bringing about environmental and behavioral changes that will improve the health of the community and its members. It often involves partnerships and coalitions that help mobilize resources and influence systems, change relationships among partners, and serve as catalysts for changing policies, programs, and practices (CDC, 1997, p. 9). Community engagement can take many forms, and partners can include organized groups, agencies, institutions, or individuals. Collaborators may be engaged in health promotion, research, or policy making"
>
> **(US Department of Health and Human Services, National Institutes of Health, 2016, para 1).**

The promise of community-engaged research is the ability to address the complex set of social, environmental, cultural, and community factors that affect health.

Evidence suggests that community engagement is an important ingredient in implementation and translational sciences, including tailoring evidence-based practices to meet the needs of marginalized communities (Kost et al., 2012; Wilkins et al., 2013; Yarborough et al., 2013). Despite the promise of community-engaged intervention efforts and increased research on stakeholder engagement, the empirical evidence on best practices for stakeholder engagement and evaluation of engagement indicating an association between the quality and quantity of engagement and research outcomes is still limited. However, the recognition and focus on community engagement as a tool to facilitate greater cultural appropriateness, community acceptance of interventions, and health recommendations remain despite the need for additional research.

WHY COMMUNITY-ENGAGED RESEARCH

The desire to address the acceptability of treatments, interventions, and health recommendations derived from research increases the importance of community-engaged research for nursing. Cleary and Hunt's (2010) call for nurses to engage in collaborative relationships with other health professionals, service providers, community-based organizations, and community stakeholders to develop the knowledge and evidence base to benefit the community follows the 2004 National Institute of Nursing Research's call for a "scholarship of engagement." There is also a strong recognition that the health and healthcare issues of today require nursing's public and civic leadership (Fyffe, 2009). To fulfill this professional agenda, nurses must understand the various categories of community engagement, the strategies and activities involved, and consider how they might affect health and healthcare goals.

To assist in facilitating and accelerating nursing's participation in community-engaged research, this chapter provides an overview of key ideas, practices, and skills common to strategies under the umbrella of *community engagement*. It begins with a brief history of community engagement in health research and practice and moves to an overview of the continuum of community engagement and the nuances of the various strategies encountered under the rubric. A review of the implementation process is provided, including the preparation and planning required for the successful implementation of any engaged process. Finally, the use of logic models and other planning tools to assist in operationalizing community involvement in activities designed to achieve outcomes desired by the community is discussed.

THE HISTORY OF ENGAGEMENT

Over the decades, foundations, federal offices, and a growing number of researchers have recognized the importance and necessity of developing collaborative research strategies (National Institute of Nursing Research, 2004). One of the first government agencies to do so was the US Department of Housing and Urban Development (HUD), which established the Office of University Partnerships in 1994 to encourage and expand partnerships between universities and their local communities to promote the development of healthy communities (U.S. Department of Housing and Urban Development, 2021). By the beginning of the new century, federal funding agencies focused on health (Agency for Healthcare Research and Quality, National Institutes of Health) began recognizing, supporting, and in some instances requiring engagement in health-related research (Education Network to Advance Cancer Trials, Community-Campus Partnerships for Health, 2008; Patient-Centered Outcomes Research Institute (PCORI), 2018; Seifer et al., 2003; Sung et al., 2003; Vishwanathan et al., 2004; Westfall et al., 2007). Researchers also began to argue the benefits of community-engaged research, including greater participation rates, increased external validity, decreased loss of participants at follow-up, and increased organizational and community capacity (Vishwanathan et al., 2004).

In addition to trends driving the development of various forms of community engagement, social pressures on academic institutions and professionals have played a role in its implementation. Calls and demands for accountability from legislators and the public led to shifts in how institutions conducted service activities designed to meet public and community needs. The term engagement was introduced to describe a "two-way" approach to interacting with community partners to address societal needs (Kellogg Commission on the Future of State and Land-Grant Institutions, 1999) in contrast to the traditional "one-way" approach. The community-engaged philosophy emphasized a shift away from an expert model of delivering university knowledge to the public and a movement toward a more collaborative model that allowed community partners to play a significant role in creating and sharing knowledge that was mutually beneficial to institutions and society.

To facilitate this shift, key organizations and associations have leveraged their influence to support changes in university and community relationships. For example, in 2006 the Carnegie Foundation for the Advancement of Teaching developed a new classification to recognize a category of community-engaged institutions that define themselves by their commitment to the ideals of public engagement (Purpose Institute in Partnership with the Carnegie Foundation, 2021). The Carnegie Foundation defines community engagement as the "collaboration between institutions of higher education and their larger communities (local, regional/state, national, global) for the mutually beneficial exchange of knowledge and resources in a context of partnership and reciprocity" (Purpose Institute in Partnership with the Carnegie Foundation, 2021, para 1). In addition to the Carnegie Foundation's support for engagement, the North Central Association of Colleges and Universities included engagement as a key measure of institutional quality (US Department of Education, 2006). These activities and positions provide greater legitimacy to academic commitments to public and community partnerships.

FRAMEWORKS GUIDING COMMUNITY-ENGAGED RESEARCH

Whether or not it is understood or acknowledged, most of the calls for community-engaged research are drawing on two traditions of research, frequently discussed as the Northern and Southern traditions of participatory research (Wallerstein et al., 2008). The societal crises and social movements of the 1960s, coupled with questions about the responsiveness of academia to social needs, contributed to challenges in how scientific research related to health and behavior, along with other research related to societal well-being, was conducted. These challenges led to efforts to identify new theories and strategies for conducting scientific inquiry. These new theories and approaches to scientific inquiry began to address topics such as the ownership of knowledge, the role of community participation, and the importance of power relations in the research enterprise (Wallerstein et al., 2008). The result was new participatory research frameworks and terms that linked applied social science research to activism.

The emergence of multiple paradigms was related to subtle differences in methodology. These paradigms included participatory rural appraisal and rapid assessment procedures (De Koning & Martin, 1996), constructivist strategies in evaluation research (Lincoln, 2003), and disciplinary applications of the participatory framework such as classroom action research and critical action research in education (Kemmis & McTaggart, 2000). In addition, action learning, action inquiry, and industrial action research in organizational psychology and organizational development emerged (Torbert & Taylor, 2001), as well as emancipatory inquiry in nursing (Hills, 2001). The community development and social action literature have contributed to participatory frameworks as well. Collaborative action research, participatory research, and emancipatory/liberatory research are examples from this body of work (Fals-Borda & Rahman, 1991; Hall, 1992; Kemmis & McTaggart, 2000; Park et al., 1993). Newer terms, community-partnered participatory research and tribal participatory research, focus on partnering (Jones & Wells, 2007) and an approach to work with indigenous communities (Fisher & Ball, 2003). As previously noted, the assumptions, practices, and outcomes of the various traditions are not easily discerned (Trickett & Espino, 2004), particularly as the various traditions have intermingled.

Today the terms *action research* and *participatory action research* are often used interchangeably. This likely occurs due to the similarity in the principles that guide the work of both traditions. In these frameworks the community determines the research agenda and shares in the planning, data collection, analysis, and dissemination of the research (Israel et al., 1998, 2005). The CBPR approach has gained prominence among health researchers. CBPR, like other participatory frameworks, involves research, action, and education (Hall, 1992). It results in researchers providing and sharing tools for community members to use to analyze conditions and make decisions informed by data on the actions needed to improve their lives. In addition, community members transfer information and understanding to researchers allowing academic endeavors to result in community benefit (Wallerstein et al., 2008).

The Northern Tradition of Participatory Research

Participatory frameworks that focus on collaborative research and practical goals, such as system improvement, emerge from the Northern tradition. The emancipatory research frameworks that challenge the research approaches influenced by colonialism and the control of knowledge by social or academic elites emerge from the Southern tradition (Brown & Tandon, 1983). Frameworks such as CBPR employ principles, strategies, and skills from both traditions (Wallerstein et al., 2008).

Noted psychologist Kurt Lewin is credited with the first use of the term *action research* within the Northern tradition. (Wallerstein et al., 2008). Beginning in the 1940s, Lewin advocated for the integration of research and practice that attempted to solve practical problems using a cycle of planning, action, and examination of the results of the action (Lewin, 1947). Lewin drew on sociological theory that held that social problem-solving required the knowledge, understandings, and meanings developed by those affected by a problem as they live their lives. This cyclical problem-solving process resulted in decision-making based on constantly increasing scientific knowledge that applied to important social problems. Practitioners and researchers in the fields of organizational and social psychology placed an emphasis on practitioners as coequals to researchers in the research process. For example, quality improvement work or research assumed that management and workers had equal power to affect increases in quality and productivity (Brown & Tandon, 1983). In education, teachers were encouraged to become researchers in their classrooms to address barriers to learning that had traditionally been the domain of academics (Wallerstein et al., 2008).

The Southern Tradition of Participatory Research

Since the early 1970s, the Southern tradition has influenced the practice of participatory research and variants that comingle traditions, such as CBPR. The Southern tradition initially gained importance and influence in Latin America, Asia, and Africa, pushed by the realities of underdevelopment in the context of colonialization. Brazilian philosopher Paulo Freire (2018) was one of the most significant influences on the Southern tradition. His work focused on shifting academic and community relationships from ones in which communities were the subjects of study to ones in which community members participate in developing the focus, implementation, and interpretation of the work (Figs. 10.1–10.4). Academics and researchers from the social sciences, who worked using the liberatory framework of the Southern tradition, created an

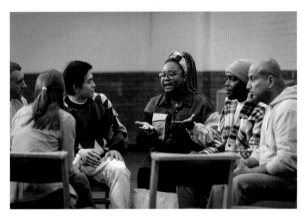

Fig. 10.1 Researcher working with community members participating in the focus, implementation, and interpretation of community challenges. (From iStock.com/SolStock.)

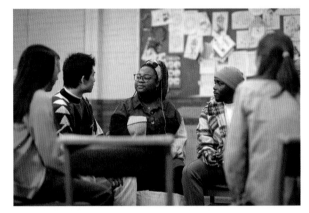

Fig. 10.2 Researcher working with community members participating in the focus, implementation, and interpretation of community challenges. (From iStock.com/SolStock.)

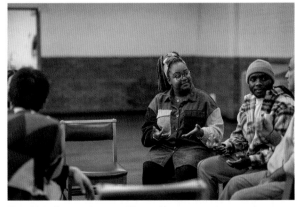

Fig. 10.3 Researcher working with community members participating in the focus, implementation, and interpretation of community challenges. (From iStock.com/SolStock.)

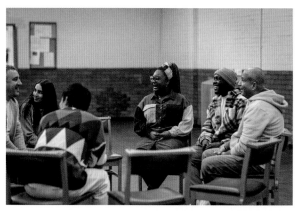

Fig. 10.4 Researcher working with community members participating in the focus, implementation, and interpretation of community challenges. (From iStock.com/SolStock.)

openness to knowledge learned from people's experiences (Fals-Borda & Rahman, 1991). Unique aspects of frameworks within this tradition are the integration of critical consciousness, emancipation, and social justice. These components encourage researchers and academics to challenge their roles in communities, noting the capacity of the poor and oppressed to create change in their own communities based on their own reflection and action. This position allows academics and researchers to be catalysts and supports of processes but not the leaders of social change (Hall, 1992). The Southern tradition has also integrated cultural and social dimensions of oppression into theories of economic and social determinism (Wallerstein et al., 2008), increasing the attractiveness of this framework in communities of color. The interest in CBPR that incorporates aspects of the Southern framework among US communities of color may be due to their recognition of a history of academic researchers undermining their traditional knowledge and ways of being.

With this history in mind, the categories of engagement practiced in academic disciplines, including nursing, are considered. Placing each framework used by health disciplines at a specific point on the continuum between nonengaged and fully engaged collaborations is difficult because the actual community-engaged practice may vary by location, context, history, and the needs and desires of community partners (Wallerstein et al., 2008). In general, however, action science, organizational action research, and the related traditions

grounded in the Lewin model fall along the end of the continuum focusing on the pragmatic use of knowledge, with cooperative and mutual inquiry close to the middle of the continuum. The participatory research and participatory action research approaches associated with Freire and the Southern tradition are generally at the end of the continuum associated with fully participatory partnerships (Wallerstein et al., 2008). Understanding these issues and tensions allows us to reflect on our engaged practice along the continuum discussed in the next section.

CATEGORIES OF STAKEHOLDER ENGAGEMENT

Community engagement is an umbrella term for a range of strategies that involve patients and family members, advocates, professionals, researchers, government and community agencies, organizations, and associations, sometimes known as stakeholders and, more recently, as partners. The strategies cover activities that fall into three broad categories: nonparticipation, symbolic participation, and engaged participation (Goodman & Thompson Sanders, 2017a). In addition, several of these categories include subcategories. When considering subcategories the engagement continuum may use descriptors that range from nonengaged, advisory, and symbolic to cooperative, collaborative, and fully engaged (Goodman & Thompson Sanders, 2017a; Israel et al., 2010; Montoya & Kent, 2011). While agreement exists on the trajectory of the continuum and the activities and strategies that represent the endpoints of full engagement, terminology and descriptions may vary at other points (Goodman & Thompson Sanders, 2017a; Israel et al., 2010; Montoya & Kent, 2011).

When thinking about the continuum of engagement, remember that the work must begin somewhere. Notwithstanding the labels used in Fig. 10.5, each point on the continuum provides an opportunity to move toward the goal of a vibrant and meaningful partnership.

Nonparticipatory Engagement

There are some who may include the nonparticipation category as a community engagement category. Although the usual purpose does not include engaging stakeholders in the planning, implementation, evaluation, and/or decision-making aspects of the treatment, project, intervention, or research, community

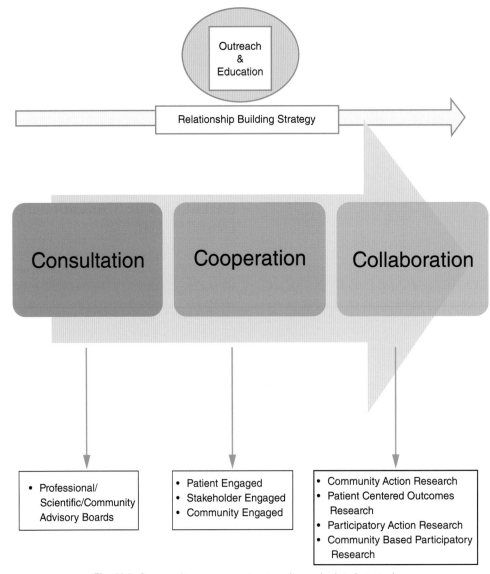

Fig. 10.5 Community engagement categories and related strategies.

stakeholders may value this activity. Nonparticipation is often represented by outreach and education. Outreach and education involve professionals and researchers joining the community of interest and educating nonacademic stakeholders about a particular topic. Key members of the target population (gatekeepers) can be engaged as advisors and assist professionals and researchers in making key connections. Although classified as nonparticipatory the strategy may be valued by the community. When done well, community members receive access to information and resources that are sometimes difficult for them to access under normal circumstances (Thompson Sanders et al., 2021). This may lead community members to value outreach and engagement over advisory or consultative strategies.

Symbolic Engagement

The next category of engagement, *symbolic participation,* begins to include community members and other relevant stakeholders. Subcategories of symbolic participation often include coordination and *cooperation*. Coordination is typically described as researchers gathering community stakeholders to assess important elements of a project, with community members providing feedback to professionals and academic researchers. In this category of engagement, community members give feedback and this feedback provides researchers with information about the community and the research proposed, but it is the researchers' responsibility to design and implement the work without a desire for or expectation of help from the community members. Researchers may also provide outreach and education as a component of engagement in this segment of the continuum. Research results may also be disseminated through community groups and gatekeepers.

Cooperation involves researchers asking community members for help with a project instead of just asking for advice. There may be activity on the part of community members in defined aspects of the project, including recruitment support, activities related to designing study questions/items and selecting measures, data collection strategies, and interpretation of outcomes. Community health partners and researchers discuss key aspects of the project. At this point on the continuum, researchers attempt to provide opportunities that improve community health partners' understanding of research and its potential importance through study participation. Importantly, when community engagement falls into the symbolic category, it is unclear whether the work will be perceived as valuable to or will benefit the community. When community members and other partners advise and help without having decision-making power, there is an appearance of full engagement. However, this category of engagement arguably lacks meaningful input.

Engaged Research

In the engaged participation category, patients, caregivers, and advocacy groups that traditionally have limited power are given shared decision-making authority along with powerful partners (e.g., hospital systems, health center leadership, and academic researchers). These partners collaboratively manage the project based on community priorities (Arnstein, 1969). Action research, CBPR, participatory action research, and community action research are all forms of engaged participation. These forms of engagement are believed to achieve their aims through a focus on bringing together

multiple partners, including practitioners, researchers, and communities, to establish trust, share power, enhance strengths and resources, and examine and address health needs and concerns with solutions developed in collaboration (American Hospital Association, 2010; Israel et al., 1998).

The engaged segment of the continuum is often described as collaboration (Goodman & Thompson Sanders, 2017a, 2017b). At this point on the continuum, the community has a major voice and role in setting the research agenda. Community health partners collaborate in decision-making and share resources throughout the study. Researchers, professionals, community members, and other partners are actively involved in the study design, recruitment, and development of study questions, selection of measures, and the interpretation of the findings. Partners may also assist with data collection and follow-up activities. The research team attempts to act in ways that demonstrate that input from partners is valuable. They also work to have partners benefit in some way from the work. For example, community partners may receive new data on issues confronting the community and resources to make change. Researchers and community members meet to discuss ways they can have respectful and trusting relationships and how they might plan to continue working together.

One type of collaboration is *patient*-centered collaboration, with patients, caregivers, and advocacy groups determining research priorities and collaborating on the design and implementation of the project activities, in addition to the interpretation and publication of findings (Patient-Centered Outcomes Research Institute, 2012). Patient-centered outcomes research assists individuals and their caregivers in having their voices heard when the outcomes that inform the value of healthcare options are assessed. Another frequently discussed collaborative strategy is CBPR (Goodman & Thompson Sanders, 2017a). CBPR "bridges the gap between science and practice through community engagement and social action," as emphasized by Wallerstein and Duran (2010, p. S40). With a goal of societal transformation (Minkler, 2003), CBPR involves community partners in all aspects of the research process, with all partners contributing expertise and sharing decision-making (Israel et al., 1998; Minkler, 2003). By promoting equitable power and strong collaborative partnerships, CBPR offers a positive alternative to traditional "top-down" research (Minkler, 2004) and is increasingly applied across disciplines as diverse as medicine, nursing, sociology, social work, psychology, and others (Israel et al., 2010).

As discussed in the previous section on the history of community-engaged research, the principles that guide these various strategies converge. However, each is different in its practices and the application of the principles. A fundamental requirement of each strategy is respect for the community and the value of incorporating community perspectives and insights into research and interventions (Sapienza et al., 2007). Each of these strategies seeks to develop meaningful relationships among academics and community partners to promote changes in policies and interventions that improve well-being through the mobilization and organization of resources, individuals, groups, and agencies (D'Alonzo, 2010; Israel et al., 2005; Viswanathan et al., 2004).

Summary

A substantial portion of CBPR work has been conducted with low-income communities and other disadvantaged populations and has attempted to provide a platform for the needs, concerns, and suggestions of "those who are most affected" by inequities to be heard (Israel et al., 2010). Here, CBPR is placing its emphasis on the active involvement of "those who are most affected" from Kurt Lewin's action research (Minkler, 2004). CBPR's emphasis on colearning is drawn from Freire's critical thinking work, providing a clear example of the influence of the Southern tradition of participatory work (KU Work Group for Community Health and Development, 2016; Minkler, 2004). Given its theoretical underpinnings of self-determinism, CBPR changes people's perceptions of themselves and what they can accomplish (KU Work Group for Community Health and Development, 2016).

To successfully prepare for implementing a community-engaged research program, professionals and academic researchers must reflect on our own positionality, the resources available to us, and our ability to adhere to the principles of engagement required of each category. This reflection helps us better understand the biases, beliefs, and practices that will support and/or undermine our efforts to conduct community-engaged research. The Student Learning Activity later in this chapter may assist you in solidifying your understanding of the strategic categories along the continuum and identifying your strengths and continuing education needs to do this work.

IMPLEMENTATION OF COMMUNITY-ENGAGED RESEARCH

Community engagement involves developing professional links across professional, advocacy, and community organizations and working collaboratively on projects with identified outcomes (Fig. 10.6). Relevant health sector partners include health and service providers, patient/consumer stakeholders, nongovernment organizations, professional bodies, and academic communities. Nurses can participate in community engagement activities encompassing a range of professional activities: consultation, media presentations, providing input into curricula, guest seminars, working on external committees and boards, and acting as reviewers for professional bodies and peer-reviewed journals. With major changes in healthcare looming, nurses must be visible leaders in the public debate on health and healthcare policies.

Ideally, implementation of community-engaged health-related activities is conducted in ways that assure that the communities and partners most likely to be affected by interactions, collaborations, and/or partnerships have involvement and voice from conceptualization of the ideas and methods to implementation of services, activities, and policies, and interpretation and dissemination of results (Minkler et al., 2003). While this approach is believed to improve community acceptance and use of interventions, services, and activities, there are frequently barriers to implementation (Cargo & Mercer, 2008). Many issues can affect the implementation of community engagement.

Relationship development that includes trust and rapport building is required for successful and sustainable efforts. This is one reason that imbalances in power and knowledge that often exist among patients, practitioners, researchers, and community partners must be addressed (Weerts & Sandmann, 2008). Additionally, equitable participation in efforts is sometimes difficult to achieve given differences in community and academic priorities (Cargo & Mercer, 2008), thus the focus on community inclusion in determining the targets of action. There are many strategies available to build the trust and relationships required for the successful implementation of community engagement, including keeping agreements, sharing information, admitting mistakes, maintaining confidentiality, actively seeking engagement and involvement in decision-making,

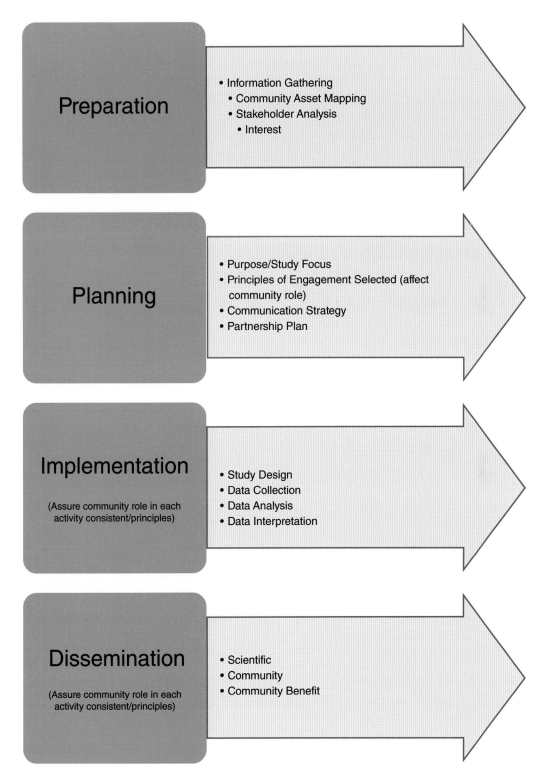

Fig. 10.6 The community engagement process.

TABLE 10.1   Eleven Key Principles of Community-Based Participatory Research in Health
• Community is defined using identity;
• The collaboration identifies and builds on strengths and resources within the community;
• The process is structured to facilitate collaborative, equitable involvement of all partners in all phases of the research;
• The process is structured to integrate and achieve a balance of all partners;
• Knowledge, activities, and interventions are structured to assure respect for and inclusion of community input;
• The processes established promote colearning, cobenefit, and capacity-building for all partners;
• The processes established involve a cyclical and iterative process;
• Health promotion is addressed from both positive and ecological perspectives, focusing on local relevance and social determinants of health;
• Knowledge, findings, and outcomes are shared with all partners;
• Dissemination of knowledge and findings involves all partners;
• The collaboration involves a long-term commitment by all partners.

Adapted from: Israel, B., Schulz, A., Parker, E., & Becker, A. (1998). Review of community-based research: Assessing partnership approaches to improve public health. *Annual Reviews of Public Health, 19,* 173–202.

acknowledging the skills of others, and working to build capacity and skills among stakeholders.

It is important to know and admit that not all forms of community engagement have been subjected to research (Table 10.1). However, systematic reviews of community-based participatory clinical trials and research efforts found that few studies involved the community in all phases of the enterprise (Cargo & Mercer, 2008; De las Nueces et al., 2012). Despite this challenge, funders, academic institutions, and communities increasingly value and see benefits in collective efforts to address complex social issues such as those affecting health and healthcare. Martin and colleagues (2005) noted that "social problems are simply beyond the range of single organizations; rather synergistic efforts are required to increase the potential impact of policies" (p. 13). In addition, Wilson (2004) noted that a potentially key feature of academic and community partnerships involves an intentional commitment to long-term engagement with community partners to solve our most pressing health and healthcare concerns. Ultimately, engagement is meant to improve the quality of health research and healthcare outcomes (Jagosh et al., 2012).

When partnering with community members and organizations, colleges and universities may develop increased trust, rapport, and credibility with the local community. However, the ultimate goal of community engagement is to form academic-community partnerships that are *mutually beneficial* such that both parties can meet their needs (Kennedy, 1999; Marullo & Edwards, 2000). In addition to faculty publishing findings from their partnership experiences and integrating their research with their teaching, community partners should gain knowledge and resources that enable and empower them to address their issues of concern (Marullo & Edwards, 2000). The tangible benefits that may emerge through university-community partnerships include access to university resources (libraries, technology, etc.), access to faculty expertise that contributes to enhanced organizational capacity to carry out their work through additional support received from faculty and students, and improved quality and rigor of program evaluations (Suarez-Balcazar et al., 2015). Realizing these goals requires time and attention to preparation and planning processes.

Preparation

Adequate preparation for community-engaged research requires information-gathering activities that can be summarized in three steps. First, it is important to understand that the term *community* means different things to different people. It is important for community-engaged scholars to clarify their meaning so they can identify the appropriate partners and be transparent in their communications with potential participants and partners.

There are several ways to define and understand community. A neighborhood may define a community, but a community can also be socially and psychologically defined. Definitions of community based on physical boundaries typically use administrative boundaries, for example, census tracks, blocks, or areas determined by natural or manmade barriers (Fig. 10.7). When community is linked to neighborhood these administrative and/or natural and manufactured boundaries may or may not be meaningful to community partners. In

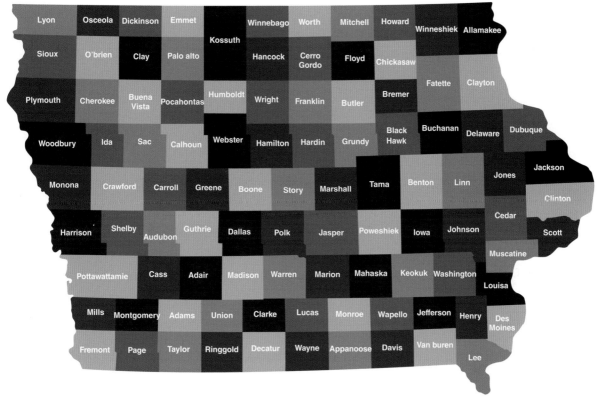

Fig. 10.7 Iowa State County divisions. (From iStock.com/bamlou.)

addition, their relevance may be due to who the partners are in the community. When community is defined psychologically and socially, the term typically reflects a social identity and/or affiliation, such as race, ethnicity, nationality, gender, social experience, a disease, age, or generational group (Fig. 10.8). Community defined based on psychological or social identities transcends physical boundaries and affects research planning.

Professionals and researchers must understand how community stakeholders understand the community. It is not just what community at what time, it is also an issue of how the "community," however defined, sees itself and how it believes others see it. The intersection of these beliefs matters with respect to the availability of resources and assets, how the community thinks about representation, and its willingness to share its time and resources.

The final consideration involved in the definition of community is an understanding of why you wish to engage this community for the project of interest. Your answers to this question may influence community response to the efforts you wish to propose. As a

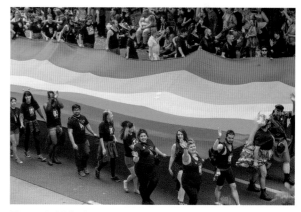

Fig. 10.8 LBGTQ+ community. (From iStock.com/carterdayne.)

researcher, be aware of reasons that are self-serving and the suggestion that you may not have community needs or interests at the forefront of the work.

The next task is to understand the history, assets, and resources of the community. If a primary tenet of community-engaged frameworks requires respect for community, it is incumbent on the researcher to begin understanding the factors that have shaped the community over time and those attributes that stimulate pride in the community. This knowledge may also influence who is asked to participate in decision-making. Just as it is not easy to answer what "community" means, who participates and may represent the community can be complicated. In addition to using archival resources to examine the history of the defined community, asset mapping is a strategy that can enrich researcher knowledge and understanding that informs decisions on research in the community and with the affected partners.

An asset may be a person, place, thing, or quality that is of value to the community/neighborhood or an organization and/or serves as a resource. Community assets come in many forms and knowledge of them promotes using a strengths-based approach to community-driven work (Kretzmann & McKnight, 1993). Researchers are encouraged to spend time visiting the community to gain insight into the organizations, institutions, and associations (schools, libraries, churches, businesses, museums, youth services, etc.) located in the community and what they contribute, as well as the physical spaces (parks, community gardens, monuments, etc.) that serve as positive points of contact that support rejuvenation and well-being. Depending on the work of interest, researchers may identify other assets that may be important to their work, including people. The Community Experiential Learning Activity at the end of this chapter provides an opportunity to explore the idea of *asset mapping* and consider including it in preparation activities before presenting your interests and ideas to the community.

The final step in preparation focuses on gathering and organizing information about potential partners. The process of identifying partners and determining those who should be asked to represent the community is linked to how community has been defined and the issue and/or work of interest to the researcher but also the community. The task for the researcher is to build on the work of asset mapping to gain knowledge of who in the community has an interest or stake in the issue, and who is currently working on the issue or related issues. As organizations, institutions, associations, and individuals are identified, contact information should be added, as well as notes on why a particular entity or individual might be interested in the work and the resources they might offer to support it.

There are several factors to consider in building a collaboration or partnership. This reality should lead to the recognition that not all potential contacts will be contacted and not all will be contacted at once. It is important to use a stakeholder analysis strategy as an opportunity to decide who should be a part of the initial planning for the research or community activity/work and whom you will reach out to as specific activities and needs emerge. Researchers should be careful to avoid simply considering the most powerful partners for inclusion. Instead, it is important to identify who will likely be most invested in the work and the key decision makers who will be important to change efforts. There is also a role for advocates and influencers who may not attend all meetings or be engaged in all activities but are important to support for and completion of the required activities and work.

The focus of your work may influence the type of engagement undertaken, which in turn affects the partners needed to support your work. Much depends on the commitments required to conduct the intervention or research to be proposed and who can make and execute them. The initial phase of developing a nursing treatment or intervention may benefit most from the input of diverse health professionals; thus a consultative engagement approach and an interprofessional scientific advisory committee might be most appropriate to the work. If your potential treatment or intervention has implications for groups or businesses related to healthcare the work might continue to benefit from a consultative approach, but the focus may shift to an intersectorial partner advisory committee that includes partners from insurance, the pharmaceutical industry, hospital administration, and diverse health professionals. Partner-engaged research becomes more valuable as the work progresses. As the need for feedback and assistance with research implementation increases, the approach to engagement may move beyond consultation, and you might move to a cooperative engagement strategy. This will require adding patients, patient advocates, and members of relevant advocacy groups to your advisory committee. In addition, stakeholders involved may become more active in the work.

From a collaborative engagement perspective the effort to develop solutions that address inequities requires the engagement of the voices of those members of a community who bear a disproportionate burden of poor health and associated outcomes. Therefore the composition of the stakeholder list beyond resources, assets, and the likelihood of interest in a partnership requires special attention. A history of ongoing racism, classism, and residential segregation has engendered mistrust among communities that have experienced discrimination and marginalization and the institutions meant to serve them (e.g., police, medical, and social services) and may reduce the willingness to participate among those most important to the work (Hurt, 2009). Therefore, outreach and attention to the inclusion of members of communities often excluded are required and should receive attention at the beginning of planning efforts. This signals sincere appreciation of the values of their voices.

Final Considerations in Preparation

Once you understand the landscape of the community, its assets, and stakeholders with the potential for collaborative interaction, you are ready to conduct initial outreach to them. If you, as the researcher or another researcher planning to join the work, have a good relationship with someone at or in a key organization, it is probably best to build on that relationship. If there is no key contact, it may be best to begin by sending a letter with accompanying information on you, your work, and your interest in meeting. It may be necessary to follow the letter with a phone call, when you can try to determine a mutually agreed upon next step, perhaps an informational call or meeting. Remember that positive contact is the main path to building relationships.

Informational meetings will allow you to understand how community is defined among potential partners and how this fits your definition and interests. You will also add to your list and understanding of community assets. Most importantly, these meetings will allow you to gradually convene those partners who will join you in the planning phase of community-driven work. The Community Experiential Learning Activity at the end of this chapter also provides an opportunity to think through stakeholder analysis.

Planning

Planning processes are important for any activities that seek the engagement of diverse partners to identify, address, and support the changes required to improve community well-being or system/intervention effectiveness. Once you have identified key stakeholders and community partners, you may begin to develop the components that will become your partnership plan or memorandum of understanding (MOU). The partnership plan or MOU will ensure that all partners have a common understanding of the purpose of the collaboration/partnership and the form it will take. The advisory end of the continuum tends to focus on MOUs while the collaborative end of the continuum focuses more on partnership plans. Regardless of which document is used the document will guide the implementation of the activities necessary to address the purpose of the work and meet identified goals. In addition, the document serves as the basis for determining the success of the collaboration/partnership and/or the need to refine the plan as work proceeds (Table 10.2).

Coplanning with partners is key to developing a successful collaboration/partnership. Having identified key stakeholders and partners, you can begin to nurture your community relationships and build trust. If you are focused on CBPR, a key aspect is the engagement of partners in all phases of the work and a collaborative process that recognizes the strengths and assets of partners, which makes coplanning even more essential to the process.

Fundamental to community engagement is respect for the community and incorporating community attitudes, beliefs, and insights on needs and problems when developing research and interventions (Sapienza et al., 2007). When communities are fully engaged in the process the academic community is better positioned to assist in facilitating changes in programs and policies that improve well-being through the mobilization and organization of resources, individuals, groups, and agencies (D'Alonzo, 2010; Israel et al., 2005; Viswanathan et al., 2004). The time you allot to coplanning may signal your level of respect for the community.

There are four key constructs to consider when engaging multilevel partners in the research process: (1) commitment of partners to the process and the goals of the project; (2) capacity of partners to participate in the process and engage in research activities; (3) commitment of researchers to meaningfully engage partners; and (4) trust among researchers and partners (Goodman & Thompson Sanders, 2017a; Hamilton et al., 2017; Jones & Wells, 2007). It is important to allow sufficient planning time for partners to get to know each other, hear, understand, and consider each partner's perspective on the issue(s), and for partners to consider how their perspective might allow them to contribute to the effort. These activities also permit trust building between researchers and partners, as well as among partners.

Transparency matters in community engagement. It is important to share key information that may affect partner decisions about their support of and participation in the work. Researchers often overlook institutional and funder

TABLE 10.2   Outline of Partnership Agreement/Memorandum of Understanding
Partners:
(List organizations, agencies, and partners participating, and contact information.
1.
2.
3.
4.
Principles guiding the processes of the partnership:
(Indicate the community engagement/CBPR principles that the partners see as important to maintaining the partnership. Describe the application of the principles to the activities of the partnership.)
1.
2.
3.
4.
Goals:
(What is the partnership to accomplish? Use specific, measurable, achievable, realistic, time-bound goals.)
1.
2.
3.
Activities:
(What will the group do to accomplish the goals of the partnership?)
1.
2.
3.
Responsibilities (What will each partner do for each goal and activity related to that goal. What resources are expected from and provided to each partner?)
Organization A agrees to:
Stakeholder B agrees to:
Agency C agrees to:
Signatures_____   Date_____

requirements and limitations when treatment, intervention, and research are discussed with community partners. For example, what partner needs and requests will grant funds cover? This varies depending on the funder, and community expectations may be based on their experience with funders. Typically, federally funded grants cannot be used to cover the cost of food for meetings. If partners host meetings on your behalf, will or how will they be reimbursed? How do community members feel about the funder's requirements to provide unrestricted data access to other researchers at the end of the project period? Are your partners aware of journal requirements for authorship? The failure to disclose and plan for funding, data, and authorship concerns may harm researcher and partner relationships via unmet expectations.

The second phase of the work is to discuss community concerns and needs with the goal of developing the focus and purpose of the project/intervention or work. At the nonparticipation end of the continuum, researchers simply share their plans for the project and seek advice that they may or may not use. As researchers seek to move along the continuum of engagement, they must be prepared to respond to partner feedback. At the participatory end of the spectrum, identifying the focus and purpose requires open and honest sharing among group members. It is hoped that the interaction required is facilitated by the initial phase focused on developing trust and a sense of relationship. Action and participatory researchers should also consider the facilitation process. The partner with the strongest facilitation skills should take on this role and may not be the researcher or a member of the research team. Permitting a partner to facilitate may be a researcher's first lesson in equitable relationships and respect for the knowledge and skills of all partners.

The planning process requires adequate time be allotted for sharing and consensus building. The agenda and meeting facilitation must promote the inclusion of all voices. This may mean developing strategies to ensure the representation of key partner voices, even in their absence (virtual participation, webinars, electronic voting, etc.). In addition, consideration of strategies that build on community strengths and assets is important. To this end, time should be devoted to a group review of the asset map to determine the need for additions, deletions, and the most useful assets for the work. This will facilitate the group working from a strength-based perspective, fostering a community sense of developing and building on its most valued assets.

Once the purpose is determined, project outcomes should be developed based on this purpose, community context, and use of data to inform outcomes. Discussion of the purpose, goals and outcomes should consider how the selected outcomes and activities serve the patient or community population, further highlighting the importance of their inclusion among key partners. Partners must also be able to access and review data important to decision-making with enough time to question and supplement the data, and discuss how it might affect the project, intervention, or research purpose (Goodman & Thompson Sanders, 2017a; Hamilton et al., 2017). The need to share data and information in a timely manner may be the researcher's second lesson in equitable partnership. Sharing data with and allowing community partners to question and challenge the data, and facilitating the addition of community knowledge, is a demonstration of respect for the knowledge and input of all partners.

With a purpose and/or outcomes in mind, the third task for professionals and researchers interested in engagement at the cooperative and collaborative levels is to have the group review the principles for community engagement discussed in the literature. The group must develop consensus on the principles most important to its functioning. Table 10.1 lists the 11 principles most often encountered in literature. It is unlikely that engagement focused on the consultative end of the continuum will include many of the principles listed, while collaborative engagement efforts might include most of the principles considered.

At the collaborative and participatory levels, rather than doing research "on" or "in" the community, researchers should be committed to conducting research *with* the community as equal partners (Israel et al., 1998). As shared decision-makers, community partners are valued and recognized for their strengths, assets, resources, and

experiential knowledge (Minkler, 2004). Last, community-engaged scholars should embrace colearning, which attempts to ensure that all involved parties gain insight and skills from one another (Wallerstein & Duran, 2006). The principles selected should, at a minimum, reinforce these expectations. Partnerships focused primarily on research will consider principles focused on data sharing and disseminating findings more often than partnerships focused on treatment or service provision. As the relationships and activities of the collaboration develop, there may be a need to revisit the engagement principles selected to guide the work. As stated at the beginning of this section, it is important to recognize the need to revisit agreements made early in the process.

Planning for communication is critical to the smooth implementation of the collaboration. Ongoing communication and opportunities for discussion are important to managing a project or research program. Because the process is iterative and subject to change, flexibility is required for all partners. This plan must ensure sustained communication, decision-making, shared vision, and change management fundamental to engaged processes. Optimally, a communication plan is developed that identifies a schedule for reviews of project milestones during the planning process. Strong communication plans identify the responsible parties who share information on progress, challenges, and successes linked to the project goals at periodic intervals. Finally, the partners should determine responsibility for documentation of the method and timeline for sharing decisions and outcomes.

As the planning continues, participants should determine the resources required to complete each activity. Time is a critical resource in the healthcare environment, particularly for nurses, and acknowledgment and planning for its allocation is critical. The ability of the team to obtain needed resources for the project, intervention, or research can determine if activities and desired outcomes are realistic. As stated, as activities are decided and refined, the responsibilities of each partner, the timeline for completion, and the resources provided, received, and/or shared by each partner should be identified and recorded. These elements are important to developing the partnership plan/MOU. Table 10.2 provides a template for the partnership plan/MOU.

Beyond the names and contact information for partnering organizations the agreement should include the following components: The purpose of the partnership and how it contributes to or benefits the community should be clearly stated. The agreement should identify the outcomes or specific results of the work and the activities required to achieve them. Finally, logistical details, such as the resources needed to support the partnership, the role of each partner in each activity, and the work plan and schedule for activities, are required. The information in the partnership plan/MOU should be written using plain language.

Planning Tools

Two planning tools are useful in developing a partnership plan or MOU. It may be helpful for researchers and partners to develop a *theory of change* document that captures the key ideas guiding their work. The document begins with a statement describing the problem, and the information and key assumptions that led to a focus on this problem. It identifies the group, population, community, and so on whose needs or concerns may be addressed by the work, with notes on the data, information, and key assumptions that informed research decisions. The next two questions relate to the plan to reach the focal group, and the activities required to bring about change. Again, data and key assumptions are important to include. Document the measurable effects of the work, the wider benefits, and the long-term goal or change you hope to see. Once these questions are addressed, a second planning tool, the *logic model,* can be used.

Logic models are helpful to teams and assist in developing and documenting objectives, inputs, activities, outcomes, and timelines. They also serve as a mechanism for accountability and evaluation, are useful for keeping partners informed of progress on the work, and allow all partners to see where the project is successfully meeting goals and where additional thought and effort may be required. Remember that as the partnership changes, expands, or contracts, activities will shift, as will other elements of the logic model.

The logic model provides a sequence of statements that each lead to the next step in planning the group's work. The statements require the group to determine the resources needed to complete the activities that will contribute to achieving the established goals. Two sets of measurable outcomes are developed based on the activities and goals of the work. Outputs assist the group in tracking the implementation of the activities and progress of the work. Outcomes allow the group to determine if the activities lead to the changes expected (developed to be consistent with the theory-of-change steps needed to bring about change and measurable outcomes). Fig. 10.9 provides examples of considerations that are helpful in completing this planning tool.

Implementation

Once the planning phase is complete, the proposed treatment, service, intervention, or research may begin. The theory of change, logic model, and partnership plan or MOU must be shared with all partners. These documents should be reviewed to ensure they remain current in addressing expectations for the timing, location, activities, and logistics that are needed moving forward. The plan or MOU should include a section that establishes the method of communicating information and meetings required for ongoing updates on and revisions of the work. This section should address communication about tasks and next steps, along with responsibilities and resource needs and how these might be addressed.

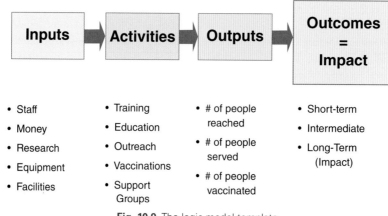

Fig. 10.9 The logic model template.

The meeting schedule is important and can provide opportunities for ongoing input and suggestions as the work progresses. During implementation, adherence to the communication plan and the partnership plan/MOU requires strong facilitation skills. Bringing people to the table is not enough to sustain engagement. Meeting, agreeing on a purpose, and setting goals is not the end game. Data and resource sharing are laudable but will not ensure success. The goal is to change the social, economic, educational, health, and well-being of community members so all can live, work, play, and reach their full potential. Achieving this outcome requires partner commitment and accountability.

Meetings should be guided conversations that make space for all partners while adhering to the timeline for periodic review and reporting of the work (Fig. 10.10). An agenda will permit organized meetings that acknowledge and encourage interaction and positive conversations. It may be necessary to politely interrupt very vocal partners to ensure all partners have time and an opportunity for input. The facilitator should be comfortable addressing conflict among partners. Meetings should be documented via minutes and shared with partners. Minutes facilitate monitoring for task completion.

Conflict and challenges are to be expected and must be addressed rather than avoided. Acknowledge challenges while avoiding win-lose and blaming frameworks upon presentation. The next step is to identify the facts, specifics, and most important issues involved. The group should be encouraged to ask questions to learn about the issue under consideration. The group can then discuss issues using shared knowledge. In addition, the solicitation and presentation of solutions may also prove helpful in resolving concerns. The time allotted to process challenges and conflicts is dictated by the group's sense of the issue's importance. Quality decisions are facilitated by polling the group when attempting to build consensus because it allows the group to assess the amount of support for actions or proposed decisions. Again, record decisions in the minutes for monitoring and accountability.

Community partners may need encouragement and support to feel comfortable participating in some phases of the research process, particularly data analysis and interpretation (Komaie et al., 2018). It should be clear to partners that they need not conduct analyses to comment on whether testing certain relationships makes sense. Researchers may need to plan and provide training to ensure adequate preparation, skill, and confidence for those partners interested in these activities (Coats et al., 2015; D'Agostino McGowan et al., 2015). If participation involves work that is also completed by staff, the principle of equity suggests the need to ensure community partners and members receive compensation comparable to staff employed by the researcher. It should also be clear that engagement does not require participation in every activity by every partner but does require that all partners have the opportunity to participate in all phases of the work based on their skills, capacity, and availability.

There will be other barriers to implementation as the work continues. However, your asset map and stakeholder analysis will facilitate your ability to meet challenges. The community infrastructure to support the work, and the capacity and ability of different stakeholders to participate, may be challenged. However, current partners may be willing to assist or supplement the efforts of partners unable to meet commitments. In addition, this may be the time to reach out to partners not included in the original plan or MOU. The partners may be willing to provide supplemental resources and support. Similarly, capacity, infrastructure, and gaps in information may be addressed through resources offered by your institution, including the Office of Community Engagement, a Clinical and Translational Science Award Program Community Engagement Core, or the capacity efforts of larger, more established community-engaged research teams. Creative solutions are required to engage isolated areas and communities and those reluctant to participate due to issues of mistrust. Mobile vans may be deployed to communities, meetings and events can be scheduled in the community, and

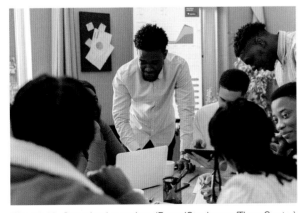

Fig. 10.10 Organized meeting. (From iStock.com/ThreeSpots.)

participation in civic events and activities may reduce or address the barriers encountered.

A final issue that affects the inclusion of all community partners and stakeholders is accessibility. Accessibility may be facilitated by asking participants to share their needs. Inclusive meetings involve consideration of language access, the food and drink offered given dietary needs and restrictions, the physical space related to sensory conditions, transportation and mobility, scheduling assistance, and resources to support full participation.

Accessibility involves the meeting or activity location. Has the partnership considered whether meeting and activity locations provide physical and transportation access for all participants and do they have the resources needed to conduct the meeting in an accessible manner? It is important to assess the sound conditions to ensure all can hear, and visual conditions to ensure all can see. The partnership should have a plan to meet language needs, including American Sign Language (ASL) translators and materials in required languages. Review materials for readability and jargon that might reduce access and participation. Is a refrigerator available for lactating individuals and individuals who must have access to refrigerated medication? How are the needs of participants with children who are not school-aged addressed? How these issues are addressed signals the desire to be inclusive.

Dissemination

The final stage of the engagement process is dissemination. The primary issues of this phase should have been addressed during the development of the partnership plan/MOU. The format, timing, type, and level of data disaggregation should be based on community input and preferences. The dissemination phase is an opportunity to revisit data ownership, clarifying any funder-dictated obligations to place data in a repository or make it available to other researchers. The community partners and stakeholders should assist in planning the method of sharing study findings with the community. Researchers should revisit the method of and format for data sharing appropriate and feasible for each interested partner.

The research team should set aside time to discuss planned papers and presentations and determine partners' interests in participating in their preparation and authorship. As noted in the planning section, academic researchers should share authorship requirements for each journal under consideration. Consistent with the principle of shared decision-making, community partners should be included in journal selection decisions. Again, participation in dissemination activities is not required but should be available to all interested partners.

CONCLUSION

Community-engagement strategies are believed to promote participation in treatment, interventions, and research among members of marginalized communities. Community engagement seeks to bring together academics, professionals, researchers, and communities to examine and address needs and health concerns identified by the community through a process that establishes trust, shares power, fosters colearning, enhances community strengths and resources, and builds capacity (Israel et al., 2005). The failure to include the voices of those most impacted by the inequity observed in the community is likely a missed opportunity to improve the quality and outcomes of health-promotion activities, disease prevention initiatives and health-related research studies (Jagosh et al., 2012; Minkler, 2004). As noted, the adoption and implementation of community engagement strategies have been variable. This may be partly due to the time and resources required to engage respectfully and equitably.

The expectation of shared decision-making and participation throughout the research effort, including recruitment, development, and delivery of the intervention, data collection, and analysis, may be daunting for community members. A systematic review of CBPR clinical trials showed that most CBPR studies reported that involvement varied by level and type of activities, such as identifying study questions, recruitment efforts, development and delivery of the intervention, and data collection methods (De las Nueces et al., 2012). One strategy proposed to improve the implementation of multiple-stakeholder engagement is attention to capacity-building efforts for patient, community, and health stakeholders. Partnerships have successfully developed, implemented, and evaluated training programs for increasing research literacy among community health stakeholders (Coats et al., 2015; D'Agostino McGowan et al., 2015; Goodman & Thompson Sanders, 2017b). This initial commitment by researchers may encourage and support partnership development, as it seems to increase stakeholders' confidence in their ability to make meaningful contributions to benefit their communities. It also illustrates that with time and resources there are solutions for any barriers to community-engaged research.

STUDENT LEARNING ACTIVITY

Now that you have read about the categories of engagement that occur along the continuum of community engagement consider the scenarios that follow. Reflect on your learning and try to identify the category of engagement described. As you reflect, note the elements of the description that suggest that level of engagement.

Study framework: "Comparing the Use of Evidence and Culture in Targeted Colorectal Cancer Communication for African Americans" (Thompson Sanders et al., 2010).

This study focuses on the effects of culturally targeted colorectal cancer communication strategies among African Americans. The study is a two-arm randomized control study of cancer communication effects on affective, cognitive processing, and behavioral outcomes over a 22-week intervention. The primary aim is to compare the effects of peripheral + evidential and peripheral + evidential + sociocultural cancer communication strategies' effects on affective reactions to the publication, cognitive reactions, and processing (motivation to process, sense of relevance, and identification), perceived benefits and barriers and intent to screen. The authors engaged the community as described in the following scenarios.

Scenario 1: The project team engaged patient advocates from the healthcare center to review and rank research priorities for the team. These advocates have expertise in cancer prevention, treatment, and care. This enabled the researchers to identify the categories of research most critical to patients. These priorities stimulated this research. Building on this work, the authors will engage a community advisory board (CAB) and patient advisory team (PAT) in all phases of the proposed study (planning, drafting study materials and protocols, recruiting participants, study implementation including data collection, participant retention, data interpretation, and helping share findings in both scientific and community-friendly formats). The CAB includes decision-makers and program staff from a healthcare center and two supporting hospitals. The PAT includes patients with cancer and their parents/caregivers/spouses/partners whose lived experience represents the community and people likely to be affected by this study.

Scenario 2: The researchers will work with decision-makers and program staff from a healthcare center and two supporting hospitals. These individuals are knowledgeable about the target population. They will advise on study materials and protocols, recruiting participant recruitment, study implementation, and data collection. The researchers plan to seek their assistance if they encounter puzzling findings.

Scenario 3: The researchers will engage a CAB in the developing aspects of the proposed study (reviewing study materials and protocols and helping with plans and recruitment of patients; study implementation including encouraging participation and retention, and reviewing and commenting on findings). The CAB includes decision-makers and program staff from a healthcare center, two supporting hospitals, and patients with cancer or their parents/caregivers/spouses/partners. These individuals are knowledgeable about the community and have already experienced cancer screening and/or care.

Scenario 4: The researchers will work with community-based organizations focused on health. The leaders of these organizations have agreed to host events where researchers can share information on rates of colorectal cancer in the African American community, describe the study, and increase awareness of the study. Some organizations will allow the setup of recruitment tables at their health fairs and events as long as educational cancer materials are provided. The leaders of these organizations are knowledgeable about the target population and some share identities with intended study participants.

CORRECT RESPONSES AND RATIONALE

Scenario 1. This is an example of collaboration. Patients, patient advocates, and other partners are members of the research project team. Community members participate in decision-making, particularly in areas that require a deep understanding of community needs and desires. *The keys to identifying this category of community engagement are community partner participation in study development from the beginning, including problem identification, and participation as members of the research project team who participate in decision-making throughout the process.*

Scenario 2. This is an example of consultation. An advisory board exists but shared decision-making is absent, and there is no attempt to be inclusive of community partners or representatives of the intended participants. *A key factor in identifying this category of engagement is that the advisory board has a limited role in the study, which primarily involves advice on study materials, recruitment, and retention during study implementation.*

Scenario 3. This is an example of cooperative community engagement. An advisory board exists that is inclusive of a variety of community partners. The advisory board members provide active guidance and assistance on research materials, recruitment and retention, and interpretation of the data to the research team. In addition, they may comment on the findings. *A key*

difference between this level of engagement and collaboration is that the CAB members do not share in decision-making. However, they advise on most aspects of the study design and implementation. In addition, the CAB members were not involved in identifying the study focus and planning.

Scenario 4. *This is not community engagement; it is outreach and education.* While not community engagement, these activities can build community relationships. In addition, community members and leaders often find participation in these events meaningful and beneficial to their ongoing efforts to encourage healthy lifestyles and well-being.

COMMUNITY-SPECIFIC EXPERIENTIAL LEARNING ACTIVITY

Community engagement requires knowledge of the community and its assets, relationship building, and planning. In this activity, you will combine asset mapping and stakeholder analysis as you engage in relationship building. Use demographic and health data to identify a population and/or community experiencing health inequities that interest you or your team. Once you have identified a population and/or community, begin the planning process by completing each task that follows.

Task 1. Asset mapping to support community-engaged research

Asset mapping is a strategy used in community-engaged or community-driven projects and research (Kretzmann & McKnight, 1993). Community assets are qualities, people, places, and things that are resources or valued by a community or neighborhood. Assets help people be hopeful and see the promise of their community. You can use assets to motivate work to enhance and/or build a community.

Take a tour (you and/or your research/project team) of the community or neighborhood that you have identified. You may drive, but walking may allow you to meet community members, which can be informative. If your focus is a population, tour the neighborhood(s) and communities where members of the population live. As you tour, identify resources that might support the work you hope to complete. You are attempting to

identify associations (community development organizations, block units, neighborhood watch, etc.), institutions (churches, schools, libraries, health centers, etc.), and physical spaces (community centers, parks, community gardens, wide streets, sidewalks, bike lanes, etc.). Write down names that you encounter as you complete the tour. Describe how this asset contributes to the community.

Task 2. Stakeholder analysis

Upon completing the task, you must identify leaders or workers at the organizations and institutions that you encountered on your tour. Research these associations, institutions, and organizations. Next, organize your information about potential stakeholders related to your community research or project. List the name of the key contact at each organization. As you go through your analysis, identify the stakeholders who are most important to the work. Note why the organization might be interested in the project. To do this, you may want to assign stakeholders to key categories. Consider categories related to business, government (elected officials, aides), nonprofit and school administrators, youth-serving organizations, and community (leaders, volunteers, neighborhood association members). Finally, note what resources this stakeholder might have to offer. Construct a table using this example:

Category	Stakeholder	Contact person	Why project of interest to stakeholder?	Resources to offer?

Task 3. Key informant interviews

Based on your stakeholder analysis, select your top five potential partners and schedule interviews with your contacts. Be prepared to provide a clear and succinct statement of your interest in the community/neighborhood or population. Seek information on the partner's mission, vision, and current activities, and their current partners. This interview should also yield information on the partner's perspective on community assets, concerns, and needs. This information should allow you to refine your list and identify the partners that might best serve as members of your project/research team.

A NURSING CASE STUDY IN COMMUNITY-BASED PARTICIPATORY RESEARCH IN PUBLIC HEALTH NURSING

This case study highlights nurses applying the CBPR framework in an ethnographic study focusing on culture and African American infant health. Using this approach allowed the nurse researchers to engage in full partnership with community members and stakeholders. Within the case study, one can see how the nurses applied the principles of CBPR, such as building trust within the community, collaborating with multiple stakeholders, maintaining scientific excellence, and adhering to the appropriate ethical protocols when conducting CBPR. In addition, the case study demonstrates how the community was an equal partner in all aspects of the research process, from recruitment of participants, decision-making about research protocols, data collection and analysis, and reaching an agreement on the findings.

Data from Savage, C. L., Xu, Y., Lee, R., Rose, B. L., Kappesser, M., & Anthony, J. S. (2006). A case study in the use of community-based participatory research in public health nursing. *Public Health Nursing, 23*(5), 472–478. https://doi.org/10.1111/j.1525-1446.2006.00585.x

REFERENCES

American Hospital Association. (2010). *Committee on research. AHA research synthesis report: Patient-centered medical home (PCMH)*. American Hospital Association.

Arnstein, S. R. (1969). A ladder of citizen participation. *Journal of the American Planning Association, 35*(4), 216–224.

Brown, L. D., & Tandon, R. (1983). Ideology and political economy in inquiry: Action research and participatory research. *The Journal of Applied Behavioral Science, 19*(3), 277–294.

Cargo, M., & Mercer, S. L. (2008). The value and challenges of participatory research: Strengthening its practice. *Annual Review of Public Health, 29*, 325–350.

Cleary, M., & Hunt, G. E. (2010). Building community engagement in nursing. *The Journal of Continuing Education in Nursing, 41*(8), 344–345.

Coats, J. V., Stafford, J. D., Sanders Thompson, V. L., Johnson Javois, B., & Goodman, M. S. (2015). Increasing research literacy: The community research fellows training program. *Journal of Empirical Research on Human Research Ethics, 10*(1), 3–12. https://doi.org/10.1177/1556264614561959.

D'Agostino McGowan, L., Stafford, J. D., Thompson, V. L. S., Johnson-Javois, B., & Goodman, M. S. (2015). Quantitative evaluation of the community research fellows training program. *Frontiers in Public Health, 3*, 179. https://doi.org/10.3389/fpubh.2015.00179.

D'Alonzo, K. T. (2010). Getting started in CBPR: Lessons in building community partnerships for new researchers. *Nursing Inquiry, 17*, 282–288. doi: 10.1111/j.1440-1800.2010.00510.x.

De Koning, K., & Martin, M. (1996). *Participatory research in health: Issues and experiences*. Zed Books.

De las Nueces, D., Hacker, K., DiGirolamo, A., & Hicks, L. S. (2012). A systematic review of community-based participatory research to enhance clinical trials in racial and ethnic minority groups. *Health Services Research, 47*, 1363–1386. doi: 10.1111/j.1475-6773.2012.01386.x.

Education Network to Advance Cancer Clinical Trials, Community-Campus Partnerships for Health. (2008). *Communities as partners in cancer clinical trials: Changing research, practice, and policy*. Education Network to Advance Cancer Clinical Trials, Community-Campus Partnerships for Health.

Fals-Borda, O., & Rahman, M. A. (1991). *Action and knowledge: Breaking the monopoly with participatory action research*. Intermediate Technology/Apex.

Fisher, P. A., & Ball, T. J. (2003). Tribal participatory research: Mechanisms of a collaborative model. *American Journal of Community Psychology, 32*(3–4), 207–216.

Freire, P. (2018). *Pedagogy of the oppressed*. Bloomsbury Publishing.

Fyffe, T. (2009). Nursing shaping and influencing health and social care policy. *Journal of Nursing Management, 17*(6), 698–706.

Goodman, M. S., & Thompson Sanders, V. L. (2017a). The science of stakeholder engagement in research: Classification, implementation, and evaluation. *Translational Behavioral Medicine, 7*(3), 486–491.

Goodman, M. S., & Thompson Sanders, V. L. (2017b). *Public health research methods for partnerships and practice*. Taylor & Francis Group.

Hall, B. (1992). From margins to center? The development and purpose of participatory research. *American Sociologist, 23*, 15–28.

Hamilton, A. B., Brunner, J., Cain, C., Chuang, E., Luger, T. M., Canelo, I., & Yano, E. M. (2017). Engaging multilevel stakeholders in an implementation trial of evidence-based quality improvement in VA women's health primary care. *Translational Behavioral Medicine, 7*(3), 478–485.

Hurt, T. (2009). Connecting with African American families: Challenges and possibilities. *The Family Psychologist, 25*(1), 11–13.

Israel, B. A., Coombe, C. M., Cheezum, R. R., Schulz, A. J., McGranaghan, R. J., Lichtenstein, R., Reyes, A. G., Clement, J., Burris, A. (2010). Community-based participatory research: A capacity-building approach for policy advocacy aimed at eliminating health disparities. *American Journal of Public Health, 100*(11), 2094–2102. doi: 10.2105/AJPH.2009.170506.

Israel, B. A., Eng, E., Schulz, A. J., & Parker, E. A. (2005). *Methods in community-based participatory research for health.* John Wiley & Sons.

Israel, B. A., Shulz, A., Parker, E. A., & Becker, A. B. (1998). Review of community-based research: Assessing partnership approaches to improve public health. *Annual Reviews of Public Health, 19*, 173–202.

Jagosh, J., Macaulay, A. C., Pluye, P., Salsberg, J., Bush, P. L., Henderson, J., Sirett, E., Wong, G., Cargo, M., Herbert, C. P., Seifer, S. D., Green, L. W., & Greenhalgh, T. (2012). Uncovering the benefits of participatory research: Implications of a realist review for health research and practice. *Milbank Quarterly, 90*(2), 311–346. doi: 10.1111/j.1468-0009.2012.00665.x

Jones, L., & Wells, K. (2007). Strategies for academic and clinician engagement in community-participatory partnered research. *Journal of the American Medical Association, 297*, 407–410.

Kellogg Commission on the Future of State and Land-Grant Institutions. (1999). *Returning to our roots: The engaged institution.* National Association of State Universities and Land-Grant Colleges.

Kemmis, S., & McTaggart, R. (2000). Participatory action research. In Denzin, N. K., & Lincoln, Y. S. (Eds.), *Handbook of qualitative research* (pp. 567–605). Sage.

Kennedy, E. M. (1999). University-community partnerships: A mutually beneficial effort to aid community development and improve academic learning opportunities. *Applied Developmental Science, 3*(4), 197–198.

Komaie, G., Goodman, M., McCall, A., McGill, G., Patterson, C., Hayes, C., & Thompson Sanders, V. L. (2018). Training community members in public health research: Development and implementation of a community participatory research pilot project. *Health Equity, 2*(1), 282–287.

Kost, R. G., Reider, C., Stephens, J., & Schuff, K. G. (2012). Research subject advocacy: Program implementation and evaluation at clinical and translational science award centers. *Academic Medicine, 87*(9), 1228–1236. https://doi.org/10.1097/ACM.0b013e3182628afa.

Kretzmann, J. P., & McKnight, J. (1993). *Building communities from the inside out.* Center for Urban Affairs and Policy Research, Neighborhood Innovations Network.

KU Work Group for Community Health and Development. (2016). Chapter 36, Section 2: Community-based participatory research. Retrieved February 29, 2016, from http://ctb.ku.edu/en/table-of-contents/evaluate/evaluation/intervention-research/main.

Lewin, K. (1947). Frontiers in group dynamics: II. Channels of group life; social planning and action research. *Human Relations, 1*(2), 143–153.

Lincoln, Y. S. (2003). Constructivist knowing, participatory ethics and responsive evaluation: A model for the 21st Century. In Kellaghan, T., Stufflebeam, D. L. (Eds.), *International Handbook of Educational Evaluation. Kluwer International Handbooks of Education,* vol 9. Springer, Dordrecht. doi: 10.1007/978-94-010-0309-4_6.

Martin, L., Smith, H., & Phillips, W. (2005). Bridging "town & gown" through innovative university-community partnerships. *The Innovation Journal, 10*(2), 1–16.

Marullo, S., & Edwards, B. (2000). From charity to justice: The potential of university-community collaboration for social change. *American Behavioral Scientist, 43*(5), 895–912.

Minkler, M. (2003). *Community organizing and community building for health.* Rutgers University Press.

Minkler, M. (2004). Ethical challengers for the "outside" researcher in community-based participatory research. *Health Education & Behavior, 31*(6), 684–697.

Minkler, M., Blackwell, A. G., Thompson, M., & Tamir, H. (2003). Community-based participatory research: Implications for public health funding. *American Journal of Public Health, 93*, 1210–1213.

Montoya, M. J., & Kent, E. E. (2011). Dialogical action: Moving from community-based to community-driven participatory research. *Qualitative Health Research, 21*(7), 1000–1011. https://doi.org/10.1177/1049732311403500.

National Institute of Nursing Research. (2004). Roadmap implementation meeting. Integration of NINR areas of science with the NIH roadmap. Retrieved March 30, 2021, from http://ninr.nih.gov/assets/Documents/RoadmapImplementationMeeting01.2004001.doc.

Patient-Centered Outcomes Research Institute. (2013). Establishing the definition of patient-centered outcomes research. Retrieved from https://www.pcori.org/research-results/about-our-research/patient-centered-outcomes-research.

Patient-Centered Outcomes Research Institute (PCORI). (2018). The value of engagement. Patient-Centered Outcomes Research Institute. Retrieved March 6, 2023, from https://www.pcori.org/engagement/value-engagement.

Park, P., Brydon-Miller, M., Hall, B., & Jackson, T. (Eds.). (1993). *Voices of change: Participatory research in the United States and Canada*. Bergin & Garvey.

Purpose Institute in Partnership with the Carnegie Foundation. (2021). Community engagement classification. Retrieved March 21, 2021, from https://public-purpose.org/.

Sapienza, J. N., Corbie-Smith, G., Keim, S., & Fleishman, A. R. (2007). Community engagement in epidemiological research. *Ambulatory Pediatrics, 7*, 247–252.

Seifer, S. D., Shore, N., & Holmes, S. L. (2003). *Developing and sustaining community-university partnerships for health research: Infrastructure requirements*. Community Campus Partnerships for Health.

Suarez-Balcazar, Y., Mirza, M., & Hansen, A. M. (2015). Unpacking university-community partnerships to advance scholarship of practice. *Occupational Therapy in Health Care, 29*(4), 370–382.

Sung, N. S., Crowley, W. F., Genel, M., Salber, P., Sandy, L., Sherwood, L. M., Johnson, S. B., Catanese, V., Tilson, H., Getz, K., Larson, E. L., Scheinberg, D., Reece, E. A., Slavkin, H., Dobs, A., Grebb, J., Martinez, R. A., Kom, A., & Rimoin, D. (2003). Central challenges facing the national clinical research enterprise. *Journal of the American Medical Association, 289*(10), 1278–1287.

Thompson, V. L. S., Kalesan, B., Wells, A., Williams, S.-L., & Caito, N. (2010). Comparing the use of evidence and culture in targeted colorectal cancer communication for African Americans. *Patient Education and Counseling, 81*(S1), S22–S33. https://doi.org/10.1016/j.pec.2010.07.019.

Thompson Sanders, V. L., Ackerman, N., Bauer, K. L., Bowen, D. J., & Goodman, M. S. (2021). Strategies of community engagement in research: Definitions and classifications. *Translational Behavioral Medicine, 11*(2), 441–451. https://doi.org/10.1093/tbm/ibaa042.

Torbert, W. R., & Taylor, S. (2001). The practice of action inquiry. In Reason, P., & Bradbury, H. (Eds.), *Handbook of action research: Participative inquiry and practice* (pp. 250–260). Sage.

Trickett, E. J., & Espino, S. L. R. (2004). Collaboration and social inquiry: Multiple meanings of a construct and its role in creating useful and valid knowledge. *American Journal of Community Psychology, 34*(1–2), 1–69.

US Department of Education. (2006). *A test of leadership: Charting the future of U.S. higher education*. Washington, DC.

US Department of Health and Human Services, National Institutes of Health. (2016). Community engagement. Retrieved March 25, 2021, from https://www.nih.gov/health-information/nih-clinical-research-trials-you/community-engagement.

US Department of Housing and Urban Development. (n. d.). The Office of University Partnerships: About OUP. Retrieved March 21, 2021, from https://archives.huduser.gov/portal/oup/home.html.

Vishwanathan, M., Ammerman, A., Eng, E., Garlehner, G., Lohr, K. N., Griffith, D., Rhodes, S., Samuel-Hodge, C., Maty, S., Lux, L., & Webb, L. (2004). Community-based participatory research: Assessing the evidence. *Evidence Report/Technology Assessment (Summary), 99*, 1–8.

Wallerstein, N., & Duran, B. (2006). Using community-based participatory research to address health disparities. *Health Promotion Practice, 7*(3), 312–323.

Wallerstein, N., & Duran, B. (2010). Community-based participatory research contributions to intervention research: The intersection of science and practice to improve health equity. *American Journal of Public Health, 100*(S1), S40–S46.

Wallerstein, N., Oetzel, J., Duran, B., Tafoya, G., Belone, L., & Rae, R. (2008). What predicts outcomes in CBPR. *Community-Based Participatory Research for Health: From Process to Outcomes, 2*, 371–392.

Weerts, D. J., & Sandmann, L. R. (2008). Building a two-way street: Challenges and opportunities for community engagement at research universities. *The Review of Higher Education, 32*, 73–106.

Westfall, J. M., Mold, J., & Fagnan, L. (2007). Practice-based research "blue highways" on the NIH roadmap. *Journal of the American Medical Association, 297*(4), 403–406.

Wilkins, C. H., Spofford, M., Williams, N., McKeever, C., Allen, S., Brown, J., Opp, J., Richmond, A., Strelnick, A. H., & CTSA Consortium's Community Engagement Key Function Committee Community Partners Integration Workgroup. (2013). Community representatives' involvement in clinical and translational science awardee activities. *Clinical and Translational Science, 6*(4), 292–296. https://doi.org/10.1111/cts.12072.

Wilson, D. (2004). Key features of successful university-community partnerships. In Pew Partnership for Civic Change (Ed.), *New directions in civic engagement: University Avenue meets Main Street*. University of Richmond

Yarborough, M., Edwards, K., Espinoza, P., Geller, G., Sarwal, A., Sharp, R., & Spicer, P. (2013). Relationships hold the key to trustworthy and productive translational science: Recommendations for expanding community engagement in biomedical research. *Clinical and Translational Science, 6*(4), 310–313. https://doi.org/10.1111/cts.12022.

RESPONSES TO STUDENT REFLECTION QUESTIONS

CHAPTER 2

1. Individual choices do play a role in a person's relative position on the socioeconomic ladder. Still, for most people, other factors can contribute to SES that may lie beyond the person's control:
   - Housing insecurity can happen when individuals and communities become displaced due to urban revitalization resulting in gentrification.
   - When there is no legal mandate for small companies to offer health insurance or sick leave, a person may have to quit their job due to health reasons.
   - When previous criminal offenders must check the criminal record box on employment applications, it lessens their chances of obtaining gainful employment.
2. A UBI would provide income and revenue to meet basic needs.
   - Having an added income could reduce the poverty rate.
   - When those at the bottom of the economic ladder accrue more income, the gap in income inequality can begin to decrease.
3. When working in the community, nurses can address the social and healthcare needs of populations by working across sectors such as with faith-based organizations, homeless shelters and transitional housing, community-based transportation programs to help communities have access to healthcare, grocers, pharmacies, and a host of other resources needed to promote and maintain health.
4. There is no correct answer to Question #4. Instead, reflect on how you felt when deciding how to expend your limited funds.

EXPERIENTIAL LEARNING: POVERTY SIMULATION

Experiencing Poverty

Poverty simulations are one way to help students understand how poverty impacts health and gain insight into another person's plight. Simulation exercises help students learn about poverty, the social and structural determinants of health, and social justice. In brief, nursing faculty at a southern university designed scenarios to help students understand the challenges associated with poverty. Students were to read each scenario and, in groups of three to five, go out in the community to acquire the resources the individual needed in the given scenario. The students would later reflect on their experience, discuss the challenges encountered, lessons learned, and how the experience would impact their future nursing practice. Read the scenarios, determine how you would gather resources if you were the person in the situation, and how the experience might change your view on poverty.

- A woman in her 50s who is new to town lives out of her car, is unemployed and uninsured, has several chronic conditions, and recently ran out of medication.
- A low-income family of six has no access to healthy, affordable food and is concerned about obesity among their four young children.
- A mother of two is trying to escape domestic violence and has no car, money, or essential documents to secure employment or assistance (e.g., birth certificates).
- After discovering she was pregnant, a homeless adolescent mother was beaten and kicked out of the house by her drug-abusing parent.
- A young veteran got out of the military and is suffering from posttraumatic stress disorder.
- A legally blind woman in her 70s lives in a rural area with limited public transportation and needs to travel for a medical appointment.
- A single undocumented mother who has a disabled child needs to find a clinic for immunizations and a school to accommodate the child's special needs.

From: Johnson, K. E., Guillet, N., Murphy, L., Horton, S. E., & Todd, A. T. (2015). "If only we could have them walk a mile in their shoes": A community-based poverty simulation exercise for baccalaureate nursing students. *The Journal of Nursing Education, 54*(9), S116–S119. https://doi.org/10.3928/01484834-20150814-22. Reprinted with permission from SLACK Incorporated.

POVERTY RESOURCES		
Resource	Description	Website
Experience Living in Poverty	Poverty simulation that allows students to role-play the lives of impoverished families.	https://www.communityaction.org/povertysimulations/
The Poverty Simulation	Community Action Poverty Simulation is an interactive experience that immerses the student in the realities of poverty.	https://www.povertysimulation.net/about/

From: The Poverty Simulation. (n.d.). Why a simulation? Retrieved from https://www.povertysimulation.net/about/.

CHAPTER 3

1. Limited educational attainment, limited employment opportunities, and occupying the lower rungs of the socioeconomic ladder are all potential impacts.
2. Higher levels of educational attainment correlate with better health, better employment opportunities with increased financial security, and more opportunities and resources across the life trajectory.
3. Use plain language strategies, use CLAS standards as appropriate, employ the use of an interpreter if necessary, and determine whether the provider has language concordance.

CHAPTER 4

1. Nurses should consider the impact of the physical, natural, and built environment on an individual's health, as it can create barriers to safety, employment, socialization, physical activity, healthcare, and education.
2. Living in a clean, safe, and well-designed built environment can increase physical activity, promote access to healthy food, and decrease exposure to harmful climate exposures.
3. Nurses are positioned to collaborate with other leaders in the community to advocate for increased access to healthy foods, improved walking paths, and community health screening events.

CHAPTER 5

1. Nurse-led clinics can offer healthcare services in underserved communities, thereby improving access with the goal of improving health outcomes and keeping people in their community rather than being hospitalized. In addition, nurse-led clinics and CHWs collaborate to sponsor CHW programs that emphasize health promotion and health education for those populations in the community. Additionally, the clinics are centered in the environments where people live, thus providing the nurse awareness of the needs, resources, and conditions of the community.
2. Voting can have a significant influence on health. Voting determines the distribution of resources within communities, including many aspects of the lived experience, such as minimum wage laws, employee benefits, work conditions, and the availability of social assistance programs, the local school systems, and child development resources. Voting and community engagement provide individuals with mechanisms to have their voices heard.
3. There are direct correlations between the conditions of living environments and health. Unhealthy social environments have been associated with higher risks of disease. Conditions in the social environment weigh heavily on the health of the individual and community, including the level of violence in the community, the physical or built structure of the community, how the community is designed, and whether the design is health enhancing. Mounting evidence has demonstrated that high crime rates, delinquency, levels of education, psychological stress, and various health problems are affected by the environments within which one is born, lives, plays, works, and ages.

CHAPTER 6

1. There are no right or wrong answers to question 1. Responses require a personal look inward after one has read the chapter, and reflection on how anyone, including yourself, can be characterized as in a social group depending upon variances in physical

characteristics such as skin and hair color and/or other facial features.

2. *Health inequities* are differences in health status and resources related to and fueled by power, money, and displacement of people.

Health disparities are critically uneven health outcomes, such as maternal and infant mortality, life span, and death from cancer.

Racism is a SDOH, a system of beliefs and practices that anchors power and well-being of dominant races at the expense of historically excluded races. Its purpose is to dehumanize, exploit, and/or eliminate the "other."

Race is a socially constructed term used to group people hierarchically according to certain variances in physical characteristics.

3. *White privilege* is the unearned and invisible race-based advantage of being considered a White person in the United States.

White supremacy is a set of beliefs, or doctrine, that White people are a superior race and dominate society; this doctrine forms the basis of laws and actions that control and dehumanize people.

White fragility is the denial, awkwardness, and often defensiveness expressed by a White person during race-based conversations.

4. *Health equity* is the fair and just opportunity for each person to live the healthiest life possible. Nurses can advance health equity at the personal, institutional, and structural or systems level.

5. *Antiracist actions* are any efforts to recognize and exterminate racism by decisively appraising and reforming systems, institutional structures, policies, and language to reallocate power and resources equitably.

6. *Racial justice* is the systematic and fair treatment of all people resulting in racial equity—equitable outcomes and opportunities for all. As our society becomes more ethically, historically, and culturally aware, the doctrines and stereotypes it holds about people are informed by/through this awareness, and this positive change moves toward a more racially just society. An individual does not stay unchanged during the process, but will be affected by it, one way or another.

7. The *groundwater metaphor* describes organization-linked actions that target the political, economic, and environmental social determinants of health.

Upstream determinants are any toxic or social stressors that influence health in a community, family, or group, such as scarce housing, lack of jobs, or food deserts.

Midstream determinants are the learned and reinforced human behaviors, like smoking or alcohol abuse, that increase risk for chronic diseases.

Downstream determinants are the practices by medical and nursing professionals to identify and effectively treat those with chronic disease, the underserved, and the uninsured, and include follow-up care.

8. *Difficult conversations* are honest, respectful dialogues about discrimination, racial biases, stereotyping, microaggressions, and untested, unchallenged assumptions about people.

9. Question 9 can only be answered by internal self-examination and understanding of *White privilege,* which is described in Question 3.

10. The term "takeaway" means the key points or key message(s) contained in a presentation. In this case it means the most important information about *race, racism, discrimination,* and *privilege* in nursing that you will carry with you and use after reading this chapter.

The news item that is used as the basis of the following Case Study first appeared in the January 27, 2021 *Chicago Tribune* newspaper (Hawthorne, 2021a, p. 8) with follow-up a week later (Hawthorne, 2021b, p. 3). It brings several areas of the city together: two opposing neighborhoods; the Mayor's and Governor's offices; the Illinois Environmental Protection Agency (EPA); the Department of Housing and Urban Development; the United Neighbors of the 10th Ward citizen's group, which is fighting the project; and a major industrial manufacturing business, in hearings to block the company from moving to a low-income Southside Chicago neighborhood. Read the Case Study and respond to the questions posed using what you have learned from this chapter on race, discrimination, and bias in the United States. You can do this independently or as part of a group effort. All quoted materials are from pages 8 and 3 of the articles published in January and February of 2021, respectively (Hawthorne, 2021a; Hawthorne, 2021b).

CHAPTER 7

1. Make sure your op-ed contains the following: An opening statement with a hook, the main point including why the topic is important and why readers should care, a compelling case, evidence-based research, and an ending with a solid call to action. Be sure to cite references. You also should acknowledge the opponent's view and the advantages and disadvantages of their position.

2. Before you start, research the topic thoroughly and incorporate the following guidelines by the CDC (2021a): Clearly define your objective. (Do you want to highlight content, spark action, or encourage awareness on the issue?) Determine your intended target audience. Keep your content to the maximum character limit of 140 characters. Determine if your tweet requires more posting on the matter. Is there a schedule of times to post that should be set up to keep your audience engaged? Evaluate your Twitter experience. (What were your metrics, and what lessons did you learn from this experience?)
3. Conduct a force field analysis of the issues, state the matter of concern, identify driving and restraining forces, and identify stakeholders; reflect on why those stakeholders may be for or against the proposed issue.
4. The NCC advocates for policies that improve care for patients, families, and communities by advancing research and strengthening the nursing workforce.

CHAPTER 8

1. Conduct a self-assessment to reflect on your various social identities. Determine if you are in a position of privilege or oppression, feel included or excluded, and if you include or exclude others based on some aspects of their social identities.
2. Consider societal policies and practices that oppress marginalized groups. Explore the power dynamics between partners. Determine what skills are needed to build partnerships.
3. Success can be measured in several ways. What did the partners decide would be the measures of success? If goals and benchmarks were established in the partnership, they can be used to assess progress. All parties should be accountable for the outcomes.
4. You could describe how you view the "Six Conditions of Systems Change" evolving in a newly formed partnership.

CHAPTER 9

1. The Upstream and Downstream Thinking section enables the student to see different levels of interventions and that population-level interventions must occur at the upstream level.
2. Upstream interventions are aimed at policies and practices that change structures within systems and society that contribute to health inequities.

INDEX

Note: Page numbers followed by *f* indicate figures, *t* indicates tables, and *b* indicate boxes.